THE DRUG PARADOX

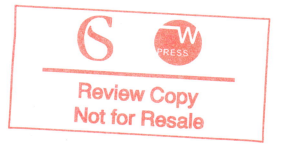

THE DRUG PARADOX

An Introduction to the
Sociology of Psychoactive
Substances in Canada

Tara L. Bruno and Rick Csiernik

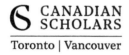

CANADIAN
SCHOLARS
Toronto | Vancouver

The Drug Paradox: An Introduction to the Sociology of Psychoactive Substances in Canada
Tara L. Bruno and Rick Csiernik

First published in 2018 by
CSP Books Inc.
425 Adelaide Street West, Suite 200
Toronto, Ontario
M5V 3C1

www.canadianscholars.ca

Library and Archives Canada Cataloguing in Publication

Bruno, Tara L., 1981-, author
    The drug paradox : an introduction to the sociology of psychoactive substances in Canada / Tara L. Bruno and Rick Csiernik.

Includes bibliographical references and index.
Issued in print and electronic formats.
ISBN 978-1-77338-052-0 (softcover).—ISBN 978-1-77338-053-7 (PDF).—
ISBN 978-1-77338-054-4 (EPUB)

    1. Drugs—Canada. 2. Drug abuse—Canada. I. Csiernik, Rick, author II. Title.

HV5840.C3B78 2018   362.290971   C2018-900760-5   C2018-900761-3

Text design by Elisabeth Springate
Typesetting by Brad Horning
Cover design by Gordon Robertson

18   19   20   21   22   5   4   3   2   1

Printed and bound in Canada by Webcom

Canada

DEDICATION

Terrance "Terry" Elliott
1953–1990
Your journey, though too short, lives on through my work.

&

Jonathan "Jon" Saumier
Even though we are miles apart, I think of you every day—you are my soul twin.
I hope this work speaks to you!

—Tara Bruno

For those sleeping rough tonight, those confined in institutions, and our
Indigenous sisters and brothers, with hope that the fears that prevent us
from listening to and understanding each other will be lessened by the words
and ideas expressed in these pages.

—Rick Csiernik

CONTENTS

PREFACE

According to social constructionists, there is nothing inherently good or bad about psychoactive drugs or psychoactive drug use. What we have been told about drugs and drug use, both good and bad, are products of social definitions and socialization. However, social definitions and socialization can be conflicting and contradictory. For example, lessons from parents, teachers, and legal authorities may be in direct contrast with the media, peers, and romantic partners. What do social patterns of substance use tell us about how people make sense of these conflicts? If psychoactive substances are merely socially constructed entities, then what is to be said of the empirical research confirming the varying degrees of risk associated with every psychoactive substance? Indeed, from an empirical standpoint, there are real dangers associated with psychoactive substances for some people under certain conditions, not all of which are attributable to the chemical substances or to individual biology or psychology. There are important social consequences, including legal, financial, and relational, that must also be considered when examining psychoactive substances. Moreover, social consequences may depend on a variety of other factors, including who is using, what substance is being used, how much is being used, the reasons for using, the environment of use, and the people surrounding the use.

Drugs and drug use are multi-faceted phenomena, requiring a biopsychosocial approach. While biological and psychological research continue to gain prominence, sociological research on psychoactive substances in Canada receives much less attention and government funding. However, sociology has a great deal to contribute to our understanding of psychoactive substances—because sociologically, psychoactive substances are puzzling. They can do so much good, yet they can also produce great individual and societal harm. There are both socially constructed and empirically validated aspects of psychoactive substance use that produce significant social harm. Meanwhile, there are many social and cultural benefits of psychoactive substances. Some substances are viewed with contempt and fear, while the users of these same substances celebrate and even promote the potential benefits. Which reality is true?

The central theme of this book is to examine the paradoxical aspects of drugs and drug use in Canadian society, while also providing a basic foundation in the sociology of psychoactive substances in the Canadian context, using a holistic biopsychosocial framework. The authors of this book have combined our respective expertise to contribute to the ever-growing and important area of substance use, misuse, and dependence in Canadian society. Though focused primarily on the sociological aspects of drugs and drug use, we incorporate existing knowledge and research from many disciplines, including sociology, biology, psychology, history, politics, law, criminology, economics, and social work.

Importantly, it is not just the substances themselves, nor individual pathologies, that can produce benefits or harms. How we respond to drugs and drug users in our society has important implications for individual outcomes and societal patterns of use. Historically, our legal responses to drugs and drug users represents what sociologist Patricia Erickson (1999: 275) refers to as a "persistent paradox." Beyond our socio-legal response to drugs and drug users, though, there appear to be many contradictory aspects to drugs and drug use in society. Why are some drugs considered normal, socially acceptable, or at least tolerable, while others are demonized? Who or what makes these definitions so widespread and who benefits from this conceptualization? To what extent are these definitions verified by empirical studies? To what extent do empirical studies help to solidify or refute societal responses to and definitions of psychoactive substances? This book offers an overview of the socially constructed and objectively verified knowledge about psychoactive substances in Canadian society and beyond.

This introduction to the sociology of psychoactive substances in Canada includes 13 chapters covering a broad range of critical perspectives and issues. The first chapter sets out the central theme of the book—that drugs and drug use are complex and often involve puzzling and contradictory discourses. We also explore core concepts, including the definitions of drugs and psychoactive substances, drug abuse, misuse, dependence, and addiction. Chapter 2 provides a brief history of and the politics behind Canada's drug laws and describes the various pieces of legislation pertaining to drugs since the turn of the twentieth century.

Chapter 3 examines the moral and medical models of drugs and addiction, while also providing a basic overview of some biological and psychological explanations. In contrast, Chapter 4 introduces several different sociological theories that have been used to explain various patterns of drug use, including initiation into drug use, different types of use, continuation of use, and quitting use. In Chapter 5, we provide a sociologically grounded overview of the psychopharmacological properties of various substances, highlighting the puzzling connections between the pharmacological and legal classifications under the eight different schedules of the Controlled Drugs and Substances Act.

Expanding on the socially constructed notion of drugs and drug use as significant social problems, Chapter 6 examines various media representations, including newspaper headlines, public service announcements, and political attack advertisements. Turning to the empirical evidence, Chapter 7 examines the various ways in which sociologists study substance use and related issues by presenting some of the most up-to-date research available from population-based studies, field-based studies, and clinical population studies. Chapters 8 and 9 expand on this by examining general prevalence rates of use in Canada, demographic correlates, and relational correlates including peers and families.

Chapters 10 and 11 present two types of responses to substance use and substance users in Canada. The first examines prevention strategies, specifically drug education within schools. The second type of response, presented in Chapter 11, critically examines various legal responses to drugs and drug use.

Finally, Chapters 12 and 13 examine various drug policies from an international perspective, then turn to Canada's approaches. More specifically, Chapter 12 provides an overview of international drug conventions, as well as some examples of countries with varied responses to drugs and drug use. Chapter 13 concludes with an overview of Canada's simultaneously punitive and pragmatic drug policies and practices, reinforcing the puzzling and paradoxical nature of our approaches towards psychoactive drugs and psychoactive drug use.

It is our hope that this book will encourage students to resist accepting the status quo and help deliver the message that drugs are part of our cultural milieu. For what other nation has both a beer and a whisky named after it? Criminal punishment and medical stigmatization are not working and have never worked. It is time to consider what we can do about drugs that is not going to continue to undermine users' physical and mental health while criminalizing a human activity that predates our written history. We hope to assist this process by having you think in a rational manner that will challenge your beliefs and perceptions, which are no doubt socially constructed rather than based on evidence. We hope you will look at social and public health aspects more, rather than simply accepting that drugs and drug use are individual problems, faults, or shortcomings.

Tara Bruno and Rick Csiernik

ACKNOWLEDGEMENTS

To the many students who continue to ask questions and challenge preconceived notions about drugs and drug users, despite their morals: you are the impetus for this book. We thank you all for keeping the dialogue going! This book is a reflection of many people's contributions and whose support and encouragement are very much appreciated. To begin, we would like to especially thank our fabulous research assistants Alyssa Holden and Jasmine Bender, who helped with so many tasks that are impossible to list briefly: you helped shape this book and the knowledge contained in it. Brikena Qamili, Shelby Lee, Stacie Williams, Kristen Pearn, and last but certainly not least Ryan Hanna: your extra assistance with putting the pieces together is also truly appreciated. To Jessica Sommers, an awesome administrative assistant, thank you for helping get everything organized in the early stages and for your great attention to detail.

We would also like to thank all the staff at Canadian Scholars for their assistance with this initiative. In particular we want to acknowledge the assistance of Susan Silva-Wayne for advocating the need for this book; Emma Melnyk, who took the project and moved forward with it immediately from the beginning; Natalie Garriga, who helped us survive the development phase; and Lizzie Di Giacomo, who supported all of the last minute changes during the final stages of production. We truly appreciate all of their hard work, patience, and flexibility as we attempted to capture the most up-to-date information on drug policy in Canada.

Finally, to our friends and families who always seem to come last but who are always first in our thoughts, thank you for everything.

1

The Drug Paradox: Canada's Conflicting Approaches to Drugs and Drug Users

1.1: WHAT IS THE DRUG PARADOX?

A paradox is defined as something that seemingly contradicts itself but can still be true. This captures the essence of psychoactive drugs, their use, and the perception of their use in Canada. The public sentiment concerning substance use is often characterized by two seemingly contradictory messages: one that promotes the fear and loathing of substances and those who use them due to the perceived and actual negative outcomes of their use, and the other that there is a limited acceptance that substance use is a part of our everyday lives with real economic benefits derived by Canadian society from the marketing and sale of drugs. These sentiments are closely linked to the legal classifications of substances, rather than the actual harm posed. Indeed, licit substances are often viewed with less contempt and are even an accepted part of our cultural activities. Illicit substances, on the other hand, are typically viewed as dangerous and malicious; however, there is often limited empirical evidence to support these claims. Based on the existing evidence, licit drugs are a far greater social and public health issue compared to illicit drugs (International Narcotics Control Board, 2014; Thavorncharoensap et al., 2009). The irony, of course, is that the notion of licit and illicit is, for the most part, a social construct.

This paradox not only exists in the minds of the public, but also exists in historic and contemporary policy responses (Erickson, 1999). Canada's National Anti-Drug Strategy, set out by the Conservative government in 2008, clearly illustrates how drug use continues to be defined as problematic in contemporary society. Using abstinence-based advertising and educational programs mainly targeting youth, the anti-drug strategy resorted primarily to fear messaging in an attempt to deter those who were considering using socially defined illicit drugs. Moreover, the advertisements and educational programs aimed at parents further encouraged adults to be alarmed, frightened, and proactive at the first suspicion that a child or youth may be using drugs (Government of Canada, 2007). However well intentioned, the negative imagery and messages in media representations of substance use, along with ongoing government campaigns aimed at not only discouraging but also preventing any substance use, contribute to the perception that substance use is a serious and escalating social problem in need of action and intervention.

In contrast to the alarmist approach of government agencies and some educators about drugs—that their effects alone "cause" addiction—the normalization approach to substance use acknowledges that individuals are active agents, capable of making both responsible and irresponsible decisions (Aldridge, Measham, & Williams, 2011; Sandberg, 2011; Erickson & Hathaway, 2010) and that substance use has been a historic component of Canadian society since colonization (Csiernik, 2016; Etienne & Brownbill, 2010). From this perspective, the social context is also seen as important in setting out standards for more or less responsible use of substances. Appropriately, attempts to demonize drugs and present substance users as deviant have been countered in policy debates by youth movements, such as Canadian Students for Sensible Drug Policy (cssdp. org), and the more historical Le Dain Commission (1973), both of which recognize the varying degrees of harm associated with different substances and different levels of use.

According to sociologist and prominent Canadian drug researcher Patricia Erickson (1999), Canada has a long history of public health traditions and progressive laws protecting human rights. However, when it comes to substance use and users, laws and policies have tended to reflect more punitive, stigmatizing approaches. Even more puzzling, Erickson contends, is that the laws and policies are not always followed in practice. In Canada, methadone maintenance and treatment have expanded, safe injection sites have been protected by the Supreme Court, and a large number of municipalities offer various harm reduction programs, including needle exchange, crack pipe distribution, training in how to reverse heroin overdose using freely dispensed naloxone (Narcan) kits, safe consumption sites, and assistance in responding to illicit substance use issues.

These competing positions of criminalization and stigmatization on the one hand and a strong public health approach on the other have yet to be considered as the source of Canada's inability to address substance use and misuse in a progressive and pragmatic way. What is needed is a greater public awareness, based on empirical evidence, that acknowledges not only the problems but also both the hedonistic and functional aspects of psychoactive substance use. At a societal level, it must also be recognized that there are economic and social realities of licit drug and prescription use that cannot be ignored. Once this public awareness is strengthened, the status quo can be questioned more rigorously and the laws and policies reformed from an evidence-based standpoint rather than from an ideological perspective.

However, changing people's beliefs about drugs is a challenging task given the historic fearmongering that has accompanied the arbitrary determination of the legality of various psychoactive agents. This paradox itself is firmly rooted in contradictions regarding the competing interests of science and morality, with morality remaining the more prominent in terms of policy creation. What is both interesting and noteworthy about these two separate domains is that the distinction between science and morality has been particularly and seemingly purposefully blurred when it comes to illicit versus licit drugs and drug users (Reinarman, 2005).

Substance use and misuse is a complex and interdisciplinary field of research. The current understanding of substance use and its outcomes evoke a vast range of cultural, political, biological, pharmacological, psychological, and social implications, all of which inevitably influence both interventions and policies. Canada's approach to drugs and drug use is simultaneously progressive and oppressive, which has left the general public in our country in a state of utter confusion and uncertainty about the nature of drugs and drug use. Until there is a better acceptance and understanding of drugs and drug users, policies, programs, and public perceptions will continue to contradict one another, creating paradoxical approaches.

This chapter introduces the tension between official definitions of drugs and drugs use and some existing research on drugs and drug use in Canada, including the current social reality of drugs and drug-related harms in Canada. The following section begins by delineating several key terms mentioned throughout the text that are often misrepresented or misunderstood in everyday conversation—and sometimes even the existing academic literature.

1.2: DEFINING THE CORE CONCEPTS

The term *drug* can be defined in several different ways. For some, the idea of drugs denotes medicines prescribed by doctors to benefit ill patients. Others view drugs as over-the-counter medications used for the relief of either acute or chronic ailments. Still others use the term to refer to illicit substances, while some include licit substances such as tobacco or alcohol in their definition, with a minority also correctly including solvents and inhalants in this categorization.

Psychoactive drugs are substances that alter our central nervous system (CNS), including our thoughts, emotions, and behaviour. They can also affect our autonomic nervous system, and thus have the potential to either balance our systems or, more typically, disrupt core biological functions including the cardiovascular, endocrine, respiratory, immune, and digestive systems. They also have the ability to disrupt our ability to sleep and dream, which in turn affects our mental health (Csiernik, 2014a). Thus, *drug* refers to any psychoactive substance, licit or illicit, that is used for the intended or unintended purpose of altering one's mind and bodily functions.

In sociological terms, drugs are more than pharmacological or biochemical substances that alter the human body and mind. "In addition to their inherent pharmacological properties, drugs are also taken *in certain ways, by certain people, for certain reasons*; moreover, they are also social, cultural, political and symbolic phenomena ..." (Goode, 1999: 27; emphasis in original). For the purposes of this book, *drugs* will be used broadly to include all of these references as they pertain to psychoactive substances. Throughout, the term *substance* will also be used interchangeably to refer to psychoactive drugs that have the aforementioned potentials. Using these terms synonymously will hopefully send a clear message that "drugs" are not necessarily bad in the way that we have come to attach particular meanings to the term; they are simply substances, just like the more widely accepted uses of alcohol and tobacco.

Just as people define drugs differently, there is considerable debate and confusion regarding the differences between drug use, drug abuse, drug dependence, and drug addiction. Some people use these terms interchangeably, suggesting there is no distinction between the person who used cannabis one night at a party and the person who feels the need to drink excessively every night of the week despite experiencing negative personal and social consequences. However, these two scenarios are obviously quite distinct. The former refers to an instance of drug use, whereby the individual may or may not ever use the substance again. If the individual does use the substance again, this would still be considered drug use and not drug abuse, dependence, or addiction, as some might suggest or believe.

It is not surprising that the general public and researchers alike use these terms interchangeably. Even the institutional supports for drugs and drug users remain inconsistent in the use of certain terms. For instance, the Canadian Centre on Substance Abuse (CCSA)[1] and the Centre for Addiction and Mental Health (CAMH) both engage in similar types of research, yet as the institutional names suggest, the former appears to be concerned with substance abuse, while the latter focuses on addiction. This lack of consistency and precision only creates greater confusion and misconception in society, leading people make inaccurate and harmful judgments about substance use and substance users.

The concept of *drug abuse* has a more nuanced definition, as the proper definition of drug abuse differs from drug use in most cultures (Faupel, Horowitz, & Weaver, 2010). In some cases, drug abuse refers to the misuse of substances leading to negative personal, family, vocation, health, social, community, and societal outcomes. This can include the use of substances for reasons other than the originally intended purpose, such as the use of prescription medications for non-medicinal reasons, or even the use of someone else's prescription without consulting a medical professional. More commonly, drug abuse refers to the use of any substance that is not condoned by the broader society or culture. So, for example, the use of any socially defined illicit drug in Canada may be classified as drug abuse, while the licit drug alcohol would be considered *haram* (forbidden) among many Muslims living in Canada, and for some Mormon groups even a sip of a caffeinated beverage would be considered drug abuse as well.

Of course, the medical or disease model of drug abuse differs from the above social understandings of substance abuse. According to previous versions of the American Psychiatric Association's (2000) *Diagnostic and Statistical Manual of Mental Disorders* (DSM-IV-TR), substance abuse was characterized by any one of the following four criteria:

1. The inability to fulfill major role obligations.
2. Engaging in physically hazardous activities.
3. Recurrent legal problems.
4. Continued use despite persistent or recurrent social or interpersonal problems.

The second major classification of substance use disorders according to the medical or disease model is *drug dependence*. This classification of drug use was controversially used for several years in the medical community to refer to the physical and psychological aspects of substance use. According to some researchers, substance dependency is really just a sub-component of the more commonly used term *addiction* (Csiernik, 2016). Nevertheless, previous versions of the DSM (American Psychiatric Association, 2000) defined drug dependence as consisting of any three or more of the following seven criteria:

1. Tolerance—the need for increased amounts of the substance to achieve the desired effect or a diminished effect when using the same amount of the substance.
2. Withdrawal—physical discomfort with the discontinuation of use or the substance (or another similar substance) is used to avoid the physical pain accompanied by a discontinuation in use.
3. Increase in the amount consumed in either a single episode or over a longer period of time than was intended (binging).
4. Desire to cut down or control use.
5. Excessive amounts of time are spent engaging in activities to obtain, use, or recover from the effects of the substance.
6. Quitting or reducing important social, occupational, or recreational activities because of the drug use.
7. Use is continued despite negative consequences.

The American Psychiatric Association's fifth edition of the DSM (2013) no longer refers to substance abuse and substance dependence as the two major classifications of substance use disorders. Instead, substance abuse and substance dependence are collapsed into one disorder with mild, moderate, and severe categories. Interestingly, the actual criteria have remained relatively unchanged, with a few exceptions. Recurrent legal problems related to substance use have been removed and craving or strong desire to use has been added to the newest version. Aside from these relatively minor changes, there were no other significant changes made to the symptoms of what was once referred to as *substance abuse* and *drug dependence*, yet the new terminology, according to the DSM-V, is *substance-related disorders* and *addictive disorders*.

The renaming of substance use disorders in the medical community seems to be a relatively arbitrary process, with scant evidence to support the replacement of one term over another (Courtwright, 2011; O'Brien, 2010). Where the term *addiction* and its variations had been avoided for several years in medical diagnostics, we are now seeing a return to its usage with no significant changes to the way in which the concept of addiction will be measured and diagnosed. Instead, there are a series of substance-specific disorders, including: alcohol-related disorders; caffeine-related disorders; cannabis-related disorders; hallucinogen-related disorders; inhalant-related disorders; opioid-related disorders; sedative-, hypnotic-, or anxiolytic-related disorders; stimulant-related disorders; tobacco-related disorders; and other (or unknown) substance-related disorders. Included in this diagnostic scheme is the single non-substance-related disorder of gambling, which historically was associated with mental health disorders such as compulsive fire setting (pyromania) and compulsive hair pulling (trichotillomania); again, this indicates the difficult nature of conceptualizing this complex phenomenon. Each of these disorders can be further classified as mild (characterized by the presence of two to three of the symptoms), moderate (characterized by the presence of four to five of the symptoms), and severe (characterized by the presence of six or more of the symptoms). It is also worth noting that in order to be diagnosed as having an addictive disorder, substance-related or not, a person only requires two symptoms to be present.

Not surprisingly, *drug addiction* or *addictive behaviours* are probably the most misused and confused terms in public and academic discourses on drugs. The origin of *addiction* comes from the Latin word *addictus*, which means to be passionately committed, bound, or devoted to a practice. This appears not to be a bad pursuit. However, once the term became associated with individuals pursuing intoxicating substances with passion and commitment, or behaving against the norm while intoxicated, pejorative meanings emerged of the originally harmless and even desirable state of being (Levine, 1978). Moreover, the term has entered common vocabulary in the past few decades to refer to a multitude of behaviours. For instance, it is not uncommon to hear people proclaim they are addicted to a reality television program or to shopping at a particular store. Most would admit that there is a significant difference between these types of "addictions" and the related consequences compared to psychoactive substance-related addiction. Moreover, most people would agree that the public perception of the compulsive desire to watch a television show or shop does not hold the same negative connotation as a heroin or cocaine addiction.

History plays an important role in how addiction is conceptualized and perceived today. Prior to the nineteenth and twentieth centuries, addiction, or rather habituation, was not deemed a significant social problem. Drunkenness was merely taken as a normal and accepted part of social and political life. With the onset of the Industrial Revolution in North America, the temperance movement and prohibition connected the concept of individual addictive behaviour, alcoholism in particular, with both morality and workplace productivity (Csiernik, 2014b; Levine, 1978). As stated by sociology Craig Reinarman (2005: 312), "it is a notion that made sense and took hold at a point in history and in those societies in which social life was organized such that individualism had become the taken-for-granted frame of reference." During this period in time, there was a significant paradigm shift, shaped fervently by Dr. Benjamin Rush, where addiction became known as an indiscriminate disease caused by the substance itself, and individuals unable to control their urges were deemed morally culpable. The only solution or cure for this problem, according to Dr. Rush, was complete abstinence (Levine, 1978). This shift marked the beginning of the medical or disease model of addiction that still retains a prominent place in public and academic discourse.

More than two centuries after Dr. Rush's proclamation that addiction is a disease that can only be treated with abstinence, there remains strong support among neuroscientists and other biologically orientated scientists (Cruz, 2011; Hagele, Friedel, Kienast, & Kiefer, 2014; Tang & Dani, 2009). However, researchers from other academic disciplines have actively challenged these broad and factually contentious claims (Alexander, 1987; Briones, Cumsille, Henao, & Pardo, 2013; Enoch, 2011; Reinarman, 2005). As Reinarman (2005) argues, harms do not always occur from substance use, and when harms do occur, often the negative outcomes cannot be attributed to the substance alone. Social psychologist Stanton Peele's (1985a) discussion on heroin-using mothers demonstrates how multi-faceted issues such as addiction are often confounded with other possible explanations. In the case of heroin-using mothers, Peele argues that the negative effects observed in their newborns are often observed as a consequence of knowing that the mother uses heroin. Additionally, he asserts that when women in their role as mothers are labelled using the oppressive term *addict*, it often goes unacknowledged that there are multiple other factors that are more than likely contributing to the negative effects on their babies, including not only poor physical and mental health but also often poverty. Nevertheless, blame continues to be placed solely on the effects of the drug and the mother's choice to use drugs because these are the most widely accepted and simple explanations for addiction.

Finally, it is imperative to mention the sociological significance of the two classic biological markers of addiction: tolerance and withdrawal. According to Peele (1985b), even tolerance and withdrawal are conditioned by psychological and sociological factors. Similarly, Robin Room (1997) contends that the concepts of tolerance and withdrawal do not exist in societies that have never acknowledged their existence. Peele (1985a) set out a similar argument, suggesting that most persons using psychoactive drugs do not experience the conventional symptoms of withdrawal and tolerance; in fact, those who report having experienced elevated tolerance and terrible withdrawal are those who have brought attention to themselves and their "problem" in the first place, and are only a small self-selected sample of people who experience addiction. He concludes that many individuals neither seek help, nor do they ever experience the classic symptoms. Rather, the process of drug use is played out, whereby individuals go through periods of problematic consumption and controlled use, without seeking the help of others or resorting to complete abstinence, as is advocated by those who think the disease lies within the drug or the individual.

In essence, *addiction* is a holistic concept that encompasses biological, psychological, and sociological factors. As Peele (1985a: 20) stated three decades ago:

> Addiction exists fully only at a cultural, a social, a psychological, and an experiential level. We cannot descend to a purely biological level in our scientific understanding of addiction. Any effort to do so must result in omitting crucial determinants of addiction, so that what is left cannot adequately describe the phenomenon about which we are concerned.

While the disease model of addiction supports a medicalized approach to substance use and misuse, a second approach to addiction, known as the moral or free-will model, suggests substance use and any problems resulting from substance use rest within the individual's moral agency. According to the moral model of addiction, the individual is solely responsible for making pro-social or asocial choices regarding substance use. Many of our policies and programs remain rooted in this moral model; however, such individualized framing of the problem fails to acknowledge the sociocultural influences that are just as important, if not more important, than the individual.

Even the medical or disease model, which was intended to be less stigmatizing and founded exclusively on the biological basis of addiction, is problematic. This model is evidenced in the criteria set out in both the past and present versions of the DSM, where there is a lack of experiential, social, and cultural factors taken into consideration when diagnosing an individual with a pathological disorder. In fact, according to the objectives of the DSM-V, criteria were explicitly revised to ensure that the symptoms would be relevant across various cultures. If diagnostic criteria are going to be the benchmark for identifying persons in need of treatment, then it is imperative that the criteria actually reflect the experiences of the individuals biologically, psychologically, and sociologically.

1.3: THE SOCIAL REALITY OF DRUGS AND DRUG USE

The sociological significance of drugs and drug use are often ignored or vastly underestimated in both the moral and disease models of addiction. Yet the social relevance and social consequences of drugs and drug use are central to our understanding of drugs, drug users, treatment, prevention, and policy development. For instance, the social costs of drugs are far greater for alcohol and tobacco than all of the illicit drugs combined. According to the Canadian Centre on Substance Abuse's most recent analysis, the social cost of substance abuse in Canada in 2002 was almost $40 billion (Rehm et al., 2006). Tobacco accounted for approximately $17 billion, followed by alcohol with just under $15 billion; all of the illegal drugs (including cannabis) accounted for just over $8 billion. These estimates include both the direct and indirect social costs associated with tobacco, alcohol, and illicit drugs. The direct costs assessed in this study included health care, law enforcement, prevention, and research. The indirect costs of the use of these substances included the cost for short- and long-term disability, as well as premature mortality.

Productivity losses, an indirect cost, were the largest expense to Canada, with approximately $24.3 billion, 61 percent of the overall costs of substance use. The second highest cost was for health care, amounting to $8.8 billion, which is 22 percent of the overall costs. The third most expensive cost was for law enforcement, which amounted to $5.4 billion or about 14 percent of the overall costs. Of this amount, almost one third was alcohol related, whereas approximately 22 percent was attributed to illicit drugs. The remaining costs, which were minute by comparison, went towards research and prevention efforts.

In the same study, researchers estimated the number of deaths attributed to alcohol, tobacco, and illegal drugs. Interestingly, for alcohol there were both deaths caused and deaths prevented by its use: the net deaths from the use of alcohol were 4,258; there were 8,103 deaths caused by alcohol and 3,845 deaths prevented by the moderate use of alcohol. The same calculations were not made or even considered for illegal drugs, even though several illegal drugs are used for self-medication purposes. Nevertheless, 1,695 deaths were attributable to all of the illegal drugs combined, 44 percent of that attributed to alcohol. Even more striking is the number of deaths associated with tobacco according to this report: 37,209 in 2002. This is one part of the drug paradox in Canada: public perceptions and policy decisions are rarely based on facts or empirical evidence; instead, the existing moral and medical views of addiction still prevail over a more encompassing, empirically based biopsychosocial model of addiction.

Relatively speaking, there are certainly greater social costs for tobacco and alcohol. However, a paradox emerges here as well, as the general public and policy-makers alike still believe that illegal drugs are far worse than alcohol, while the evidence clearly indicates the opposite. This is partly attributable to the kinds of government research being conducted and the manner in which it is being presented to the public. The general public trusts that the information they are being given is unbiased and accurate, especially when it is disguised as being representative of the population. However, this is not necessarily the case. The Harper Conservatives heavily influenced the types of research that were disseminated to the public via the media through the firing and muzzling of scientists, and by processing evidence through a bureaucratic vetting process that was adhered to by all government scientists during their time in power (Gatehouse, 2013). The result was that scientific evidence contrary to government mandates was actively repressed (Turner, 2013).

Even when reports were released to the public, there were still issues with the manner in which evidence was presented. For instance, according to the 2012 findings of the Canadian Alcohol and Drug Use Monitoring Survey (CADUMS; Health Canada, 2012), approximately 2 percent of illicit drug users reported experiencing harms connected to their drug use in the past year. This could include harms in any one of the following domains: physical health, social life, finances, home or marriage, work or school, legal issues, problems learning, and housing. So how does this compare to the harms reported by alcohol users? Unfortunately, the report did not include this; thus, it is unknown whether these issues were of greater or lesser significance. Instead, when examining the problems associated with alcohol use, the 2012 CADUMS asked about harms that may have been related to other people's alcohol use. Interestingly, approximately 14 percent of people reported being harmed physically, verbally, and/or emotionally because of someone else's drinking.

This is not to suggest that illegal drugs do not pose significant harms, though again, the notion of licit and illicit is a social construct rather than an objective fact. There are certainly significant damages to society and the individual when illegal drugs are consumed, manufactured, and trafficked. However, the problems associated with illegal drugs could be significantly reduced if evidence-based research and practice was being delivered and disseminated to the public, rather than continuing to provide morally biased and ideologically driven programs and laws (Des Jarlais, 1995).

Regardless of the legal or moral status of a substance, drugs, drug use, and drug misuse cannot be fully understood from within a single framework or discipline. Though the disciplines of biology and psychology have historically dominated the discourse surrounding drugs, sociology also has extensive insight and evidence to offer in providing an understanding of drugs in society. It is not only the psychoactive substance and the individual user that need to be accounted for and understood, but also the social environment and broad social patterns of substance use that are vital to understand when developing a holistic understanding of the complex phenomenon of addiction. Certain groups of people, under particular circumstances, are often subjected to more or less formal and informal social control (Goode, 2008). These social variations cannot be understood in terms of drugs and their influence on the human mind and body alone. Indeed, the mechanisms of social control are largely a reflection of society's preconceived notions about particular groups of people and the threats they may pose to society if not adequately controlled. Thus, a sociological approach encourages us to consider not only the social status of people who are using substances, but also the social conditions that encourage or control use.

Central to developing a sociological understanding of substance use and misuse in society are gender, age, social class, sexual orientation, sexual identification, and racial and ethnic origins. Historically, oppressed populations have used and misused psychoactive drugs to greater degrees because they are othered. Although these differences can be influenced by biology and psychology, social factors amplify or attenuate these known vulnerabilities (Csiernik & Rowe, 2017).

The remainder of the book will provide an introduction to an evidence-based account of drugs and drug users in Canada, while considering the origins and implications of the subjectively created drug problems that exist in society. As stated before, Canada's drug paradox is complex. Individual lives are involved and society is inevitably impacted by the outcomes of various approaches to drugs and drug users. When we continue to see drugs only through a criminal or medicalized lens, rather than a social or public health lens, this leads us towards an individual-based, punitive stance on drugs. Thus, we must challenge the status quo, and learn more about the complex reality of drugs and drugs use in Canada beyond the criminalized and stigmatized views that currently dominate. This approach will require you to adopt a critical perspective, which in turn may lead you to examine the sources of your beliefs in the context of new facts and ideas. Even if you do not change your perspective entirely through this introduction to the sociology of psychoactive substances, we hope you will weigh the evidence reflectively and thoughtfully.

NOTE

1. Noting the intentional and negative connotation of the term *abuse*, the Canadian Centre on Substance Abuse officially changed its name to the Canadian Centre on Substance Use and Addict on in May 2017. The acronym remains CCSA.

PARADOXES

1) There is a generally held view among the public and policy-makers alike that illegal drugs result in more addiction-related issues and criminal activity, while the evidence clearly indicates the opposite.
2) Licit drugs account for a greater number of physical harms, including deaths annually, than illicit drugs, yet there remains a greater emphasis on addressing illicit drug use.
3) Factors that determine if a drug is licit versus illicit are more socially than biologically defined.
4) With more knowledge about drugs currently available than ever before, anti-drug messages continue to be primarily morally based rather than scientifically grounded.
5) Canada is a leader in public health policy and practices, yet drug use remains stigmatized and criminalized.
6) Distinct biological, psychological, and sociological knowledge exists, yet rather than integrating them, these fields tend to battle to define addiction through their own unicimensional lens.
7) Both moral and medical models of addiction persist in society, yet the two models are at odds with one another, yielding confusion and contradictions when people try to discuss and understand the "causes" of addiction.

CRITICAL REFLECTIONS

1) What is your definition of addiction?
2) What social influences have shaped your definition of addiction?
3) Why have biological views on addiction become more prominent in society than sociological theories?
4) What differentiates a licit drug from an illicit drug?

5) What value is the DSM definition of drug use? What critique do you have of this approach?

6) Why do you think there is greater stigma associated with illicit drugs, despite the fact licit drugs create more health and social issues?

2 The History and Politics of Canada's Drug Laws

Despite a long cultural history of substance use to alter one's physical or mental state, the history of psychoactive drug laws in Canada is relatively short. In fact, the first official federal legislation was enacted just after the turn of the twentieth century. Even with the passing of various laws and regulations, certain drugs in Canadian society have gone through periods of tolerance and acceptance, only to be later deemed the next societal scourge. Some critics, and in fact many people in society, might believe that we have become better equipped to deal with the "drug problem" through various laws and policies because of increased scientific evidence. Some have even argued that Canada's approach to drugs and drug users is founded upon principles of harm reduction (Grant, 2009). While it is true that some policies and practices are certainly more progressive and pragmatic than those in other countries, Canada's approach to drugs is a "persistent paradox" (Erickson, 1999). In practice, while Canada has a history of public health–based approaches, when critically examining drugs, our laws are quite punitive.

Historically, Canadian drug laws have rarely reflected rigorous scientific facts (Csiernik, Bhakari, & Koop-Watson, 2017; Erickson, 1998; Fischer, 1999). Even when there appears to be empirical evidence to support a law, there is no explicit explanation offered by the government for such approaches, nor is there a clear explanation of why various drugs are classified under a particular drug schedule. Instead, it is more often the case that drug laws are founded upon political and moralistic interests, with a not-so-subtle hint of racism and oppression (Boyd, 1984; Carstairs, 2006; Duster, 1970; Giffen, Endicott, & Lambert, 1991; Marshall, 2015). Indeed, the short history of Canadian lawmaking surrounding drugs reveals an uneasy truth: drugs and drug users are not a significant social problem until they are socially created to be problematic (Giffen, Endicott, & Lambert, 1991; Goode, 1989; Jensen & Gerber, 1993). The history and politics of drug laws and regulations in Canada reflects these unfortunate realities.

Prior to the turn of the twentieth century, psychoactive substances were commonly consumed for various religious, recreational, and medicinal purposes (Dyck & Bradford, 2012; Green, 1979). There were no federal laws regulating the manufacture and distribution of psychoactive substances, so citizens were free from any legal penalties associated with possession, manufacturing, importing, and distribution. However, there was also no quality control and consumers had little recourse if the substance was inactive or toxic. For the colonists, Canadian life was relatively free and liberal.

However, with Confederation and the building of the Canadian Pacific Railway, several aspects of Canadian society began to change, and questions of morality and cultural dominance surfaced, underscored by urban-rural tensions. These issues would serve as the major foundation of Canada's first drug laws. Before any drug legislation was enacted in Canada, there were several decades of moral crusades encouraging temperance, or complete prohibition of alcohol (Malleck, 1999). The moral energy emerging from the middle class and legislative bodies was undeniable. However, during this era there was rarely a focus on substances other than alcohol that were not only readily available but openly advertised—including cocaine for toothaches, heroin for cough control, and the unrestricted growth of hemp.

2.1: PROHIBITION ERA

Unlike the United States, Canada never had full alcohol prohibition, except for a brief period between 1918 and 1920 as part of the larger War Measures Act (Malleck, 2003). Outside of that period, provinces and municipalities had the discretionary power to enact local regulations, but there was never a federal bill introduced. Much of the political decision-making under Prime Minister Wilfrid Laurier (1896–1911) is attributed to a lack of full consensus amongst the provinces, in particular Quebec's unwillingness to support a nationwide prohibition of alcohol, despite a plebiscite where the majority, outside Quebec, did vote in favour of alcohol prohibition (Hallowell, 2013). This particular era in Canada saw the rise of a Temperance Movement with a firm rural foundation, with provinces holding the legislative power to determine if alcohol could be sold and consumed by citizens within its borders. This resulted in each of the provinces having a different history with respect to prohibition, temperance, and government regulation. In Ontario, prohibition was enacted in 1916 only to be repealed in 1927, making alcohol publicly available under government control and regulation, which is maintained in a similar manner today (Malleck, 2003). Prince Edward Island was the first province to enact full prohibition in 1901 and the last province to repeal the laws in 1948 (Government of Prince Edward Island, 2002). Quebec, on the other hand, never supported prohibition, but the War Measures Act forced the province into prohibition for a brief period of time, with the province rescinding prohibition immediately after the War Measures Act was withdrawn in 1920 (Malleck, 2003).

In the Canadian Temperance Movement, the societal concern was not with alcohol so much as the people consuming the substance; thus, legislation still allowed for the manufacture and distribution of alcohol under prohibition as long as citizens were not purchasing and consuming it (Malleck, 2003). Thus, even in this era, alcohol was always available either by prescription from doctors or in the form of beverages containing less than 2.5 percent alcohol, as it was believed it was not possible to become intoxicated at such low levels.

As a result of these concessions, Canada became an important source for bootlegging and illegal distribution of alcohol in North America (Schneider, 2009). The history of alcohol prohibition worldwide is often cited as one of the main contributors to organized crime, labelling particular groups of people as morally abhorrent. The decision to prohibit or enforce widespread temperance is perhaps one of the greatest historical examples of the inability of law enforcement to completely eradicate substance use and abuse (Nadelmann, 1989). Despite the early signs that prohibition did not work for alcohol, several different Canadian drug laws were enacted and amended beginning early in the twentieth century with the same outcomes.

2.2: THE OPIUM ACT (1908)

The Opium Act of 1908 was the first official federal drug legislation in Canada (Green, 1979). As the name suggests, there was only one substance of concern under this law: opium. The particulars of the legislation were relatively limited in scope, but it made it an indictable offence to import, manufacture, possess, or sell opium for purposes other than medicinal use. People violating these provisions could face up to three years in prison and/or a fine ranging from $50 to $1,000 (Government of Canada, 1908a). By today's legal standards, it is clear that the sanctions associated with the Opium Act carried much shorter prison terms and smaller fines. This would eventually lead to the revision, expansion, and renaming of the legislation in only a few short years.

While many would like to believe that the passing of federal legislation concerning opium was founded upon significant evidence and proper consultation with officials, this was not the case (Mosher, 1999). As mentioned before, Canada's history of drug laws, including the debut of the Opium Act in 1908, was almost exclusively socially constructed. Giffen, Endicott, and Lambert's (1991) in-depth historical analysis reveals four social factors that collectively contributed to the successful and virtually uncontested passing of the inaugural Canadian psychoactive drug legislation.

The first condition that contributed to the passing of the act was the moral reformist movements that existed in Canada, and North America more generally. In Canadian society, the primary moral concerns centred on maintaining the dominance of Anglo-Saxon colonizers and their notions of moral behaviour. Central to these beliefs was the inappropriateness of drunkenness, prostitution, gambling, and other hedonistic pursuits. With this came the not-so-subtle concern of the sexual mixing of races. Opium was primarily associated with Chinese labourers, and the concern of the reformists was that drugs were being used to sexually exploit non-Asian women. Moral reformists of the time, usually fundamental or evangelical Protestants, pushed for legislation to criminalize immoral behaviour, including opium-related activities. There is relatively little evidence to suggest that these moral reformists were concerned about the actual effects of opium use or the prevalence of misbehaviour amongst these newer immigrants; instead, they were more concerned about how these groups, who were culturally different, might undermine the economic and moral superiority of the more powerful white Europeans.

A second (and related) factor that allowed for the initial opium legislation to be passed uncontested was the intense racial hostility towards Asian immigrants in the latter part of the nineteenth century and the early twentieth century. It was believed this group and other new immigrants posed a significant threat to the established dominance of white Europeans. Given that opium was a common cultural practice amongst some members of the Chinese population, proposing legislation that criminalized these vulnerable groups ensured that the existing status quo was maintained. Targeting one of their cultural practices, and a major source of economic subsistence for many, reinforced the minority status of Asian immigrants in Canadian society.

The third factor adding to the strength of the legislative momentum was the international anti-opium movement. North American and European leaders believed that the economic and social successes of their countries were evidence of the natural dominance of Caucasians. Accordingly, they believed it was their civic duty to denounce abhorrent behaviour and impose the proper and noble way of living on other less developed nations. In Canada, the anti-opium movement was legitimated in part because it was believed it would help relieve the problems China was experiencing with opium if Canada took a strict stance on the issue. The irony is that opium became a prominent drug in China only after England defeated China in the aptly named Opium Wars of the nineteenth century, forcing the importation of the drug after China had prohibited it.

Finally, the widespread lobbying for anti-opium legislation was the fourth condition that contributed to the eventual enactment of Canada's first drug law. Interestingly, the lobbying efforts to impose restrictions on opium in Canada were not confined to the more dominant Anglo-Saxons and political elites. Many Asian immigrants supported the anti-opium legislation and lobbied the government to enact legislation that would immediately suppress the manufacture, distribution, and sale of opium, as it was also affecting the well-being of their communities (Giffen, Endicott, & Lambert, 1991).

2.3: PROPRIETARY OR PATENT MEDICINE ACT (1908)

In the same year that the Opium Act was passed, Parliament also passed the Proprietary or Patent Medicine Act (Government of Canada, 1908b). This legislation prohibited the use of medicinal cocaine, limited the amount of alcohol that could be contained in medicinal preparations, and required pharmaceutical companies to label ingredients if heroin, morphine, or opium was used. The important distinction between this act and the Opium Act was not the substances being controlled as much as the criminal status attached to the offences and the notable differences in the penalties (Giffen, Endicott, & Lambert, 1991). Under the Opium Act, violations were treated as criminal infractions carrying the potential for significantly more jail time—a maximum of three years—and a much more substantive monetary fine of up to $1,000; the same was not true if the substance was created for medicinal purposes and violated the regulations set out in the Proprietary or Patent Medicine Act. In addition to potentially losing the ability to register a product for sale, the maximum fine under this act was only $100, while the maximum jail time was 12 months (Dion, 1999).

2.4: THE OPIUM AND DRUG ACT (1911)

As mentioned, the Opium Act was limited in its scope, focused solely on opium and not its derivatives or any other substances that were deemed a threat to the social order. Aside from this limitation, it did not take long to realize that it was ineffective in curbing smuggling between provinces and across national borders (Giffen, Endicott, & Lambert, 1991). Labour Minister Mackenzie King, who was aiding Prime Minister Wilfrid Laurier with investigating the effectiveness of the Opium Act of 1908, proposed three reasons for introducing a new bill:

1. the Shanghai Commission, which was the first international attempt to make collaborative recommendations concerning opium imports and exports (United Nations, 2009);
2. the panic in Montreal caused by cocaine use, which was believed to be spreading through all segments of society (Murray, 1987); and
3. the need to grant special powers to the police to ensure that the Act could be enforced effectively (Giffen, Endicott, & Lambert, 1991).

The 1911 Opium and Drug Act attempted to address these emergent issues and the shortcomings of the 1908 act by extending the focus of the legislation to include opium, cocaine, and derivatives of these substances (Government of Canada, 1911). The number and types of offences were also extended to include greater regulation of medical and scientific uses of the substances, as well as greater restrictions on who was authorized to manufacture, possess, and distribute the drugs. Some of the most notable changes included extending the list of offences to include possession for the purpose of using; introducing greater police power to search and seize; making it an offence to be in a dwelling or building containing narcotics[1]; and introducing the reverse onus clause, where individuals had to prove that they were not involved with or intending to use the drugs if they had been accused. This final change was in direct contrast to the legal principle of innocent until proven guilty, which applied to all other criminal offences.

Whereas the 1908 act treated violations as indictable offences, the 1911 act carried less severe penalties, though the main targets for criminal enforcement still remained users and traffickers. Based on these significant changes, the 1911 legislation is argued to be the true beginning of Canada's national drug prohibition and the legislated, and thus socially-constructed, standpoint that drug use was a criminal act as opposed to a medical or social issue (Giffen, Endicott, & Lambert, 1991).

By the 1920s, several additional amendments were added to the 1911 act (Government of Canada, 1920). In 1921, drug penalties were expanded to seven-year sentences for crimes committed under the act (Government of Canada, 1921), while whipping and deportation became penalties for convicted offenders in 1922 (Government of Canada, 1922). Interestingly, in 1923, cannabis was added to the list of prohibited substances (Government of Canada, 1923). There was no parliamentary debate provided, nor any objections to adding this new, relatively unheard of or used substance to the act. This placed Canada among the first nations to prohibit cannabis, making use and possession of this substance a criminal offence.

Much of the impetus for this change was the work of pioneering Canadian feminist activist Emily Murphy, whose book *The Black Candle*, published in 1922, claimed marijuana turned its users into homicidal maniacs. This tactic would be used a decade later in the United States, though the rationale for prohibition there was primarily economic, not moralistic as in Canada. Nevertheless, this minor and simple addition to Canada's list of prohibited substances has had tremendous consequences both individually and socially over the past century, and the moralistic view from 1923 continued to dominate the debate regarding the use of cannabis for medical and recreational purposes for nearly a century.

2.5: THE OPIUM AND NARCOTIC DRUG ACT (1929)

By the end of the 1920s, the drug laws shifted towards an even more punitive stance against drugs and drug users, further criminalizing this behaviour. Some have attributed the support of this movement to the ongoing racist media propaganda of Emily Murphy (Mosher, 1999), while others have argued that Murphy was not the sole figure responsible for the initial criminalization of cannabis (Carstairs, 2006; House, 2003). Murphy was not responsible for the harsh sanctions that the government would introduce in the Opium and Narcotic Drug Act of 1929, though there is likewise no evidence to suggest that she was opposed to the harsh punishments.

Indeed, there were several social forces operating at the time cannabis debuted in Canada's drug legislation. Amongst these influences were the enforcement agencies, members of parliament, politicians from the United States, and perhaps most importantly an ignorant public. The major focus of the 1929 act was on harsher drug penalties. The most notable changes from the previous legislation included an extension of whipping to include *all* convicted drug offenders, increases in the minimum fines for smoking opium, double-doctoring,[2] and fraudulent trafficking[3] (Government of Canada, 1929).

Ultimately, when new and harsher penalties were introduced, there was widespread support in parliament and little public resistance (Mosher, 1999). The only noted concerns were with the potential mistreatment of doctors and other medical professionals under the legislation. Nevertheless, the act was passed.

Over the course of the next three decades, there were few changes to the legislation, though there was a continued effort to revisit the penalties and impose stricter sanctions on both traffickers and users, especially in the mid-1950s (Mosher, 1999). These issues would emerge again when a Special Committee on the Traffic in Narcotic Drugs in Canada in 1955 was launched to investigate the narcotic drug situation in Canada (Solomon & Green, 1982). Though there were no legislative changes that directly resulted from the Senate committee, not surprisingly the public and political sentiment was to stiffen the existing penalties, as the moral model of substance use was the dominant lens through which drugs continued to be viewed. Some people suggested including the death penalty for higher-level trafficking, while others suggested extending the minimum penalty for trafficking to 14 years in prison. For simple possession offences, it was suggested that there be a mandatory minimum sentence of six months in jail. However, the Senate committee's final report indicated that there was no longer an overwhelming consensus about what to do about drugs in society. Education and treatment started to slowly emerge as possible alternatives to the criminal justice approach that had been embraced since the beginning of the century.

There were also external forces that led the Senate committee in this direction and to make certain recommendations. Perhaps most important was Canada's adoption of the Single Convention on Narcotic Drugs through the auspices of the United Nations in 1961 (United Nations, 1972). This was an important point in drug legislation history, as it consolidated the existing international drug laws into a single convention, formally replacing the 1912 Hague Convention. Undoubtedly, this single convention influenced the introduction of the next federal drug legislation, as it was necessary for Canada to ensure that our domestic laws were consistent with international agreements.

2.6: THE NARCOTIC CONTROL ACT (1961)

In response to the findings of the Senate committee and the need to comply with the Single Convention on Narcotic Drugs, the Narcotic Control Act of 1961 was introduced. This body of legislation would become the primary instrument of Canadian drug control for over 35 years. A puzzling feature of this legislation is that its name refers only to narcotics, not other psychoactive substances or drugs that do not have the properties of a narcotic. However, the actual content of the law included these previously criminalized substances: the pure form or a derivation of opium, cocaine, and cannabis (Government of Canada, 1961). While the impetus behind the legislative change seemed promising, again, the emphasis was on enforcement strategies rather than more pragmatic approaches through education and treatment. The major changes to the legislation included the removal of a minimum six-month jail term for possession. The maximum seven-year sentence for possession still remained, and the minimum and maximum penalties for importing remained unchanged, with the minimum penalty being seven years and the maximum being a life sentence (Government of Canada, 1961).

Throughout the 1960s, however, there were increasing numbers of young people using cannabis in Canada. With the strict enforcement strategies contained in the Narcotic Control Act, many otherwise "respectable" young people were now being charged with indictable offences. In 1969, at the urging of Minister of Health and Welfare, John Munro, the act was changed to allow for cannabis users to be fined and processed summarily (Mosher, 1999). In the same year, the historically significant Le Dain Commission was struck with the task of examining psychoactive drugs and non-medicinal drug use in Canada. The interim report released in 1970 recommended that possession of any illicit substance should not result in a fine greater than $100. This recommendation toward a more lenient and pragmatic approach to drugs and drug users was further echoed in the 1973 final report from the committee, with a recommendation specific to cannabis possession that penalties associated with simple possession should be eliminated. This would have been Canada's first challenge to the Single Convention on Narcotic Drugs.

However, despite the extensive scientifically grounded background research conducted by the Le Dain Commission, the recommendations for a change in focus from law enforcement to prevention and treatment have yet to be fully realized in Canadian drug policy, and even the United States is now moving ahead of Canada in terms of pragmatic approaches (Mosher, 2011).

While there was an appearance of a decline in the prohibitionist approach to drugs from 1969 into the 1980s, laws and lawmakers remained relatively silent on the issue (Erickson, 1992).

The late 1980s, however, saw a wave of intense media and political campaigns to eradicate drugs once and for all under an enhanced "War on Drugs," just as HIV/AIDS was becoming a prominent health and societal issue. Overnight, prohibition was back in full force, especially in the United States, with drug users again being demonized and calls for those with AIDS to be socially and geographically isolated, as lepers had been centuries ago. Though the most recent War on Drugs formally began during the 1970s under the Nixon administration, it was during the Reagan years when policy was simplified under the banner of "Just Say No," which suddenly became a reasonable practice model. This "war" escalated during an era when the United States was involved in no other major global conflict, other than invading Grenada, and was more prominent and costly in the United States than in other countries.

Despite the highly promoted public relationship between Prime Minister Mulroney and President Reagan, the support for a War on Drugs was not widely supported amongst Canadian citizens, nor did it become immediately established in Canadian practices (Erickson, 1992). Jensen and Gerber (1993) argue that there are several reasons why Prime Minister Brian Mulroney's declaration of a "War on Drugs" did not incite panic in the Canadian public. First of all, Mulroney's popularity was actually on the decline when he attempted to follow the United States blindly into this war. Undoubtedly, Mulroney thought he could use drugs to bolster his popularity, but in fact, the actual rates of illicit drug use were on the decline in Canada at the time, so there was no real threat to pursue. Another reason why the drug war did not take root in Canada is because there was little support from the opposition parties to uphold Mulroney's claim. Unlike in the United States, where both the Republicans and the Democrats were fighting over who was going to better deal with drug issues, Canadian opposition parties had no interest or concern in psychoactive drugs as a major party policy platform. Thus, there was no real heightened concern, even within Parliament, at the time. Finally, despite historically being leaders in prohibitionist policy in North America, during this period Canadian citizens had paradoxically become more liberal than American citizens with respect to illicit drug use. Thus, despite a relatively punitive law enforcement approach to drugs from a government-control standpoint, the Canadian public was not in general fixated on the fear of societal collapse arising from individual possession or personal use of illicit substances.

2.7: CONTROLLED DRUGS AND SUBSTANCES ACT (1996)

From the 1960s to the end of the twentieth century there was a significant amount of scholarship from Canadian sociologists and other social scientists surrounding drug policy and its effects on society and users (Erickson, 1998). In the early 1990s, when new drug legislation was being tabled, over three decades of evidence had been collected using both large-scale surveys and qualitative, community-based studies. However, the evidence did not inform the end result. As Erickson (1998) stated, Canadian research had ultimately been "neglected and rejected" in the formation of the Controlled Drugs and Substances Act (CDSA).

In 1997, under Prime Minister Jean Chrétien, the CDSA became Canada's new federal drug control statute (Government of Canada, 1996). Repealing the Narcotic Control Act and Parts III and IV of the Food and Drugs Act, the CDSA contained eight schedules of controlled substances and two classes of precursors— substances used in the manufacture of synthetic or semi-synthetic drugs (Fischer, Erickson, & Smart, 1996).[4] Under this act, amendments can be made to any one of the schedules at any given time if it is deemed necessary for the public interest (Collin, 2006).

While there is no way to ascertain why existing evidence on the harms of prohibition were not considered in this legislation, some compelling explanations have been offered (Boyd, 1998; Erickson, 1998; Fischer, 1999). Erickson (1998) outlines several potential reasons for the disappointing enactment of the CDSA. When the Narcotic Control Act of 1961 was being considered for revision and replacement in the early 1990s, no federal government leader expressed any interest in changing the status quo. Enforcement and punitive control had been a mainstay of Canadian drug legislation for almost a century, and the introduction of a new approach was not on any political party's agenda. This was, in part, because there was no real electoral advantage for Prime Minster Chrétien to take a different approach, or, as was the case historically with other leaders, he had personal and political beliefs that were more conservative than liberal. Even though it was clear that the public did not support Conservative Prime Minister Mulroney's initial attempts to create a moral panic concerning drugs (Jensen & Gerber, 1993), neither was there a substantive push from citizens for any reform when Liberal Prime Minister Chrétien came to power. Thus, when presented with evidence that did not support the existing status quo, government bureaucrats had no vested interest in hearing it. Added to this is the significant undermining of the value of science and evidence in informing policy, especially with such moralized issues as drugs and drug users. Finally, Erickson (1998) suggests that Canadian drug policy with respect to illicit substances suffers because of an ongoing trade-off with more liberal and tolerant policies towards legal substances such as alcohol and tobacco.

An alternative viewpoint reflects the influence of other countries on Canadian drug policy. Drug policy expert Benedikt Fischer (1999) referred to the 1980s and early 1990s as a "window of opportunity" for Canada to shift its focus from a prohibitionist approach to a public health approach, as adopted in many parts of Europe. However, he argues that Canada's inability to approach drugs more pragmatically was primarily a result of our close economic, geographic, and social ties to the United States. The political climate in the United States remained moralistic and prohibitionist during this perceived opportunity for drug law reform in Canada. Thus, it appears that Canadian politicians had too much to lose by challenging the existing drug legislation, which is further reflected in their current ambiguity regarding medical marijuana, derived from the cannabis plant.

2.8: MARIHUANA FOR MEDICAL PURPOSES REGULATIONS (2013)

Cannabis is part of the hemp family of plants. While hemp has many commercial, agricultural, and industrial uses, its most renowned psychoactive strain, marijuana, has a variety of documented therapeutic uses. This includes producing relief from nausea and vomiting produced by chemotherapy; increasing appetite among people with HIV and other terminal illnesses; aiding in the treatment of glaucoma; relieving muscle spasms associated with spinal cord injuries and multiple sclerosis, as well as decreasing seizures for some forms of epilepsy; and alleviating gastrointestinal disorders, depression, anxiety, tension, and chronic pain (Elikkottil, Gupta, & Gupta, 2009; Ogborne, 2000; Walsh et al., 2013).

Beginning in 2000, court challenges to the prohibition of cannabis on medical grounds began to be heard and won. For over a decade, judges ruled that the prohibition on cannabis was unconstitutional, as it did not contain any exemption for medical use and thus violated citizens' rights to liberty and security in a manner that was not in accord with the Charter of Rights and Freedoms. Finally, on April 1, 2014, the Marihuana for Medical Purposes Regulations (MMPR), was introduced, allowing access to marijuana for medical purposes in Canada through licensed producers if prescribed by a physician (Government of Canada, 2014). Individuals requesting use of the drug would no longer have to apply through Health Canada, though physicians were still required to complete a medical document enabling patients to purchase the appropriate amount related to their conditions directly from a licensed producer approved by Health Canada (Health Canada, 2013b; Health Canada, 2015). Despite this progressive move forward, by keeping the legal classification in place and ensuring that only Health Canada–approved producers were used, this ensured that a degree of stigma surrounding marijuana use, even for medicinal purposes, was maintained.

2.9: ACCESS TO CANNABIS FOR MEDICAL PURPOSES REGULATIONS (2016)

Under the Liberal government elected in 2015, cannabis use for medicinal purposes has already seen significant changes. Though many believe these changes arose at the directive of the newly elected prime minister, the reality is that the former MMPR legislation was repealed as a product of a federal court ruling in a 2016 case involving four people using marijuana for medicinal purposes. The new legislation essentially allows people who have been granted permission by a licensed doctor to produce a limited amount of cannabis for their own consumption, rather than being forced to purchase the medicine from government-licensed producers. The legislation also allows users to have someone else produce a limited amount for them, if they do not wish to produce it themselves. However, the new legislation is a temporary solution to the limitations of the MMPR, until the government's formal legislation to legalize and regulate cannabis is enacted in 2018.

2.10: A FRAMEWORK FOR THE LEGALIZATION AND REGULATION OF CANNABIS IN CANADA (2016)

During the latter part of 2016, a multidisciplinary task force consulted with municipal, territorial, provincial, and Indigenous governments, as well as community organizations, youth, patients, and medical experts, to develop a plan for the legalization and regulation of cannabis. The objective of this task force was to investigate the multitude of positions on cannabis and propose an evidence-informed framework for Canada to legalize and regulate cannabis (Health Canada, 2016). The task force's recommendations focused on five thematic areas: (1) minimizing harms of use; (2) establishing a safe and responsible supply chain; (3) enforcing public safety and protection; (4) medical access; and (5) implementation. Among the key recommendations were:

- A national minimum age of 18 to purchase cannabis, with provinces and territories having the latitude to set limits above 18 to coincide with alcohol and tobacco age requirements.
- Restrictions on advertising and promotion similar to those applied to tobacco products, including the prohibition of products that mix cannabis with other substances, such as tobacco or alcohol.
- The use of tax revenues derived from sales to fund education, research, and enforcement of not only cannabis use disorders but also underlying risk factors such as mental health and social disadvantages.
- Development of a public education campaign to begin immediately to educate the public, especially youth, parents, and vulnerable populations, about cannabis and the proposed legislation (Health Canada, 2016).

The anticipated date for the official enactment of the proposed cannabis act is the summer of 2018. Appendix A (see pp. 262–263) provides a summary of the provincial and territorial regulations for cannabis legalization prepared by Ottawa lawyer Trina Fraser, partner at Brazeau Seller Law, at the time of publication (Fraser, 2018).

2.11: CONCLUSION

Until its defeat in 2015, the Conservative-led federal government continued to view cannabis as a major public threat. As well, even though the Supreme Court of Canada, the ultimate arbitrator of the constitutional validity of legislation, has consistently struck down proposed legislation to close safe injection sites and invoke mandatory minimum sentencing, there was still a significant moralistic push from the Conservative government to eradicate drug use and drug users through punitive enforcement strategies (Hyshka et al., 2012). This disconnect between the social conservative agenda under the leadership of Steven Harper and the more centralist position of the Canadian courts led by the Supreme Court of Canada underscored the paradox of drugs and drug use in Canada. However, this would take a dramatic turn with the election of the Liberal Party of Canada under the leadership of Justin Trudeau in 2015.

As it stands, the drug laws for illicit substances in Canada are still punitive, having minimal regard for cost to users and society. As a result, a significant number of Canadians are charged each year for drug offences, mostly for possession and cannabis-related offences (Statistics Canada, 2014)—a trend that has been increasing, not decreasing. After over a century of lawmaking in Canada's Parliament, the existing state of the laws regressed to the draconian legislation of the early 1900s under the Harper Conservatives, despite proposed legislation continually being overturned by appeals in both provincial and federal courts. Much has been debated in the past two decades since the enactment of the CDSA, yet little progress has been made towards a more effective approach to legislating drugs and controlling those who use them.

Thus far, breakthroughs in our understanding of how psychoactive drugs work and how to better treat addiction have had minimal impact on decision-making in Parliament. It seems a different approach needs to be taken to create a meaningful change for Canada. As Erickson (1998) suggested at the close of the last century, social scientists and drug researchers need to continue to spread their knowledge and expertise to the greater Canadian community. Canada is a democracy, where citizens have the right, and obligation, to resist policies that are not in the best interests of the country. The more knowledge the public has about the realities of drugs and the harms of punitive drug policies, the greater the possibility that legislators will have no choice but to change those policies.

In the meantime, there are small glimmers of hope for Canadian drug legislation. The Liberal Party of Canada's proposal to legalize cannabis by the summer of 2018 has sparked promise for a new approach to drugs and drug users in Canada. Yet there are still several uncertainties, including Canada's role in challenging or withdrawing from international drug conventions, or if these are even relevant anymore (Hoffman & Habibi, 2016).

While the proposed changes to cannabis legislation are certainly welcomed and long overdue, there is still no indication that any discussion surrounding changes to domestic legislation for other illicit psychoactive substances is being considered. Hopefully, once the cannabis legislation is tabled and implemented with no undermining of Canadian values and principles, Parliament can begin a careful and evidenced-based review of all psychoactive drugs, so that our policies and practices in the twenty-first century are based in fact, not fear.

NOTES

1. Scientifically, narcotics refer to opium-based drugs; legally, any drug that was banned became a narcotic. Thus, cocaine, which has the opposite pharmacological and behavioural effects than opium, suddenly became legally classified as a narcotic.

2. *Double-doctoring* refers to the practice of individuals attempting to obtain two or more doctors to prescribe the same substance during the same period of time.

3. This was implemented to ensure that only authorized persons in the medical and dental community were allowed to send narcotics through the mail.

4. The specific schedules and penalties under the CDSA are detailed in Chapter 5.

PARADOXES

1) While Canada has a history of public health–based approaches, drug laws remain generally regressive and oppressive.

2) After the Le Dain Commission presented the most progressive scientifically based review on psychoactive drugs in the world for its time, the report was tabled and Canada would focus on punitive, non-scientific policy initiatives for the next four decades.

3) Cannabis was legal during the era of alcohol prohibition, yet shortly after reinstating legal use of alcohol, cannabis was attached to federal legislation that prohibited the possession of heroin and cocaine.

4) The prohibition of cannabis did not result in any formal charges for over a decade, yet the substance remained prohibited for unknown reasons and continued to be prohibited for recreational use well into the twenty-first century in Canada.

5) Despite being among the first nations in the world to prohibit cannabis, Canada was among the leaders to allow its use medically and to enact legislation to formally legalize recreational use.

CRITICAL REFLECTIONS

1) What are the factors driving drug prohibition?

2) What utility is there in the prohibition of psychoactive drugs?

3) What limits attempts to legalize a psychoactive substance once it has been prohibited?

4) What factors contribute to the disconnect between knowledge and policy with respect to psychoactive drugs?

5) If history is any indication of how laws surrounding illicit drugs are created and maintained, how might current attempts to legalize recreational cannabis use be prevented?

3 Explaining Substance Use I: Biological and Psychological Theories

Addiction is a multidisciplinary field of study. As such, several different disciplines have contributed to the ongoing debate about the nature of substance use and substance dependence. There is no one field of study that can completely explain who will use and who will eventually become dependent on psychoactive substances. While focused on the two major areas outside sociology, this chapter begins by examining the longest running debate in the addiction field: is substance use or dependence an issue of individual morality or is it a medical problem? Biological and psychological explanations of substance use tend to support the notion that it is an individual issue, though not necessarily one of morality. Each of these fields have also come to varying conclusions about what is most important to consider when trying to understand substance use and dependence. From the outset, it is important to acknowledge that both biology and psychology play important roles in understanding substance use and dependence, but that by themselves offer an incomplete understanding of this complex phenomenon. Given that this text is sociologically focused, it is beyond its scope to provide an in-depth account of all biological and psychological explanations; however, a basic understanding of these perspectives and some of the debates in these fields is essential if one is to develop a holistic understanding of this area of study.

3.1: THE MORAL MODEL VERSUS THE MEDICAL MODEL

The history and politics of substance use and substance users offer significant insight into the various explanations or theories that are still widely contested today. Significant advancements in research have helped to empirically discredit historical views of the stereotypical drunkard or addict, and people working in the substance use field rarely use these terms that were once common even amongst researchers. However, these pejorative terms remain regularly used in public discourse. These inaccurate ideas persist in part because the historic debate rages on about whether substance dependence is a moral failing or a disease, despite the total inadequacy of the first view and the scientific shortcomings of the second. However, it is because of the prominence of the moral model that such staunch disease model advocates remain. The fact that the dialogue remains so focused on this debate significantly limits the theoretical advances made in the field. This debate is central to the drug paradox: the moral model perpetuates fear and disdain for users, and is readily employed during national elections in Canada; the medical model, while appearing to absolve users of responsibility, likewise negates any examination of larger structural and societal issues that contribute to the development of substance use and abuse (Csiernik, 2016; Hammersley & Reid, 2002). Even in the field of medicine, where the disease model would naturally be widely accepted, the beliefs of physicians still reflect some elements of morality (Lawrence, Rasinski, Yoon, & Curlin, 2013).

The moral model is the most historic approach to substance use and misuse, and thus the most established. Its influence can be witnessed through public perception, government policy, and the way in which we treat substances users. According to the moral model, substance use and misuse is a matter of personal choice and personal weakness. While the rise of the moral model is associated with individualism and the "free society" of the eighteenth and nineteenth centuries, which was accompanied by the expectation that people were responsible for their own immoral behaviour (Reinarman, 2005; Levine, 1978), its origins are associated with religious teachings intent on the well-being and survival of the faithful (Csiernik, 2016). Accordingly, blame for the failure to conform to the widely held belief that intoxication is immoral is placed solely on the individual (Room, 1997). Those who use illicit drugs, or use licit psychoactive substances beyond an acceptable social threshold (of which there is no agreed upon definition), are considered morally repugnant and responsible for their own negative outcomes.

For most illegal substance use, whether it is beyond a threshold or not, individual users are viewed with a significant amount of fear and disdain.

However, as Judith Blackwell notes (1988), the social response and legal repercussions under a moral model not only depend on the substance being used but also the social status of the user. Thus, the heroin user who engages in petty theft to procure the next fix is treated much differently than the CEO who drinks excessively and then physically abuses his or her family. Admittedly, the heroin user is more publicly visible and socially marginalized than the alcohol-dependent CEO, but as far as morality is concerned, there is little justification for why the CEO is rarely held accountable for seemingly more damaging criminal acts. This is partially explained by our less punitive stance towards alcohol in the Western world, as well as our beliefs about what is acceptable behaviour while intoxicated and what is not. There seems to be far greater acceptance of misbehaviour while intoxicated by alcohol than most other illicit substances.

Accountability under the moral model takes two forms. One method is to criminalize individuals through the use of *formal sanctions* such as laws, regulations, and punitive punishment. The stricter the laws become, the more socially marginalized individuals are for their behaviour. If individuals violate the prescribed rules they will be held fully accountable for their actions, if not under the law then at least in the way the public perceives them. The second method of accountability under the moral model is known as *informal social sanctions*. There are varying degrees of informal social sanctions, ranging from minimal responses such as expressed disapproval of behaviour by family and friends to more substantive responses such as losing a job or being rejected for treatment for not meeting the specified objectives of abstinence-based programs.

In Canada, law enforcement and criminal justice approaches, following a moral model orientation, continue to be in conflict with the medical model, which advocates for more treatment-based strategies to deal with substance dependence—though both remain individual rather than structurally focused. This latter approach originated during the late nineteenth century in the United Kingdom and the 1930s and 1940s in the United States, when a seismic shift in thinking about addiction occurred. This paradigm change had a profound effect on how people with substance dependence were viewed and treated in society, enabling for the first time medical and therapeutic communities to take hold of the issue, which held promise for a more compassionate and less blame-centred approach (Blackwell, 1988). Under this new paradigm, the disease or medical model framed substance dependence and individual users in an entirely different manner than the moral model. Rather than the individual being wholly responsible for substance dependence, the disease model is founded upon a more humanitarian approach that assumes individuals who become addicted or dependent on a substance are victims: they have lost control, due to some type of biological condition or brain disorder that can be treated, making rehabilitation possible and necessary.

According to this model, substance use itself is not a disease; only uncontrollable or harmful use is deemed worthy of the disease label. It is important to clarify that, despite the attempts of the pharmaceutical and medical industries to cure addiction during the twentieth century, the "disease" concept is not founded in scientific fact, and is therefore more of a metaphor for a loss of control than it is a specific biological condition. Our scientific understanding of substance dependence is still limited by the research that is being funded and conducted on substance dependence, which focuses mostly on biological explanations. Yet as sociologist Craig Reinarman (2005: 312) states: "After decades of diligent scientific labour we still await a truly uniform set of symptoms and a distinct site, source, and course of pathology that are necessary and sufficient for the presence of the disease of addiction." In essence, substance dependence as a disease has effectively been socially constructed, not empirically validated.

It would be misleading to suggest that the shift from a moral model to a medical model was a result of truly compassionate efforts in the medical field. Instead, as Blackwell (1988) documents, the shift from a moral model to a medical model had more to do with physicians and the medical community having a greater presence and more powerful position in society. Rick Csiernik (2016) further argues that there were and still are significant economic and political incentives that support the continued belief in the medical model.

Compared to the moral model, where individuals are met with punishment and stigmatization, the disease model emphasizes the importance of treatment by medical professionals or the widely practiced 12-step program of Alcoholics Anonymous and related mutual aid groups. From this perspective, individuals are viewed as being sick or unable to control the urge to consume and in need of help. However, research has shown that this may also be counterproductive. When individuals believe their substance dependence is a disease this removes individual autonomy and the self-confidence to control or change one's situation (Wiens & Walker, 2015). As a disease, substance dependence is seen as a lifelong condition that can only be controlled through complete abstinence. People never recover: they spend their lifetimes in recovery guarding against a return of the disease. However, social psychologist and staunch critic of the disease model Stanton Peele (1985a) argues that many individuals neither seek help nor do they ever experience the classic biological symptoms of tolerance and withdrawal. Rather, individuals can go through periods of problematic substance use to controlled substance use, without seeking help or resorting to complete abstinence. This suggests that individuals do have the capacity to control or change their substance use. If it were a disease that can only be controlled through abstinence, individual agency would not change the behaviour.

While there is great value in viewing substance dependence in a more humane and compassionate manner, the disease model has never been able to fully explain substance dependence; the most dominant form of assistance that arose in parallel under this model, the 12 steps of Alcoholics Anonymous, has also not been able to effectively address the complexities of substance dependence (Peele, 1985a). Moreover, the disease model fails to remove the feelings of shame and stigma that continue to promote the idea that those with substance dependence issues must remain anonymous to avoid personal and professional persecution (Wiens & Walker, 2015).

Thus, both the moral model and disease model have substantive weaknesses, and yet the public debate around substance use and dependence continues to revolve around two incomplete, inadequate, simplistic views. In the interim, other perspectives arose within the scientific community in response to this dominant discourse. Broader biological and psychological theories emerged, taking different though retrospectively still limited standpoints. These ranged from individuals being entirely governed by their biology or psychological state, with no individual agency, to predispositions that may or may not be fully realized depending on environmental influences and individual choices.

3.2: BIOLOGICAL EXPLANATIONS

Over time, a range of biological theories pertaining to substance use and substance dependence arose beyond the disease model. For ease of presentation, the following sections divide biological explanations into three sections: nature/drive theories, genetic theories, and neurobiological theories. Some of these theories have been widely refuted by existing evidence, others have re-emerged, while others have just begun to take a prominent place in the debate about the biological bases of substance dependence. Whatever the explanation, however, there is one common theme amongst all biological theories of substance dependence: individuals do not choose to become substance dependent, so they should not be stigmatized nor imprisoned for their condition, but instead treated and rehabilitated.

Nature and Drive Theories

The basic premise of nature- or drive-based theories is that everyone has the potential to use and become dependent on psychoactive substances because humans are naturally compelled to alter their state of consciousness (Weil & Rosen, 2004). A historical account of humans seeking out or creating psychoactive substances anecdotally supports the notion that psychoactive substance use, as a form of consciousness alteration, may be a universal phenomenon (Mosher & Akins, 2014). However, this by no means supports the contention that altering one's state of mind through substance use is a human drive. Not all humans in all places have used or desired to use psychoactive substances. To argue that something is based on human nature or an instinctual drive means that everyone would engage in the same behaviour as a matter of survival and dismisses the functionality of substance use. Consuming psychoactive substances is not analogous to eating, drinking, or even engaging in sexual behaviour. With only a few exceptions, such as the use of barbiturates to prevent fatalities from epileptic seizures or the use of antidepressants to prevent people from self-harm, psychoactive substance use is not necessary for human survival.

While altering consciousness may be deemed desirable, and certainly temporarily pleasurable, particularly during adolescence when individuals are seeking to create an individualized sense of self, there are many different ways in which this can be achieved. For instance, meditation is a form of altering one's state of mind, as is vigorous physical activity, but neither pose the health concerns that psychoactive substances do, but rather have beneficial outcomes. Thus, to suggest that substance use is rooted in our human nature is misleading, deterministic, and even fatalistic.

According to the nature theories, there is nothing inherently or biologically different about those that develop substance dependence issues and those who do not. If everyone has the potential to become dependent on substances, it is important to ask what social factors increase or decrease the risk of becoming dependent on a substance. Moreover, if all people exhibit the same propensities to alter their consciousness, then we cannot suggest that substance use or dependence is pathological or morally wrong. This should help to remove the stigma attached to psychoactive substances, though this has yet to occur.

While nature theories have not received widespread empirical support, there is evidence to support that there are biological explanations for substance dependence that suggest there are certain inheritable attributes, as well as differential brain chemistries and neural pathways, that are connected to persons who initially seek out substances and eventually become substance dependent. Unlike nature theories, however, genetic and neurobiological theories suggest there is something different about people who initiate and continue to use psychoactive substances.

Genetic Theories

Genetic theories of substance dependence are founded on the assumption that there is some inheritable gene, or more likely combination of genes, that can be used to explain why some people are more susceptible to substance dependence than others. According to genetic theories, certain inheritable traits affect the way our bodies metabolize and/or experience different substances, making us more or less susceptible to substance dependence (Mosher & Akins, 2014). For instance, Eng, Luczak, and Wall (2007) reviewed the genetic evidence for alcohol dependence amongst certain subgroups of Asian people and found that some groups are more vulnerable to negative reactions from alcohol consumption because their bodies metabolize certain enzymes, alcohol dehydrogenase and aldehyde dehydrogenase, in a manner that influences the effects that alcohol has on their bodies. This genetic connection supports several different surveys that found that people of Asian ancestry have the lowest rates of substance use and dependence. Similar genetic findings have also been found for African Americans, who metabolize alcohol rapidly and therefore do not experience the relaxing and calming effects of alcohol that many find desirable (Scott & Taylor, 2007). The assumption behind this line of research is that the negative effects experienced by those who ingest alcohol serve as a deterrent to developing further problems, because people are less likely to continue to use alcohol once they have experienced negative effects.

However, the same type of genetic evidence has not been found for the increased risk of alcohol problems often associated with Indigenous populations, who are often found to have higher rates of alcohol use and dependence (Ehlers, 2007). There are several environmental factors that also contribute to ethnic differences that cannot be accounted for in the genetic variations that have been observed. In fact, some researchers argue that cultural influences have the ability to overcome genetic influences (Boyd, 1983; Peele, 1985a; Waxman & Csiernik, 2010).

In addition to cultural research in genetics, a substantial body of research has examined the longstanding observation that substance dependence, in particular alcoholism, tends to run in families. The majority of this research is founded upon adoption and twin studies, which have made important contributions to our understanding of the biological bases of substance dependence. Based on the existing adoption and twin studies, Agrawal and Lynskey (2008) estimate that the overall effect of genetics on substance use ranges between 30 and 70 percent, with variations largely a function of the substance being used, gender, age, and cultural characteristics. On the one hand, this is quite remarkable, as there is such a significant amount of variation in substance use patterns that can be explained through genetics. On the other hand, the fact that 100 percent of the variation is not explained through these studies indicates other factors need to be considered.

Adoption studies, as a form of natural experimentation, examine the extent to which genes or the environment can predict substance use and dependence (Ball, 2007). The premise behind these studies is that we can determine if there is a genetic component underlying substance dependence if an individual born to a parent with substance dependence is then raised by an adoptive family. If the adoptee develops a substance dependence problem, then genetics are a likely explanation for the outcome. However, if the adoptee does not become dependent on a psychoactive substance, then the adoptive environment is believed to be a protective factor. Early adoption studies found that having a biological parent with alcoholism significantly increased the risk of males developing alcohol problems, regardless of whether or not the child was adopted and raised away from the biological parent. Siblings raised by their biological parent showed no significant difference in their risk of developing alcoholism compared to the adoptee, suggesting that adoption does not protect individuals from substance dependence (Goodwin et al., 1974; Goodwin et al., 1977).

Though adoption studies served as an important starting point in genetic research, there are still some significant limitations. One prominent constraint is the selective placement effect. Many adoptions were historically based on matching the adoptive parents to particular characteristics of the biological parents, which could have an environmental effect on the likelihood of developing substance dependence (Heath, 1995). Also absent from adoption studies is the potential effect of being traumatized by the separation from the biological parent, which may contribute to substance use or dependence. Moreover, adoption studies cannot adequately quantify the genetic differences between siblings raised in different environments because they do not share all of the same genes, unless they are identical twins.

Twin studies offer further support for a genetic connection to substance dependence. These studies compare the differences between identical twins, fraternal twins, and the general population to determine the extent to which genetics contribute to explaining substance dependence. Identical or monozygotic twins share the same genetics, whereas fraternal or dizygotic twins only share half of their genetics. This means that if there is in fact a genetic link to addiction, identical twins will have greater rates of addiction, followed by fraternal twins and then individuals in the general population. In Agrawal and Lynskey's (2008) review of existing twin studies, they state that between 50 to 70 percent of alcoholism was inherited through the genes. Likewise, nicotine heritability ran upwards of 70 percent, with environmental factors contributing the remainder of the risk. For cannabis dependence there was a broader estimate of 34 to 78 percent attributable to genetics. One study reported that the genetic risk of becoming dependent was 26 percent for psychedelics, 27 percent for sedative hypnotics, 33 percent for stimulants, and 54 percent for heroin. However, this is where a serious caveat needs to be introduced: this latter study was conducted in the 1990s using criteria from DSM-III, which has since been revised twice in part due to inadequate measures used in conceptualizing dependency and abuse. It also speaks directly to our use of language: although one may abuse psychedelics, their pharmacological nature makes addiction or dependency impossible. Thus, while there is certainly some type of genetic influence, how dependency and abuse are defined must be carefully considered before fully accepting the degree of heritability proposed.

Undoubtedly, adoption studies and twin studies provide considerable support for the inherited component of substance dependence. Affirmative genetic research, however, does not mean that genetics can invariably determine if we will become dependent on a substance or not; rather, it helps us to understand who is most at risk of developing substance dependence once substance use has been initiated and how much of the dependence can be explained by inheritable characteristics. Despite decades of funding and research, there is no "addiction gene" that has been discovered (Csiernik, 2016). There are multiple other factors—biological, psychological, and sociological—that influence the multigenerational transmission of substance dependence besides one's genes. Nevertheless, genetic theories help to maintain the notion that substance dependence is an issue beyond the control of the individual and society. If the risk of substance dependence is in our genes, then we cannot control its biological transmission, at least not ethically, nor can we change it through the development of social policies and more appropriate social education.

Neurobiological Theories

The current area of biological study receiving the greatest amount of interest, and thus the greatest amount of funding, is neurobiology. Neurobiologists attempt to better understand how individuals process information such as learning, emotions, perceptions, and sensations. Most neurobiological explanations continue to frame our understanding of substance dependence solely in the domain of medicine and treatment, with seemingly tangential consideration of how social contexts can attenuate or exacerbate substance use patterns. While some view this as an evolving field, drawing from a combination of brain and genetic studies, critics have claimed that it is simply an attempt to return prominence to the disease model, as the refrain of most neurobiological theorists is that addiction is a brain disease.

For instance, Alan Leshner (1997) argues that addiction is a brain disease that must take into account the social context that helps to develop and maintain the pathological consumption of a psychoactive substance. However, he does not explain how and to what extent social context matters—it just does. In response to Leshner's claim, neuroscientist Neil Levy (2013) argues that addiction is *not* a brain disease. It is "a disorder of a person, embedded in a social context" (Levy, 2013: 1). To be classified as a disease, according to Levy, the condition or impairment must persist across situations. However, developmental life-course research suggests that substance use patterns change over time, depending on various circumstances.

There are a variety of areas of neurobiological research that attempt to explain substance abuse and dependence. One perspective, intracellular signalling, states that nerve cells are the dynamic component of the central nervous system (CNS) and have the ability to adapt to changes produced by external influences such as psychoactive drugs. These changes occur in equal and opposite directions to the initial effects produced by the drug, which explains the process of withdrawal. To avoid this negative rebound, a person uses more of the drug, which leads to the development of tolerance. Chronic exposure to most psychoactive drugs in turn leads to increases or decreases in the cell's natural internal signalling mechanisms (Kallant, 2009).

A second perspective, synaptic plasticity, is related to neural plasticity, which is the process through which learning and memory is created. This theory proposes that stimuli in the environment that are associated with drug use become linked to positive memories and sensations that motivate continued drug use. Coordinated signalling of two neurotransmitters, dopamine and glutamate, leads to adaptive changes in gene expression that reconfigure neural networks. The greater the physical dependency produced by a psychoactive drug, the greater the release of dopamine, which produces a pleasure response in the substance user so that drug use becomes a repeated behaviour (Tang & Dani, 2009).

However, intracellular signalling, neural adaption, and plasticity are not unique to psychoactive drugs, but are the foundation of all human biological adaption to any stimuli or environmental stressor (Kallant, 2009). This is a very reductionist theory of addiction, and sociologists in particular have criticized this theory that claims a causal link between addiction and physiological processes, for it simply cannot fully account for the complexity of human behaviour (Oksanen, 2013). The unfortunate fact is that there is a belief that neurobiological theory needs to be strongly supported, in part to counter the renewed enthusiasm for a moral model approach to addiction, which was directly reflected in Canadian government legislation (Government of Canada 2015a, 2015b).

Many of the biological explanations of substance dependence may appear to undermine sociological explanations. However, it is important to recognize that when biological explanations are understood not as deterministic explanations but as predispositions, they are complementing rather than competing against sociological understandings of substance use. The same can be said for many of the psychological explanations of substance use, which are interconnected with biological and sociological explanations.

3.3: PSYCHOLOGICAL EXPLANATIONS

There are many different psychological theories and sub-theories relating to substance use and dependence. They all, to varying degrees, emphasize that individual behaviour can be explained by factors that are endogenous to the individual, particularly the mind. Three major categories in psychological research relate to personality theories, behaviour theories, and psychopathology.

Personality Theories

Since Freud, there have been a plethora of theories and subsequent studies examining the link between substance use and personality. One of the most widely tested and empirically validated measures is the five-factor model (McCrae & John, 1992). This model categorizes personality traits into five major categories—neuroticism, agreeableness, conscientiousness, extraversion, and openness to experience—which are believed to be consistent across time and place.

Personality research on alcoholism has attempted to identify an alcoholic personality that is consistent with the five-factor model. Many studies have demonstrated that alcohol-dependent individuals score high on neuroticism and low on conscientiousness and agreeableness (Fong, 2001), while others have shown that different levels of problematic alcohol consumption are characterized by different personality traits (Lalone, 2000). Hong and Paunonen (2009) found extraversion to be a particularly important personality trait amongst college drinkers and that for the young men in the study there was moderating effect between conscientiousness and agreeableness. Those who were less agreeable and less conscientious had the highest risk of drinking.

Other research examining the link between illicit substance dependence and personality has found some commonalities with alcohol research, suggesting there may be a general risk of substance dependence based on the inability to practice constraint and negative emotionality (Elkins, King, McGue, & Iacono, 2006). This research did not include the traditional five factors used in many other personality studies, so there is no way to ascertain if the results are comparable to other research.

In a more comprehensive longitudinal study of adults, Turiano and colleagues (2012) examined the use of tobacco, alcohol, and illegal drugs in relation to the five-factor model. They found that people who identified as being neurotic, more open, and lacking conscientiousness were at higher risk of using any substance, while being more agreeable decreased the likelihood of alcohol use and problems associated with alcohol use. Conscientiousness was also found to play an important moderating role in both alcohol use and other illicit drug use, suggesting that it is an important personality trait that can change the potential effects of other traits.

Jessor and Jessor (1977) postulate a different view: Problem Behaviour Theory (PBT). Integrating elements of the personality, environmental influences, and behaviour, they argued that substance use or misuse among youth is not a unique behaviour but one element of a problem behaviour syndrome. According to PBT, substance use of various forms, including smoking, drinking, and illicit drug use, occurs alongside other risk-taking behaviours such as delinquent involvements and sexual activity. They further argue that substance use is not as inherently negative or pathological as the name "problem behaviour theory" might suggest; rather, society labels certain behaviours as being problematic. Problem behaviours in one context may be viewed differently or more admirably in other contexts (Goode, 1999). Risk-taking, adventure, creativity, independence, imagination, and critical thinking are characteristics that society upholds and applauds in many situations, as is the case with athletes, CEOs, and both visual and music artists. However, in other situations, these same characteristics are deemed unacceptable, as is the case with substance use or misuse, delinquency, and even risky sexual behaviours.

However, there is still no consistent and universally accepted set of personality traits that significantly contribute to understanding substance dependence, or even the initiation of substance use. The amount of explanatory power that stable personality traits contribute to our understanding of substance dependence is relatively limited for two reasons. First, after decades of research, personality still only accounts for a small proportion of alcohol dependency (Mulder, 2002). Despite decades of ongoing efforts to identify a strong link, there is no such thing as an "alcoholic personality" or for that matter an "addictive personality." Moreover, there is a lack of consistency in the studies and their measurement of personality and levels of substance use. Though some studies examine the key personality traits identified in the five-factor model, other studies use different measures of personality, which may or may not be consistent with the five-factor model. Still other studies only include a few of the personality dimensions. There is no single definition of what *personality* is, leading to significant inconsistencies in the findings (Csiernik, 2016). Moreover, some studies examine any form of substance use, while others examine substance dependence. This lack of consistency, and inconsistent definitions of *personality* and *substance use*, limits the comparisons that can be made across studies and undermines the empirical validity of findings.

Although psychologists and social psychologists have been able to identify consistent traits or patterns of conduct, human behaviour is not 100 percent attributable to personality characteristics or distinct patterns of "problematic behaviour." The most extroverted person will encounter situations where more introverted traits are displayed. Likewise, a troubled young person may engage in substance use, but never commit any other unlawful acts.

Behavioural Theories

Another dominant area in psychological research on substance use and dependence is behavioural theory. Among the many different perspectives, the two most prominent theories are social learning and cognitive behavioural. Within social learning theory the two most influential views are B. F. Skinner's (1953) concept of positive and negative reinforcement and Albert Bandura's (1977) concept of imitation. In the latter case, it is believed that people learn how to use and misuse substances from watching and modelling the behaviour of others. Several different studies have examined the role of imitation from various influences, including the media and peers.

Researchers who have examined the role of media coverage on the substance use behaviour of young people have found the influence of celebrity behaviours may be oversimplified and exaggerated (Whitehead, Shaw, & Giles, 2010). According to these scientists, individuals can be critical consumers of media while not necessarily mimicking the behaviours they are exposed to through the media, even when it is a celebrity. Similarly, Atkinson, Bellis, and Sumnall (2013) found that young people do not view alcohol consumption in the media as an accurate portrayal of their own reality. In a focus group setting, young people were less inclined to report being influenced by the images and behaviours that they were exposed to in the media, suggesting that people are not simply passive imitators of behaviours they see in the media.

Beyond the traditional forms of semi-regulated media such as television, Moreno and Whitehill (2014) argue that social media such as Facebook and Twitter are also connected to drinking practices. A recent example of this was the rapid, global proliferation of "neknomination," where individuals nominated friends to have an alcoholic drink within 24 hours of being nominated and post the video to Facebook. There were numerous variations of this game, including those that escalated the behaviour. Some people chugged bottles of hard liquor, while others combined dangerous stunts with their drinking. Fortunately, this was a short-lived phenomenon on social media, but it illustrates how this form of communication can rapidly influence and alter behaviour.

Relatedly, research suggests that imitative behaviours among peers are significant with respect to substance use. In a series of experimental studies researchers found that people tend to imitate what others are drinking and the amounts they are drinking, regardless of whether or not they are in the company of same-sex peers (Engels, Overbeek, Larsen, & Granic, 2010; Larsen et al., 2010; Larsen, Overbeek, Granic, & Engels, 2012). This research suggests that people may not even be aware that they are mimicking the behaviours of those around them when they are drinking (Dallas et al., 2014), which may have important implications for educating people about monitoring their behaviour while in social settings.

Another form of learning that is frequently used to explain substance use and dependence is operant conditioning, first proposed by psychologist B. F. Skinner (1953), which involves the concepts of reinforcement and punishment. Reinforcements can be either positive or negative, and according to the theory both forms of reinforcement increase substance using behaviour. Positive reinforcement can be exemplified in many different ways, such as the acquisition of peers, relief from anxiety or pain, increased sociability or confidence, and the general pleasure that some people experience from some psychoactive substances. Negative reinforcement is simply the removal of a negative stimulus, and Skinner stated that a person would repeat any behaviour if it was reinforced in a positive or negative manner. Negative reinforcement is clearly evident in the process of withdrawal. When a drug dependent individual experiences the physical pain of withdrawal the pain is diminished, if not temporarily eliminated, by taking more of the same drug or a pharmacologically related psychoactive substance. This act of drug consumption reinforces the continuation of drug use in order to avoid the negative effects of withdrawal. Imagine the worst case of the flu that you ever had. Now you can make the pain go away in seconds by taking an injection. However, six hours later the flu symptoms return; do you take another injection to eliminate the pain? If you continue to take the injection every six hours when the symptoms return, this is an example of how negative reinforcement contributes to the dependency cycle. Another concept that is especially important to substance use and dependence research is that of extinction. Extinction occurs when the positive reinforcement for drug use gradually diminishes, leading to a decrease and then cessation of the behaviour.

Whereas reinforcement increases the likelihood of a behaviour, punishment relates to environmental responses that decrease the likelihood of a behaviour, such as being grounded for smoking underage or losing your license for drinking and driving. Punishment has the potential to weaken behaviour but is not as strong as positive reinforcement, which is why individuals continue to engage in substance use despite negative consequences. Some examples of punishment include legal consequences, such as being fined, or physical consequences, such as suffering a hangover.

Cognitive behavioural theories are interconnected with the basic premises of social learning theories. There are many treatment approaches that draw from the foundations provided by social learning and cognition theories. These concepts, which have led to empirically supported clinical therapies, are premised on the idea that behaviour is a reflection of how individuals think and feel about themselves. Furthermore, to change behaviours like substance use or dependence, the individual must learn new, positive ways of thinking.

An early example of a cognitive behavioural theory is self-derogation theory (Kaplan, 1975; Kaplan, Martin, & Robbins, 1984), based on the idea that some people develop negative attitudes about themselves as a product of their upbringing or early relationships. In response to these negative experiences, they come to associate belonging to normative groups, such as the family, school, or even peers, as being painful and thus something to be avoided. Ultimately, they seek out ways of coping that are viewed as deviant by the group that has rejected them, or non-conformist because they are seeking a sense of worth that they were unable to get from normative relationships. To restore a sense of self-worth—or to at least lessen self-derogation—individuals may decide to engage in drug using as a means of coping but also as a means of connecting with others who are not like those who had hurt them in the past.

Even though an individual may feel that they obtain a sense of self-worth from substance use and the people they associate with while they are using, once their drug use becomes problematic, the cycle of self-derogation is likely to continue. Personality studies and psychopathology have found that substance use and dependence can actually amplify rather than extinguish negative feelings, underscoring why cognitive behavioural therapy is an important avenue for substance dependence treatment.

The idea behind cognitive behavioural therapy is that becoming abstinent from drugs can be controlled by making new cognitive choices that lead to non-drug-using behaviours. It holds that an individual's problems arise from their beliefs, evaluations, and interpretations regarding life events. It is premised on the belief that by changing an individual's thoughts about themselves their drug use will likewise decrease. Skills training to break this cycle can be either intrapersonal (examining internal events) or interpersonal; in either case, the counsellor draws upon daily life examples to address both cognition and behaviour with enhanced self-efficacy, to the point where a client can once again gain control over the active decision-making processes in their life. This approach also promotes an attitude of non-judgmental acceptance as part of the process. Recovering from drug use is a learning process that takes time, for just as an addiction does not suddenly occur neither can the thoughts and behaviours that lead to drug misuse suddenly be replaced. Thus, time is needed to examine, explain, and discuss the high-risk situations that trigger drug use in order to build client self-efficacy in order to remain abstinent (Csiernik, 2016).

Psychopathology

Psychopathology refers to the scientific study of mental health disorders. Substance dependence is classified in the *Diagnostic and Statistical Manual of Mental Disorders* (DSM) as a distinct mental health condition, though substantial criticisms exist regarding the manner in which this guide has evolved and the financial conflicts of interest among its authors and the pharmaceutical industry (Cosgrove & Krimsky; 2012; Cosgrove, Krimsky, Vijayaraghavan, & Schneider, 2006).

Nevertheless, there is a substantial body of literature connecting other forms of mental health issues with substance dependence. Research examining co-existing mental health problems has been referred to as *co-morbidity* or *dual diagnoses*, though the contemporary counselling term is *concurrent disorder.*

Just as there are many different psychoactive substances, there are a myriad of mental health disorders that have been connected to substance dependence. Concurrent disorders present unique challenges for researchers and treatment providers. On the one hand, it is sometimes difficult to isolate the causal ordering of substance use disorders and mental health disorders. On the other hand, there are so many different combinations of disorders that can co-exist, making generalizations and patterns difficult to establish. Complexities aside, the Canadian Centre on Substance Abuse (2009) published a special report on concurrent disorders and declared this a significant health issue affecting Canadians, with over half of people presenting themselves for substance dependence treatment also reporting a mental health concern. Among those receiving treatment primarily for a mental health condition, up to one-fifth report also being dependent on a psychoactive substance. Some of the mental health issues that have been linked to various forms of substance dependence include attention deficit/hyperactivity disorder (ADHD), depression, anxiety, and schizophrenia (Kimberley & Osmond, 2017).

ADHD, an increasingly common disorder among both children and adults, has been linked to similar brain processes involved in substance dependence (Carpentier, 2012); not surprisingly, then, there is a high rate of concurrent substance use disorders amongst individuals with ADHD. Similarly, there is some indication that there are common or shared predispositions in one's biology or the environment that can explain the co-occurrence of depression and substance use (Canadian Centre on Substance Abuse, 2009). Others have argued that there are two other possible explanations for the link between depression and substance use: one possibility is that substance use serves as a form of self-medication for depression, while the other possibility is that substance use induces depression (Mackie, Conrod, & Brady, 2012).

According to the Canadian Centre on Substance Abuse (2009), anxiety preceded the substance use disorder in at least three-quarters of the cases where people were suffering the two concurrently. Moreover, even when substance use is stopped, a large number of people still experience anxiety. However, there are different types of anxiety disorders that tend to result in slightly different findings (Brady, 2012). Generalized anxiety disorder tends to be caused by substance dependence, whereas substance dependence co-occurring with post-traumatic stress disorder and social phobias is more likely evidence of the self-medication hypothesis (Canadian Centre on Substance Abuse, 2009). Other evidence indicates that concurrent anxiety disorders and substance use disorders is a vicious cycle with an often reciprocal relationship to one another (Kimberley & Osmond, 2017; Stewart & Conrod, 2008). What is lost in this debate, however, is that the normal human resting state is one where there is always some level of anxiety present.

Schizophrenia is one form of psychosis that has received a significant amount of attention in concurrent disorder research, especially with respect to cannabis use. Tobacco and cannabis are the most commonly used substances among people with psychosis (Canadian Centre on Substance Abuse, 2009). Tobacco use can help diminish some of the negative aspects of schizophrenia but has little impact on the progression of the mental health disorder itself. With cannabis use, however, there is evidence to support the contention that schizophrenia may be triggered or induced by cannabis use, especially amongst younger people with a biological predisposition to schizophrenia. Cannabis use can also exacerbate the symptoms associated with schizophrenia.

Research into mental health is complex, with multiple disorders being linked to various types of substance use and dependence. Added to this are issues surrounding self-medication, which can amplify or maintain both mental health and substance use disorders. In many cases, it is difficult to ascertain which came first—the mental health disorder or the substance dependence disorder. Was the person self-medicating to deal with an undiagnosed mental health disorder (Khantzian, 1997)? Or did substance use contribute to the development or triggering of the mental health disorder?

3.4: CONCLUSION

The distinct and, at times, divergent biological and psychological theories examined in this chapter serve to highlight that there is no single explanation for substance use or substance dependence. There remains a range of research actively taking place in this field, independent of studies occurring within other disciplines. The prominent reason for this is that there are multiple interrelated factors that are necessary to consider when it comes to understanding the complexities associated with substance use and dependence. Rather than debate the moral or medical, or psychological or sociological, nature of substance use and dependence, it is not only prudent but also wise to adopt a different standpoint and approach the phenomenon from a biopsychosocial perspective. The following chapter will examine sociological approaches to explaining substance use and dependence, highlighting the importance of social factors in addition to biological and psychological factors when examining substance use, misuse, and dependence.

PARADOXES

1) Social responses and legal repercussions to psychoactive drug use do not depend on the substance as much as the social status of the user.

2) There is far greater acceptance of misbehaviour while intoxicated by alcohol than most other substances, despite the fact that alcohol produces greater harm than any illicit drug.

3) While it has been established that treatment can resolve addiction issues, law enforcement and the criminal justice system continue to receive greater funding.

4) The moral model perpetuates fear and disdain for users, and is readily employed during national elections in Canada; the medical model, while appearing to absolve users of responsibility, likewise negates any examination of larger structural and societal issues that contribute to the development of substance use and abuse.

CRITICAL REFLECTIONS

1) Who benefits and who is harmed by viewing drug use through:
   i)   a moral model lens?
   ii) a disease model lens?
   iii) a biological lens?
   iv) a psychological lens?

2) What are some of the advantages and disadvantages of using biological explanations to understand addiction and drug use?

3) What are some of the advantages and disadvantages of using psychological explanations to understand addiction and drug use?

4) Given that the moral and disease models of addiction and drug use are limited, what might be a third alternative?

4 Explaining Substance Use II: Sociological Theories

As a discipline, sociology has several explanations and theories that are relevant to our understanding of substance use and substance users. Many of the theories described below are derived from sociological studies of deviance and criminology, as few explanations deal specifically with substance use as a distinct phenomenon. The theories with direct relevance to substance use include control theories, strain theories, subcultural theories, combined theories, conflict theories, and the more recent postmodern theories. As with most studies of substance use, the explanations vary in the emphasis placed on human agency and social structural constraints. Likewise, there is significant debate about the problematic nature of substance use and substance users in society.

Most of the sociological literature examines psychoactive drug use more generally, rather than through diagnostic criteria for substance dependence. In this sense, substance use and misuse are forms of risky behaviour that often occur alongside other risky lifestyle activities (Jensen & Brownfield, 1986). Substance dependence then, in light of many sociological theories, is considered an extension of substance use, whereby patterns of use have become more routinized and, for some, problematic. As well, in research involving youth, the distinction between illegal and legal substances is less common, as all substances are illegal for youth to possess and use. However, in studies comparing the legal status differences, illegal drugs are usually measured through cannabis. It is important to note that in general there is a lack of specificity in sociological theories regarding individual substances and the frequency of their use.

4.1: CONTROL THEORIES

Control theories in sociology and by extension criminology are derived from the classical school of thought, where it is argued that the "natural" state of individuals is to pursue pleasure and avoid pain (Beccaria, 1764; Bentham, 1789; Hobbes, 1651). According to this argument, there is nothing inherently different or abnormal about those who engage in substance use or even those who misuse substances; instead, what is most important to consider is what prevents "normal" people from engaging in risky behaviours, such as substance use or misuse. More contemporary theorists of this tradition, Gottfredson and Hirschi (1990), argue that all deviant behaviour is a "normal" response to the human condition of needing to pursue pleasure and avoid pain. By normal, this does not mean that the behaviour or action is acceptable by conventional standards. Rather, the normalcy of such response is merely something that any individual may consider as a course of action, if presented with the choice of pleasure or pain. Arguably, substance use and misuse can be seen as both pleasurable and painful, depending on the circumstances, the substance, and the individual.

Emphasizing that everyone has the propensity to deviate from conventional norms, control theories highlight the similarities between individuals rather than their differences. However, if everyone has the inclination to deviate, there must be some explanation for why many individuals conform to the conventional order; otherwise, society would be in a constant state of chaos. According to control theorists, the answer is simple: people choose to conform to the conventional order because they have a "stake in conformity" that is rooted in their relationships to significant others and society (Briar & Piliavin, 1965; Hirschi, 1969). Indeed, parents, teachers, employers, or other authorities control individual actions both directly and indirectly (Nye, 1958; Reckless, 1967; Reiss, 1951), thus preventing people from engaging in potentially harmful or anti-social behaviours.

Contemporary control theories tend to be classified into two main variants: one focuses on the social or external controls and bonds to which the individual is exposed, and the other emphasizes the importance of internalized self-control (Hirschi, 1969; Gottfredson & Hirschi, 1990). These divergent approaches are not mutually exclusive explanations of substance use. There are many instances where researchers have effectively illustrated the importance of taking into account both social and self-control.

Social Bonding Theory

Social bonds are best understood by drawing on the early work of Travis Hirschi (1969). The crux of Hirschi's argument is that if one's social bond is strong, then the individual is less likely to engage in deviant behaviour, such as substance use, because he or she does not want to compromise conventional relationships or future ambitions. However, if the social bond is weak then substance use is more likely, as there is nothing controlling the behaviour of the individual. Hirschi's social bonding theory includes four elements: attachment, commitment, involvement, and belief.

Hirschi's notion of attachment refers to the nature of the bond between an individual and others in society. If an individual has strong, nurturing attachments to others—parents, teachers, and friends, in particular—then there is less chance that she or he will engage in such behaviours as substance use, as the preservation of social relationships is of utmost concern to the individual (Hirschi, 1969). Since substance use may compromise relationships with others, individuals who have strong, pro-social attachments will be less likely to jeopardize their relationships. Alternatively, individuals lacking meaningful connections with others are more likely to use substances, as they do not have anyone they feel they would be disappointing.

The second and equally important element of the social bond is commitment. Commitment is the rational component of the social bond, where individuals must consider the costs and rewards of engaging in a particular behaviour, such as substance use or misuse. According to this concept, individuals will be less likely to engage in substance use because it is not only a violation of the law but also because they feel it may be viewed negatively by others. Moreover, individuals with a strong commitment to society will be less likely to engage in regular, heavy consumption patterns, as this is more likely to interfere with their commitment to conventional society, including their families and school. Thus, the more risk involved in violating the norms, the less likely an individual will engage in substance use. People are committed to conformity not only to preserve current relations, but also to invest in the future (Hirschi, 1969). Hirschi, and other control theorists including Briar and Pillavin (1965), refer to this as having "a stake in conformity." Individuals may have the propensity to engage in substance use, but if it is possible that future goals and relationships may be compromised, the individual may forego the pleasure and remain committed to conformity.

The third element of the social bond is involvement, whereby individuals are deterred from deviance because they are participating in more conventional activities that preclude them from having the time to engage in behaviours such as substance use (Hirschi, 1969). If individuals are involved in conventional activities with family, school, athletics, work, volunteering, and the like, there is less opportunity for them to be involved in risky activities involving substance use or misuse (Sen, 2010; Wong, 2005). However, if individuals spend a great deal of time hanging out with friends, riding around in cars, or feeling bored, then they are more likely to also be involved in substance use (Hundleby, 1987; Osgood & Anderson, 2004), partially because of opportunity and partially because of their negative attitudes towards conventional activities.

Finally, the last element of Hirschi's theory is belief, which is understood in terms of the internalization of the dominant value system. If an individual subscribes to the dominant belief system, then he or she is less likely to engage in illicit or excessive substance use. On the other hand, if the individual holds beliefs that are in opposition to the dominant system, then he or she is more likely to engage in substance use and misuse. Existing research suggests that individual beliefs about drugs are important predictors of substance use (Bachman, Johnston, & O'Malley, 1998; Johnston, O'Malley, Bachman, & Schulenberg, 2006; Perez, 2007). However, the specific nature of the role of belief is less understood. There is some evidence to suggest that perceived risk and disapproval might be significant determinants of use; however, they are not the most important factors to consider (Perez, 2007). For example, disapproval of parents and friends are stronger predictors of cannabis use. The relative strength of informal social control mechanisms in Perez's (2007) study may actually indicate an important connection between background influences and the development of certain beliefs about drugs.

Though research on beliefs about drugs and social bonds is currently lacking, there is a substantial body of literature that examines the importance of social bonds more generally in predicting substance use. Undoubtedly, positive experiences in the family and school, such as close attachments and consistent monitoring, can serve as forms of indirect and direct social control, preventing people from using substances for fear that they may disappoint significant others in their lives or compromise their future ambitions (Bègue & Roché, 2009; Branstetter, Furman, & Cottrell, 2009; Kim, 2004; LaRusso, Romer, & Selman, 2008).

Self-Control Theory

Individually based control theories argue that what prevents people from acting on their hedonistic nature and engaging in endless pursuits of deviance, such as illicit or excessive substance use, is their level of self-control. According to Gottfredson and Hirschi's (1990) general theory, crime and "other analogous behaviours" including substance use are consistent with the recreational activities in which some people engage; they are convenient and opportunistic, and of minimal long-term benefit. Thus, self-control is a key predictor of whether or not an individual will use or misuse psychoactive substances, with no distinction made between licit or illicit substances.

Importantly, according to Gottfredson and Hirschi (1990) and sociological explanations more generally, self-control is not a dispositional characteristic of the individual that is inherent at birth; instead, self-control is best understood as an individual barrier that is influenced by opportunities and other constraints, such as agents of socialization. In this sense, self-control is a characteristic of the individual that is instilled through adequate parental monitoring and discipline in the early years of one's life. Thus, adults have an important role to play when it comes to teaching healthy levels of self-control. People who are never taught to moderate their behaviour are likely to develop lower levels of self-control, which places them at higher risk of substance use later in life.

4.2: STRAIN THEORIES

While control theories argue that substance use is a normal response to the human desire to pursue pleasure and avoid pain, strain theorists argue that substance use is a normal response to stressful or disadvantaged circumstances embedded in the social structure or the more immediate environment of the individual. The underlying assumption of strain theories is that individuals are pushed or pressured into substance use because of external forces, not because there is a weakening of controls. By extension, this means that there must be some motivation or pressure that evokes a culturally nonconformist response like substance use. The two main variants of strain theory in sociology are Robert Merton's (1938) anomie theory and Robert Agnew's (1992) general strain theory.

Anomie/Strain Theory

The central tenet of Merton's (1938) anomie theory is that individuals in North American society share a common set of values and goals centred on the pursuit of material success and wealth. However, not everyone has access to the conventional, institutionalized means of achieving these universally accepted goals. Adapting to one's circumstances through alternate means or developing alternate goals relieves the frustration and tension that is experienced when one cannot achieve culturally valued goals through legitimate means. As such, Merton outlines five potential adaptations in his theory (Table 4.1).

Table 4.1: Robert Merton's Adaptations to Anomie

Adaptation	Shared Cultural Goals	Access to Institutionalized Means
Conformity	+	+
Innovation	+	−
Ritualism	−	+
Retreatism	−	−
Rebellion	+/−	+/−
Source: Adapted from Merton (1938: 676).		

The first adaptation, conformity, is when individuals share the culturally approved goal of material success and wealth, while also having access to the institutionalized means to achieve those goals. This group of individuals is not of much interest to studies of deviant or criminal behaviour, as they are law-abiding, conventional individuals.

The second adaptation in Merton's typology is innovation. An innovator shares the universal values and goals of material wealth and success; however, he or she does not have access to the culturally approved institutionalized means of achieving these goals. In this case, when an individual does not have access to higher education or lucrative employment, the person innovates and finds new ways of achieving the goals. This is the group Merton highlighted as the most likely to engage in criminal pursuits, such as becoming involved in the drug trade.

A third adaptation, referred to as ritualism, focuses on individuals who do not share the cultural values or goals of material wealth or success, but they still engage in the traditional institutional means of achieving success. For instance, a ritualist may not believe in wealth as a measure of success, but he or she may still pursue an education and possess a good job; rather than accumulating wealth and possessions, these individuals may donate money to causes of personal importance.

Merton's fourth adaptation, retreatism, is an important group for studies of substance use. This group refers those individuals who do not share the cultural goal of material wealth and success and they do not possess the means to achieve these goals. It is not the case that this group has never shared the cultural goals; instead, when they were faced with the realization that they did not have the means to achieve the goals, or they failed when pursuing them, they felt defeated. Not wanting to adapt through illegitimate or criminal means, like an innovator, they escape or retreat. This group is withdrawn from society, and otherwise known as outcasts. Using the language of his era, Merton stated that this was the group occupied by "chronic drunkards" and "drug addicts," alongside with "psychotics," "vagrants," "vagabonds," and "tramps" (1938: 677). While these terms are not politically correct by today's standards, it can be argued that the most frequent substance users, particularly of illicit substances, are still classified amongst the most socially marginalized groups in society and are still often described using this oppressive language.

The last adaptation that Merton identifies is rebellion. This group is characterized as the most revolutionary of all the adaptations. They do not share the cultural goals of material wealth and success, nor do they feel they need to achieve these goals through traditional institutionalized means. This adaptation can be illustrated using the case of medical marijuana use. The traditional forms of medicine advocated by doctors and pharmaceutical companies have come under intense scrutiny. Those who embrace the use of medical marijuana are seen as rejecting the authority of Western medicine and adopting an alternative set of goals to embrace healing from a more natural source, despite it being a criminalized substance. However, not everyone has access to this alternative form of medicine. Medical professionals still have the authority to determine who can and cannot use marijuana for medical purposes. In recent years, we have seen a dramatic shift in policies that allow doctors to prescribe and patients to legitimately use marijuana for a variety of different ailments. This shift can be attributed in part to the revolution or rebellion led by citizens in support of different approaches to health and illness.

General Strain Theory

Robert Agnew's (1992) general strain theory (GST) incorporates the element of failure to achieve goals that is central to Merton's theory; however, he makes the theory more generalized, and socio-psychological, by suggesting strain can also be induced through the loss of or threat of removal of positively valued stimuli, or the presentation of or threat of negative stimuli. Central to Agnew's theory is the assumption that strain does not lead directly to negative adaptations, such as substance use. Instead, strain that is followed by a negative emotional state, such as anger, is most likely to influence negative coping strategies.

According to Agnew's (1992) conceptualization, there are three potential sources of strain that can lead to a negative affective state, which in turn can increase the chances of an individual trying to adapt through various means, such as substance use. The first source of strain is the failure to achieve goals. Departing from the Merton's (1938) conceptualization, Agnew argues there are three ways in which an individual may experience strain from the failure to achieve goals: (1) when aspirations and expected achievements are disconnected; (2) when expected achievements and actual achievements are disconnected; and (3) when just or fair outcomes and actual outcomes are not the same.

The second major source of strain, according to Agnew (1992), is the removal of positive stimuli. This removal of positively valued stimuli may be actual or anticipated. Some examples of positively valued stimuli being removed might include the loss of a parent, a relationship break-up, or loss of property or employment. Similarly, Agnew argues a third major source of strain is the presentation of negative stimuli, in either actual or anticipated forms, such as physical or emotional abuse or a negative school or work environment.

4.3: SUBCULTURAL THEORIES

Cultural deviance theorists believe that subcultures are the true social explanation for behaviour. According to these theories, subcultures have different definitions or beliefs about drugs and drug use when compared to more dominant subcultures. What makes individuals deviant is not the inherently immoral nature of the behaviour they are engaging in, but the way in which their behaviour has been defined as problematic by a more powerful or dominant group in society (Becker, 1963; Goode & Ben-Yehuda, 1994). If an individual is socialized into a subculture with values and norms that condone behaviour that is condemned by the legal system, then they are considered deviant. Indeed, according to cultural deviance theorists, deviants are conformists to a separate subculture that is less powerful than a more dominant cultural group (Kornhauser, 1978). Thus, subcultures are deviant—not the individual—and subcultures are only deviant to the extent that they have been defined as such. According to these culturally based approaches, it is implied that the individual cannot be held fully accountable for his or her behaviour because circumstances and influences are the cause of one's deviance, not the individual per se (Becker, 1963; Goffman, 1963: Gottfredson & Hirschi, 1990; Matza, 1964; Sutherland, 1947).

Labelling theories (Becker, 1963; Goffman, 1963), differential association theories (Sutherland, 1947), and social learning theories are examples of subcultural theories. These theories attempt to address what encourages an individual to engage in substance use, focusing on social influences and situations. While there are variations in the extent to which each of these theories emphasize the individual as a product of his or her immediate situation, the underlying assumptions of these approaches suggest that the individual is often pushed or persuaded into becoming deviant by influential role models.

Labelling Theory

Labelling theorists derive their understanding of substance use and substance users from the symbolic interactionist tradition, drawing on the social constructionist perspective. According to this approach, there is nothing inherently deviant or problematic about substance use or substance users. Rather, it is problematic only because we have defined it as such (Goode, 1999).

For the people who use drugs, defining drugs as immoral or problematic can lead to negative consequences for one's identity, in turn influencing not only how individuals perceive themselves but also how society perceives them. According to Erving Goffman (1963), when an individual is labelled negatively, he or she possesses a stigma. Examples of this may include labelling someone as a pothead, druggie, crack whore, or drunk. These labels have a powerful, stigmatizing effect on the individual's perception of themselves. Moreover, the use of such labels legitimates negative treatment by others in society, reinforcing the dominant social order of a "them versus us" mentality (Goode & Ben-Yehuda, 1994).

Similar to Goffman's notion of stigma, Howard Becker (1963) argues that when we label people in derogatory ways, we are creating a "master status" for these individuals, which in turn influences how others in society view and treat them. At the individual level, this forms the basis of one's identity. If an individual believes they are nothing more than a pothead or a drug whore, then their behaviour will reflect this belief. In this sense then, labelling theories are not concerned about behaviour so much as the reaction to certain behaviours. It is the reaction that elicits certain behaviours. For example, most of us know someone whose parents are overly suspicious or concerned about their adolescent using drugs or alcohol. While the individual may never have used these substances, if they are accused of it on a regular basis, eventually they might use it just so that their behaviour is congruent with their parents' beliefs and reactions.

Differential Association Theory

Some critics argue that differential association theory is a pure form of cultural deviance or subcultural theories, which suggests that individuals are wholly products of their environments, and thus incapable of making individualized choices (Kornhauser, 1978). However, others have argued that differential association theory can be thought of as a sociological variation of social learning theory that accounts not only for one's current involvement in a particular group or culture but also past associations that the individual may have experienced (Akers, 1996). Accordingly, the individual and the situation influence one another. Ultimately, the individual is capable of making choices about which situations or activities he or she is willing or wanting to pursue, but those situations and influences can have an independent effect on the outcomes. As stated by Sutherland:

> Person and situation are not factors exclusive of each other, for the situation which is important is the situation as defined by the person who is involved. The tendencies and inhibitions at the moment of the criminal behaviour are, to be sure, largely a product of the earlier history of the person, but the expression of these tendencies and inhibitions is a reaction to the immediate situation as defined by the person. (1947: 5)

This suggests that an individual's response to their situation is not only a result of past experiences and social influences, but also dependent on how often they are presented with the opportunity to engage in deviance.

Sutherland (1947) argues that it is important to consider how behaviour is learned through interaction with others, especially within small group interactions. There are three particularly important elements of differential association theory that are necessary to consider: (1) the influences of others, such as peers and siblings; (2) the learning of definitions or attitudes about conventional and unconventional behaviour; and (3) the frequency, duration, and intensity of one's interaction with others in situations conducive to deviance.

The people we associate with teach us definitions or specific attitudes about what is right and wrong. Definitions that are generally unfavourable toward the law are more likely to result in deviance than definitions that are more favourable towards the law. Social influences in an individual's immediate environment, such as siblings and peers, can also influence individual perceptions about substances (Martino et al., 2006). While the decision to use a particular substance may be a matter of individual choice, social influences can still impact individual perceptions about drugs and alcohol, leading to the indirect influence of others on one's decision to indulge or refrain.

Learning within intimate groups is evidenced in the early work of Howard Becker (1953). In his seminal study on becoming a marijuana user, Becker argues that there is nothing inherently rewarding about marijuana use; rather, becoming a marijuana user involves a learning process within a group setting that not only involves the techniques of use, but also the expected effects of use. If an individual does not learn how to use properly, does not learn how to achieve the supposed effects, or does not identify the drug with these perceived effects and find them enjoyable, then becoming a marijuana user is unlikely. In order to learn how to become a marijuana user, or any other substance user for that matter, the social learning that peers provide is an important influence. These findings are also echoed in Faupel's (1991) research on heroin users.

Another assumption of Sutherland's theory is that the more frequently individuals are exposed to situations conducive to substance use, the more likely they are to internalize definitions that are unfavourable towards the law, which increases the chances of further substance use. The length of time spent in situations where substances are being used, as well as the intensity of one's relationship with the users, influences the likelihood of initiating use, experimental use, and continued or problematic substance use.

Thus, according to Sutherland's differential association theory, it is necessary to demonstrate through empirical testing that the frequency, intensity, and duration of involvement in certain groups are important indicators of substance use, while also taking into consideration the influence of attitudes or definitions towards drugs.

Social Learning Theory (Differential Association-Reinforcement Theory)

Although there are many variations of social learning theories, the work of Ronald Akers is the most widely cited in sociology, especially for substance use. The sociological version of social learning, also known as differential association-reinforcement theory, was originally developed by Robert Burgess and Ronald Akers (1966). Akers later elaborated and refined the theory, referring to his explanation more generally as "social learning theory."

The purpose behind expanding Sutherland's original theory was to account for how people might become or remain involved in substance use or other socially defined deviant behaviours. Akers supported Sutherland's original argument that the definitions, beliefs, or meanings we attach to certain activities or behaviours help shape how we will respond, and that the learning of these definitions is dependent on the frequency, duration, and intensity of our interactions with others; however, what was lacking from Sutherland's conceptualization was the learning process, or how individuals learn definitions when associating with others.

Combining ideas from Sutherland's differential association theory and psychological behaviourism, Akers, Krohn, Lanza-Kaduce, and Radosevich's (1979) social learning theory is founded upon four core concepts: differential association, definitions, differential reinforcement, and imitation. Differential association refers to the groups and individuals with which one associates, or the social environmental context. In these groups, individuals learn definitions that are favourable or unfavourable toward the law. The process by which this learning takes place, according to Akers, is through differential reinforcement and imitation. Differential reinforcement can occur in the form of positive or negative reinforcements and positive or negative punishments. Positive reinforcement is usually seen as rewarding or beneficial in some way, while negative reinforcement is the avoidance of punishment. Reinforcement, both positive and negative, is thought to increase the likelihood of repeating similar behaviours; on the other hand, punishment decreases or weakens one's commitment to certain behaviours. The differential reinforcement aspect of the theory refers to past or present rewards and punishments for similar behaviours, and the rewards and punishments that are attached to alternative forms of behaviour.

In testing social learning theory's applicability to substance use and abuse among adolescents, Akers and his colleagues (1979) found that the four elements of social learning theory account for about two-thirds of marijuana use and almost 40 percent of marijuana abuse. As for drinking, 55 percent of adolescent use was explained by social learning, while about one-third of alcohol abuse was explained using the same factors. Based on these findings, it appears that social learning is more influential in explaining use rather than abuse, which is a far more complex phenomenon than sociological theories alone can explain.

4.4: INTEGRATED EXPLANATIONS OF SUBSTANCE USE

Some theories and theorists use integrated explanations, combining multiple versions of the aforementioned research under one framework. Three examples of these combination theories include Cloward and Ohlin's (1960) differential opportunity theory, David Matza's (1964) drift theory, and Cohen and Felson's routine activities theory (1979).

Differential Opportunity Theory

Combining elements of strain theory and subcultural theories, Cloward and Ohlin (1960) argued that people living in disadvantaged circumstances are not only governed by legitimate opportunities to succeed, but their choices are also guided by proscribed opportunities. Thus, if an individual is lacking legitimate opportunities, they might, as Merton argued, turn to unlawful means of succeeding. According to Cloward and Ohlin, individuals lacking legitimate opportunities can choose to affiliate themselves with one of three different types of subcultures: criminal, conflict, or retreatist subcultures. Again, these choices depend on the availability of both legitimate and illegitimate opportunities in one's immediate surroundings.

The retreatist group is of the most interest to studies of drugs and drug use, for according to Cloward and Ohlin, individuals who are unable to succeed through legitimate opportunity structures do not necessarily have equal opportunity to succeed in criminal- or conflict-based opportunity structures either. Those who are unsuccessful or who do not wish to be involved in criminal or conflict subcultures withdraw or retreat from society. Cloward and Ohlin dubbed these individuals "double failures." In order to adapt, double failures engage in substance use as a means of coping with their circumstances. From this perspective, there is a significant stigma attached to drug use as a response to one's circumstances. Individuals who belong to the retreatist subculture are viewed as the ultimate failures, unable to fit within either of the major opportunity structures in society.

Drift Theory

Responding to the inadequacies and cultural determinism of subcultural theories, David Matza (1964) advocated for a more inclusive approach to understanding deviant behaviour. Combining elements of strain, social control, culture, and situation, the underlying premise of Matza's theory is that people are not wholly committed to either conventional or unconventional behaviour. Instead, when youth are temporarily released from traditional forms of social control, they are free to drift into more unconventional activities, usually dominated by peers. Matza argues that people regularly vacillate between conventional and unconventional worlds, while never fully committing to either. In essence, Matza acknowledges that people's lives are guided by freedom and constraint. This is a noteworthy theory for substance use in particular, where the emphasis is on both individual and situational explanations.

Matza also argues that some people are freer than others when it comes to making choices. From this standpoint, he extends his theory of drift to include components of the classical school of thought. He argues that not only are individuals motivated to deviate because of their circumstances, but they are also driven by their instinctual desire to pursue pleasure and avoid pain; thus, individuals must also be controlled by their external environment. Drawing on social control theories and social learning theories, Matza argues that all youth are influenced by their elders, such as parents and teachers. Indeed, young people and, in particular, delinquents are not wholly committed to oppositional subcultures that are a reflection of their social circumstances, but are also simultaneously involved in, and aware of, conventional behaviour and expectations.

According to drift theory, the leisure involvements of young people are not always in opposition to conventional culture; instead, the nature of youthful leisure is also influenced by conventional culture. Matza argues that young people are in a unique stage in life whereby they have been released from adult controls but are not yet fully integrated into adult culture. During this stage in life, it is recognized that there is a distinct teenage culture that takes place alongside the dominant culture, whereby some practices are a clear rejection of the dominant adult system, as seen with illegal substance use, yet other practices are reflections or adaptations derived from the adult society in which young people are inevitably embedded, as witnessed with alcohol and tobacco consumption.

Internalized attitudes that reflect either pro-social or anti-social sentiments are a central element in Matza's drift theory. When young people's attitudes towards drugs are in competition or conflict with the dominant social order, this is referred to as *subterranean values*. These alternative values are what allow individuals to drift into deviant behaviour. When released from the social controls of families and schools, young people engage in a process of "neutralizing" and distorting conventional beliefs to justify their decision to engage in unconventional subcultural activities. Sykes and Matza (1957) refer to this process used by youth as *techniques of neutralization*. Ultimately, young people are aware that their behaviour is divergent from conventional society; however, to satisfy their hedonistic urges and rationalize their submission to the influence of peers and social circumstances, they must have internalized certain beliefs or definitions about their behaviour.

Though others have argued that peers are a substantial influence when explaining delinquent involvement, Matza rejects the argument that peer pressure is the reason for unconventional behaviour. Instead, he argues that youth are aware of the contradictory messages in society and are prone to moods of fatalism; thus, when an individual is given the opportunity to engage in unconventional activities, peers do not pressure—they sympathize and empathize. Ultimately, shared experiences and beliefs among youth is what results in deviant behaviour. Peers do not pressure or force a young person to behave in a particular manner; instead, they do nothing to discourage the choices that are being made and are likely to sympathetically and empathetically encourage collective involvement in unconventional behaviour because of their shared beliefs and experiences.

Routine Activities and Lifestyle Theories

Routine activities theory (RAT), first introduced by Cohen and Felson (1979), and its variations such as lifestyle theory and opportunity theory argue that certain activities or situations are more conducive to deviant behaviours than others (Bernburg & Thorlindsson, 2001; Hawdon, 1996; Jensen & Brownfield, 1986). In an attempt to theorize about the ecological nature of deviance, rather than the characteristics of the individual, Cohen and Felson argue that deviant behaviour is best understood by looking at the circumstances of particular situations, where time and space converge. There are three key components to consider when explaining the frequency of deviant behaviour: first, there must be a suitable target or situation that presents the opportunity to commit a deviant act; second, there must be an absence of a capable guardian; and third, there must be a motivated offender.

Cohen and Felson (1979) argue that a lack of any one of these key elements would decrease the chance of substance use or misuse occurring. Furthermore, the individual as a motivated offender is not meant to be a reflection of the individual, but rather inherent in the situation. Thus, if there is no one else present and an opportunity arises, the individual may at that point in time become motivated to engage in substance use. According to this argument, individuals do not necessarily seek out situations to fulfill a particular motivation; rather, individuals are inclined to act on opportunities that present themselves, especially if there is no one watching.

The routine activities approach has been expanded to suggest that it is not only opportunity but also the specific characteristics of the situation that will determine whether or not an individual will engage in deviance. For instance, according to Hundleby (1987), social behaviour that focuses on hanging out with peers results in more cannabis and alcohol consumption. Osgood and colleagues (1996) further argue that unstructured, unsupervised, peer-dominated activities are conducive to a range of deviant behaviours, including substance use. The routine activities in these approaches focus on leisure that takes place on the streets, at night, or in other settings lacking parents, teachers, or other authority figures.

In a study of peer influences and leisure activities, Thorlindsson and Bernburg (2006) examined the extent to which partying and delinquency influences the likelihood of substance use. They found that the well-established connection between peers and substance use actually depends on the types of activities in which individuals are routinely engaged. Thus, individuals whose peers hold pro-drug beliefs, as differential association theory would suggest, are not necessarily at greater risk of using substances; instead, the connection between peer influence and substance use also depends on the types of opportunities and leisure activities that individuals are involved in with their peers. Thus, situations may not have a constant effect, as suggested by routine activities theory. Instead, there are other factors that need to be taken into consideration, including the motivated offender.

An underdeveloped feature of routine activities theory (RAT) and its variations is the motivated offender. As argued by Jensen and Brownfield (1986: 88), "particular lifestyles involve the active pursuit of excitement and fun." They further critique the passive approach to lifestyles that argues individuals are only deviant if they have the opportunity and if there is a lack of guardianship. Instead, they contend, individuals wanting to deviate will seek out situations that lack guardians and are fun and exciting. In this sense, there will always be motivated offenders—people who enjoy risk-taking more than others.

4.5: CONFLICT THEORIES

The conflict theories in sociology and criminology focus on the macro-structural conditions that contribute to substance use. The focus is removed from the individual and instead placed on the importance of power and dominance at the institutional level. Though there are several versions of conflict theory, the common assumption is that there is an unequal distribution of power in society. Those who hold the power are less subject to sanctioning, while those who hold little or no power are subjected to severe and sometimes unrealistic sanctioning. Moreover, those who hold power are able to create and maintain rules and regulations that place those with less power in positions of significant disadvantage. This unequal distribution of power often operates alongside class, gender, sexual orientation, age, ethnicity, and race.

Conflict theories have a lot of insight to offer substance use studies. Whether the institutional power is the government, the criminal justice system, or even the media, the public is left with the impression that the unequal distribution of power is legitimate and necessary (Goode & Ben-Yehuda, 1994). Interestingly, these institutional powers often work in tandem with one another, further reinforcing the legitimacy of their actions. The classic example is the current War on Drugs, which was instituted in 1971. At the government level, the War on Drugs serves the interests of politicians, at the expense of powerless individuals, by giving them a contested moral issue on which to focus attention rather than highlighting the true sources of the problem. The government does not want the people to pay attention to issues with the economy, inequality, or a lack of social programming and government support; instead, they want people to believe that the problems of drugs and drug use are paramount. In fact, they will even go so far as to make the public believe that it is drugs and drug use creating the problems they are trying to hide. Some politicians are much more effective at this than others: for instance, Brian Mulroney's attempt to wage a War on Drugs, especially against cocaine, in the late 1980s, did not work (Jensen & Gerber, 1993); however, William Lyon Mackenzie King's crusade to criminalize opium and opium users in the early 1900s was successful and had lasting implications (Giffen, Endicott, & Lambert, 1991).

Interestingly, it is not necessarily individual politicians that can be credited with the success or failure of a message being received by the public. Often, there are important social and structural conditions that can help explain differences in outcomes. Two social conflict perspectives that can help explain different political outcomes are Marxian and Pluralist perspectives.

Marxian Conflict Theory

Central to the Marxian conflict perspective is the role of economic interests and social class in society (Quinney, 1977). Laws, according to Quinney and other

Marxian conflict theorists, are created by and intended to protect those who hold power in society. Under capitalism, those who hold the power are those with money. Thus, laws are a reflection of economic interests and those who benefit most from laws that protect the interests of the ruling class. By extension, drug laws are a means of socially controlling vulnerable and less powerful groups in society with no regard to the harms that such laws may produce for socially marginalized groups.

In his work *Code of the Street*, Elijah Anderson (1999) further explores the connection between economics and social inequality. Beyond the laws that are created to protect powerful groups in society, drug dealing, which is also against the law, is seen as a desirable source of employment in otherwise disenfranchised populations. Moreover, people living in these impoverished circumstances come to understand that the laws and police are not there to protect them or serve their interests. Unfortunately, this means that these communities are also subjected to greater police surveillance and a higher likelihood of being charged with a criminal offence for their daily means of subsistence (Chambliss, 1994). Thus, in communities where few legitimate opportunities exist for gainful employment, drug dealing becomes a means of survival and the lack of trust in the criminal justice system results in people taking matters into their own hands, usually through force and violence. Marxian theory thus directs us to examine the roles that poverty, social exclusion, and the lack of meaning in one's labour play in increasing the risk of addiction, through both the demand and supply side of the drug equation.

Pluralist Conflict Theory

Like other conflict perspectives, pluralists are interested in the role of power in understanding social inequities. Unlike Marxian and other conflict perspectives, pluralists suggest that power is evident in a variety of different structures and relationships, including but not limited to the government, media, religion, science, medicine, families, schools, and even community-based organizations (Hathaway, 2015; Mosher, 2001). Rather than focus exclusively on the economic interests and the role that capitalism has in creating and maintaining social inequality, pluralists argue that power struggles can be simultaneously, though not necessarily collaboratively, happening in various institutional and personal relations, all of which contribute to social inequalities.

Howard Becker's (1963) work *Outsiders* examines the socially constructed nature of deviance and highlights the role of power in the creation of marijuana legislation, which effectively imposed controls on a particular subculture of marijuana users that was viewed as challenging the status quo. While Marxians would argue that economic interests are central to the social construction of a problem, Becker, however, argues that moral entrepreneurs play a significant role in demonizing and advocating for the social control of people who fall outside of the norm in society. Moral entrepreneurs do not necessarily have an economic interest; instead, advocacy is often rooted in a particular issue of morality, and in this case, it was marijuana use that concerned Becker.

Though Becker's work is often thought of as originating in social constructionism and symbolic interaction, it can also be understood in terms of the pluralist approach, with moral entrepreneurs being those who hold the power to define what is acceptable and what is unacceptable. Indeed, the movement towards marijuana restrictions in both the United States and Canada is a fascinating example of how a particular issue becomes defined as a problem in need of legal control. In Canada, it was the declaration of Emily Murphy (1922) that marijuana was "the new social menace," along with the support of legislatures, parents, and community advocates, that effectively demonized marijuana. This is not unlike the more recent Mothers Against Drunk Driving (MADD) movement, which has effectively, and perhaps legitimately, created a set of laws surrounding drinking and driving that never existed historically. Part of the success of the MADD movement is its collective advocacy from various factions in society (Fell & Voas, 2006; Reinarman, 1988).

4.6: POSTMODERN EXPLANATIONS

Postmodernism denotes a significant shift in thinking from previously discussed theories and explanations. Central to postmodern thinking is challenging the existing understanding of social structures, human action, and the resulting scientific claims of what constitutes the "truth." Thus, instead of having a specific set of propositions, as illustrated with the previous theoretical traditions, postmodern explanations come in several different forms. One of the core ideas shared by postmodern thinkers is to question knowledge as it currently exists and critically assess the role of authorities, including researchers and writers in the production of knowledge (Agger, 1991).

Postmodern explanations provide a different way of thinking about drugs and drug use in society by questioning the taken-for-granted assumptions or preexisting knowledge (Fox, 1999; Kamoouh, 1996). Rather than taking the status quo as a starting point for inquiry and analysis, postmodern explanations pose questions that enable us to examine phenomena from a different perspective. How do we know what we know about drugs and drug users? Who created these truths? Who is most impacted by these existing forms of knowledge? In what ways are these existing forms of knowledge used to control or discipline people? In contemporary society, how do people govern themselves, based on the existing knowledge we have about drugs and drug use? Two examples of postmodern explanations used in the sociology of drugs and drug use include the normalization thesis and Foucault's biopower.

Normalization Thesis

Until the late 1990s, most sociological explanations focused on problematizing deviant behaviours, such as illicit drug use or excessive licit drug use. The central argument was that substance use is a problem or is deviant and by extension so are the users. But what if we were to change the terms of reference? What if substance use and users are not a problem, nor are they deviant? What if they are normal? As history has shown, substance use in its many forms has existed for centuries. Problematizing the existence of substances is not producing effective outcomes. If anything, we may be exacerbating the issues involved. In response to this long history of problematizing substance use both theoretically and practically, a new perspective has emerged: the normalization thesis.

The normalization thesis originated from a five-year longitudinal study in northwest England (Parker, Aldridge, & Measham, 1998). This study followed several hundred young people as they grew up "drugwise" in the 1990s. Drawing on both individual and structural elements, there are several important contributions to our understanding of drugs and drug users that have been derived from the normalization approach.

Parker, Aldridge, and Measham (1998: 1–2) argue that youthful substance users "cannot be written off as delinquent, street corner 'no hopers.'" The reality of people's lives, the structure of society, the expectations we place on people, and the leisure activities we engage in are all far more complex than to suggest that using substances is in some way a deviant or problematic behaviour. Pathways to use are varied and complex and individuals use a rational choice model when making drug choices. In a rather hedonistic or functional manner, individuals make and remake decisions about their substance use, some with greater consequences than others.

This complexity is illustrated in the assumption that patterns of use are not dichotomous. We cannot simply categorize people as being users or abstainers.

Four broad categories of drug use illustrate the continuum and complexity of use: abstainers, ex-users, in-transition users, and current users (Parker, Aldridge, & Measham, 1998). Abstainers are those who have never tried any illicit drugs and they never intend to try any drugs in the future. Former triers or ex-users are those who have tried an illicit drug, often experimentally, but do not intend to do so again. In-transition users are those who may not have tried a drug but think they might do so in the future. Current users have all tried drugs and nearly all will have periods of regular drug use in their biographies. Ultimately, substance use patterns are not static, but rather dependent on the stages in one's life-course. Different social experiences and opportunities can and do have an effect on individual substance-using decisions.

As well, the terms *drug abuse* and *drug abusers* are not reflective of the experiences of individuals, as they imply a moral character rather than a realistic account of their decisions (Parker, Aldridge, & Measham, 1998). Elaborating on this idea, Brain, Parker, and Carnwath (2000) argue that most individuals are psychoactive consumers, not drug abusers. To illustrate their point, they offer evidence that individual choices are derived from a rational choice-making process that involves several considerations. First, users consider the taste and strength of a substance, opting for substances that will serve their needs and desires at that particular time. Second, they will consider the image and style that is attached to different substances and variations in substances; for instance, males are more likely to drink beer, while females are more likely to drink coolers or ciders. Moreover, social class is connected to image and style choices. Given that some substances are more expensive than others, purchasing the more expensive brand signifies a different style or image that is not available to others. A third rational choice a psychoactive consumer considers is the ability of a particular substance or brand of substance to produce a high (or sense of euphoria) that the individual desires. With alcohol, for instance, certain beers have higher alcohol content than others; when the user's goal is to get drunk, then drinking a beer with a higher alcohol content would be desirable, as would drinking a greater quantity in a shorter period of time.

All of these rational choices are considered alongside a fourth factor: social control mechanisms. Brain, Parker, and Carnwath (2000) refer to these as *stake holding* and *boundaries*. Individuals have to have a reason *not* to consume substances or to moderate their use of substances; otherwise, there is no risk involved in using. If an individual lacks conventional bonds to society, as outlined by Hirschi (1969), then he or she has nothing to lose by engaging in risk-taking behaviour. Stake holding, in this sense, is similar to the notion of having a stake in conformity. Boundaries are also developed and maintained by the individual when using substances. If an individual has obligations they find meaningful, then they will moderate the amount of substances used to ensure that these obligations are not compromised. For instance, if an individual has a job, then substance use is often reserved for leisure time to ensure that the job is not lost or that workplace relationships are not undermined. Again, these choices indicate a wilful, rational decision-making process.

The normalization thesis represents a significant shift in thinking about substance use and substance users. Rather than defining individuals as inadequate or destined to failure because of their social circumstances, the normalization thesis argues that substance use is a normal "timeout" from the everyday stress of living in a postmodern society and that individuals make rational, calculated choices about when to use substances and how much they should use (Parker, Aldridge, & Measham, 1998).

Foucault and Biopower

Perhaps one of the most notable postmodern theorists discussed in sociology is French philosopher Michel Foucault (1967, 1973, 1999). For Foucault, the creation of the identity of an "addict" arises through what he terms *the process of constitution of subjects*. This occurs with the intersection of different types of knowledge, power, and authority that create distinct ways of conceptualizing the individual based upon "how things are said, who says them, and what they say and do not say, to create an order of knowledge, a taxonomy, a discourse, and so make a particular subject visible" (Reith, 2004: 288). This process not only creates the image of an addict but all types of othered individuals, including those in conflict with the law, persons with mental health issues, and sexual minorities.

Foucault's concepts of discipline and biopower—the disciplining of bodies and the regulation of populations—have been applied in some sociological research to help extend our understanding drugs and drug users (Foucault, Rabinow, & Hurley, 1997). Consistent with most postmodern thinking, researchers using a Foucauldian lens question the historical emergence or "genealogy" of our existing knowledge about drugs and drug users (Rose, O'Malley, & Valverde, 2006).

A contemporary application of biopower can be viewed through examining Philippe Bourgois's (2000) ethnography of heroin users in the United States and Canada. Bourgois critically assessed the role of methadone maintenance programs and illustrated how medical and criminal justice discourses enable the disciplining of human subjects by "declaring some psychoactive drugs to be legal medicine and others to be illegal poisons" (2000: 167). Methadone is a medically acceptable and legal substance that can be monitored and controlled through bio-medical maintenance programs that reinforce the notion that addiction is only a disease. Heroin, on the other hand, is illegal and widely discredited in the United States and many places in Canada as a legitimate treatment alternative. Though methadone maintenance treatment programs are not without controversy, there is certainly greater controversy surrounding the use of heroin maintenance programs to assist users. Historically, heroin and its users have been publicly demonized in Canada, while methadone, another opioid, has been increasingly viewed as a medically appropriate substance, especially since the emergence of AIDS and HIV in the late 1980s (Csiernik, Rowe, & Watkin, 2017).

So what makes methadone more acceptable than heroin? According to Bourgois, methadone is used and more widely accepted by medical and criminal justice systems because it does not produce the euphoria other opioids do, while simultaneously preventing the negative effects of heroin withdrawal. Moreover, methadone is not seen as a highly sought-after illicit drug on the street, though it is an addictive drug and produces withdrawal if a person stops using it. Thus, methadone maintenance serves the purpose of making people productive, healthy, and free from addiction to heroin, yet also ensuring that users do not feel good from the effects of methadone while remaining addicted to it. Medically supervised maintenance and drug testing programs ensure that people's consumption patterns are strictly controlled through dosage schedules—predetermined times when doses can be delivered—and the locations where methadone can be dispensed, while also monitoring for use of other psychoactive drugs. Essentially, methadone maintenance serves as a form of social control, ensuring users remain docile within a system that limits their capacity to question the medical and legal systems that regulate their lives and substance use choices, all while providing a regular income stream for medical professionals responsible for chemically controlling this population. However, as stated above, methadone, like heroin, produces physical and psychological dependency, and the experience of many street users does not coincide with the medical discourses that we have come to accept as reality. However, unlike heroin, it is a socially sanctioned psychoactive substance.

At the population level, strict monitoring, forced treatment alternatives, and regimented scheduling is a form of what Foucault called *biopower*. Biopower is the state's ability to legitimately control and discipline entire populations through various means of medical and legal intervention. In Bourgois's work, he effectively illustrates how the state uses methadone maintenance programs as a means of trying to produce healthy, non-addicted, functioning, and productive citizens, with the underlying assumption that the state must discipline users into docile bodies. Through the regimentation of methadone maintenance, the state effectively executes its biopower over individuals addicted to heroin and related opioids by indicating which substances are acceptable and may be used without penalty or state sanction and which are not acceptable. This biopower allows the state to actively, and legitimately, socially control an undesirable population: those who are dependent on opioids.

4.7: CONCLUSION

This chapter has focused on the social, cultural, and structural explanations of substance use and substance users. By no means is this an exhaustive list of all potential sociological explanations. Instead, the objective of this chapter was to highlight some of the relevant, though often ignored, contributions that sociological theories have contributed to our understanding of drugs and drug users. Sociology has played a far less prominent role than dominant moral, biological, and psychological discourses, which have tended to individualize and pathologize substance use and related problems.

Sociology, according to Adrian (2003), has the potential to bring both a macro- and micro-level understanding to substance use and users. In strictly sociological terms, substance use and misuse are social facts. They exist. They affect both individuals and society. Accordingly, our attention must not focus solely on the individual and the substance-specific factors often stressed in biological and psychological theories. The intention here is not to deny the relevance of individual factors, nor the independent effects that particular substances have on our bodies, but rather to emphasize the importance of a holistic approach to substance use and dependence, highlighting the relevance of sociology in this approach. The only way to account for variations in substance use, misuse, and dependence patterns is through a biopsychosocial model. We cannot reduce our thinking to a single factor model, for individuals and societal realties are far more complex. As this chapter and the preceding chapter illustrates, a variety of explanations can be used to explain different types of substances being used, the frequency with which they are being used, the environments they are more commonly used in, and the people most vulnerable to use and misuse. As Figure 4.1 illustrates, there are significant parts of substance use and dependence that can only be understood by examining sociologically relevant factors; likewise, biology and psychology have made important and independent contributions to understanding who is at risk and under what conditions.

Taking a holistic approach does not assume that biology is more important than psychology or that psychology is more important sociology. Instead, each of these domains of the human experience is equally important to consider. However, the model does recognize the uselessness of the moral model, which only casts blame and creates oppression. Under the holistic biopsychosocial model, it is understood that biological, psychological, and sociological influences will vary in their relative effects, but that all three will always be present and always be part of the process.

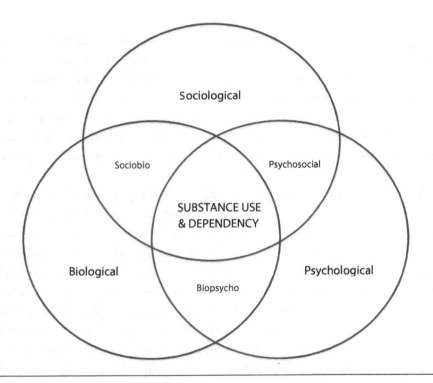

Figure 4.1: A Biopsychosocial Model of Substance Use and Dependency

Source: Adapted from Csiernik (2014a).

PARADOXES

1)   Given the divergent views on addiction from the sociological field alone, a holistic understanding of addiction is difficult to imagine when each discipline cannot even agree on what constitutes addiction.

2)   Sociology, as a discipline, is founded on individual- and societal-level explanations, yet few of the existing theories address both the micro- and macro-level forces necessary for a more holistic understanding of addiction.

CRITICAL REFLECTIONS

1)   Who benefits from and who is harmed by viewing drug use through a sociological lens?

2)   What factors do you need to take into consideration when assessing which of the sociological theories offers the best understanding of substance use and addiction?

3)   Which of the sociological explanations offer more limited insights into substance use and addiction? Can these explanations be amended to better explain substance use, addiction, and related laws?

4)   If we are to believe that addiction is a biopsychosocial phenomenon, what are the major contributions of sociological theories to this holistic conceptualization?

5)   Does the biopsychosocial model address all of the necessary elements for understanding substance use and addiction?

5 Classifying Drugs: Psychopharmacological Properties and Legal Classifications

The majority of this text focuses on the sociological aspects of psychoactive substances, meaning that the emphasis is on the external forces and societal definitions that characterize drugs and drug use. However, it cannot be denied that there are intrinsic properties of drugs that must also be considered in order to fully understand the sociological significance of drugs and drug use. The purpose of this chapter is to outline the basic psychopharmacological effects of major drug groupings that are used and misused by different segments of society, while also highlighting the legal classifications of such drugs and the penalties attached to various violations of the Controlled Drugs and Substances Act. The purpose of including the pharmacological properties and the legal classifications in the same chapter is to highlight the lack of consistency and objectivity in the current legislation in Canada. Illicit substances are rarely classified based on their pharmacological effects; instead, as will be made evident throughout, there is no pharmacological rationale that can be easily derived for the legal classifications.

5.1: WHAT IS PSYCHOPHARMACOLOGY AND WHY DOES IT MATTER TO SOCIOLOGISTS?

Generally speaking, *psychopharmacology* refers to the study of the effects of psychoactive drugs on the human mind and body. The psychological aspect is what distinguishes psychoactive drugs from other substances, in that their primary affect is upon the central nervous system (CNS), which means they all alter thinking and behaviour to varying degrees. What also makes these drugs more problematic is that they also all have secondary effects upon the peripheral nervous system, and thus produce varying degrees of physical change that a user cannot control. The pharmacological element refers to the chemical structure of the substance and the expected effects of a particular substance based on its chemical structure. From this perspective, it is important to recognize that there is no such thing as a good drug or a bad drug; there is no moral element to the chemical nature of psychoactive drugs (Hart & Ksir, 2015). Instead, it is how people behave or interact socially when using a psychoactive drug that is defined as good or bad, as these substances have all come to hold distinct moralistic meanings within specific cultural contexts. Almost all psychoactive drugs have both positive and negative effects. For example, heroin, cocaine, and cannabis, which may be thought of as bad or unacceptable, at one time were all legal substances in Canada and were used medicinally. Currently, codeine, Ritalin, and Valium may be viewed as good or acceptable, yet all have side effects that can harm users when used excessively and can lead to addiction. In Canada alcohol is legal, while in Saudi Arabia, Somalia, and Sudan it is illegal. Khat is legal in Ethiopia, South Africa, and Yemen, but illegal in Canada. In each of these examples, it is important to recognize that supposed bad drugs can have benefits, and likewise drugs viewed as good can have substantial risks associated with their use. In order to understand the socially defined good and bad nature of psychoactive substances, it is necessary to have a basic understanding of how different drugs effect the human body.

There are several different ways in which psychoactive drugs can be classified, depending on the substances being examined and the overall objectives of the classification. The objective of this chapter is to illustrate the properties of various psychoactive substances and their legal classifications under the Controlled Drugs and Substances Act. Table 5.1 highlights the psychopharmacological classification of psychoactive drugs as modified from the work of Charles Faupel, Alan Horowitz, and Greg Weaver (2010), while Table 5.2 provides the most recent version of Canada's Controlled Drugs and Substances Act

(CDSA) (Government of Canada, 2015a). The psychopharmacological classification system categorizes substances into seven groupings: opioids, depressants, stimulants, hallucinogens, cannabis, psychotherapeutic agents and performance enhancing drugs. Notably, there is no direct correspondence between these pharmacological groupings and the eight drug schedules under the CDSA. Thus, one of the objectives of this chapter is to illustrate the paradoxical relationship between the effects of drugs, their relative harms and their legal classification.

Table 5.1: Psychopharmacological Classifications of Psychoactive Drugs

Type of Substance	Effect	Examples
Opioids (narcotics) (natural, semi-synthetic, synthetic)	Slows down the central nervous system, with analgesic and calming effects Produces euphoria	Codeine, fentanyl, heroin, methadone, morphine, opium, oxycodone, and other synthetic analgesics
Depressants	Slows down the central nervous system Produces euphoria	Alcohol, barbiturates, benzodiazepines, GHB, and inhalants/solvents
Stimulants	Speeds up the activity in the central nervous system Produces euphoria	Amphetamines, bath salts, caffeine, cocaine, khat, methamphetamines, and nicotine
Hallucinogens	Produces sensory distortion and cross-sensory stimulation, producing a disconnect between the physical world and the user's perception of it	Ecstasy (MDMA), ketamine, LSD, mescaline, PCP, and peyote
Cannabis (marijuana)	Can have a slight CNS depressant effect Can produce mild euphoria. Can produce distorted sensory perceptions	Cannabis, hashish, hash oil, and shatter
Psychotherapeutic agents and	Levels moods or reduces extremes of emotional states; moves a user towards homeostasis.	Antidepressants, antipsychotics, and mood stabilizers
Performance-enhancing drugs	Enhances physical performance; no psychoactive effect on the CNS.	Proteins, steroids, and other hormonal agents

Source: Modified from Faupel, Horowitz, & Weaver (2010: 68).

5.2: OPIOIDS (NARCOTICS)

We begin with opioids, probably the most widely confused and mislabelled family of psychoactive substances. In medical and legal communities, as well as in popular culture, opioids, also known as narcotics, are used to refer to many different types of drugs. At one time, under Canadian law, cannabis and cocaine were classified as narcotics. It is only since the Controlled Drugs and Substances Act that this misclassification has been somewhat addressed. While the legislation itself no longer refers to these substances as narcotics, there are still many who confuse the meaning of *narcotic* with the more general term *psychoactive substance*, when *narcotic* was originally intended to refer to only opioids. Even in the medical community, there seems to be confusion as to what constitutes a narcotic. At some local medical centres, signs are posted stating: "Doctors in the afterhours clinics do not prescribe narcotics." In this case, the signs are referring to more than narcotics in the form of opioids; instead, it is intended to include any physical dependency–producing substance that should be carefully monitored by a knowledgeable medical professional. It is not surprising that, with wide misuse of the term *narcotic* in both medical and legal communities, the general public has also developed a misunderstanding of what constitutes a narcotic. The word *narcotic* is derived from the Greek word *narkotikos*, meaning "to be numb," an accurate description of the pain-relieving properties of opioids. However, given the widespread confusion and misappropriation of the term, the more pharmacologically inclusive term *opioid* will be used here.

Pharmacologically, opioids can be derived from the opium poppy or synthesized with a similar chemical structure (Faupel, Horowitz, & Weaver, 2010). Opioids have a depressant effect on the CNS, while also masking the human response to pain (Csiernik, 2014a). Even though other psychoactive substances may have similar characteristics, opioids can be distinguished from other categories of drugs based on three characteristics: (1) their ability to produce physical and psychological dependency; (2) the analgesic effect; and (3) the intense euphoria that the majority of opioids produce (Faupel, Horowitz, & Weaver, 2010). Opioids have the ability to quickly produce physical dependency if they are not used properly and even if used as prescribed. Of all substances known, opioids have the greatest pain-blocking ability, which makes them extremely useful and desirable in both the medical community and amongst individuals attempting to self-medicate (Khantzian, 1985). The overwhelming euphoric effect that is initially experienced by users of the most potent opioids, such as heroin, fentanyl, and crushed OxyContin pills, makes the substance desirable and produces even greater potential for developing dependence. However, as is the case with many other substance dependencies, the most desirable effects of opioids—euphoria and pain relief—are rarely felt by those who become chronic users (Levinthal, 2014).

There are several different types of opioids, which can be broadly categorized into three groups: natural, semi-synthetic, and synthetic. Each of these groups is defined below along with some examples of specific substances that are used in medical and/or recreational communities.

Natural Opioids

Sumerian writings suggest that humans have used natural opioids, in the form of opium, since as early as 4000 BCE (Csiernik, 2016). Natural opioids are derived directly from the poppy plant, *Papaver somniferum*, and do not involve the mixture of other chemicals or substances. Naturally derived opioids are also referred to as *opiates*. The term *opiates* is less inclusive and refers only to those substances that are natural opioids, while the term *opioids* includes both natural, semi-synthetic, and synthetic forms of opioids (Csiernik, 2016). Three of the most common natural opioids are opium, morphine, and codeine.

Opium is the raw milky substance that is extracted from the unripe seeds of the poppy plant. The name, *opium*, is Greek for "poppy juice." Recreationally, opium is smoked using a pipe. Medically, opium is not traditionally used unless a person cannot tolerate the effects of morphine (Csiernik, 2016). There are several other natural, semi-synthetic, and synthetic substances that have replaced opium in the medical and recreational communities. Nevertheless, it remains the first substance to be regulated and controlled under Canadian law in 1908 and still appears at the top of the list on Schedule I of the Controlled Drugs and Substances Act.

German pharmacist Friedrich Wilhelm Adam Sertürner is credited with the original discovery and naming of morphine around 1805 (Stolberg, 2009). Named after the Greek god of dreams, Morpheus (Pasternak, 2009b), morphine is the primary active ingredient in opium. It is 10 times stronger than opium and serves as a powerful natural analgesic (Hart & Ksir, 2014). After its discovery, morphine became widely used for many different ailments, including pain, menopause, depression, nervousness, asthma, and angina (Gulmatico-Mullin & Cross, 2009).

After the discovery of morphine in the early nineteenth century, other derivatives of opium were sought; one such discovery was codeine. Its name comes from the Greek translation for "poppy head" (Hart & Ksir, 2014). Similar to other opiates, codeine is used medically for its analgesic effects and also as a cough suppressant and antidiarrheal agent (Pasternak, 2009a). One of the major advantages of codeine is its effectiveness when taken orally and its ability to be combined with other non-opioid analgesics, including ibuprofen, acetaminophen, and aspirin (Smith, 1996). On the street, codeine is not as popular as other opioids, as it is not nearly as potent as morphine or other semi-synthetic and synthetic opioids.

Semi-Synthetic Opioids

Semi-synthetic opioids combine naturally occurring opioids with other chemical substances (Faupel, Horowitz, & Weaver, 2010). They are sometimes referred to as opiates because they are partially derived from opium, though they are more technically opioids, as they contain synthetic elements that are not derived directly from opium. Two of the most common semi-synthetic opioids are heroin and oxycodone/OxyContin.

The most prohibited opioid globally is heroin (diacetylmorphine or diamorphine). Named after its perceived heroic powers, heroin was developed in 1874 in Germany (Rothwell, 2011). It is classified as a semi-synthetic opioid because it is partially derived from morphine and partially from two chemicals with properties similar to vinegar. The result of this combination is an opioid that is three times more potent than morphine and whose active metabolite is morphine (Hart & Ksir, 2014). It was initially believed that heroin did not produce a physical dependency and would help with withdrawal symptoms from morphine, but within a short period of time, the extremely dependency-producing properties of heroin were noticed and it became illegal for sale and consumption globally (Rothwell, 2011). The drug has not been used medically in the United States for over a century, but in Canada and the United Kingdom it is legally available among select clinical populations who have opioid addictions but do not respond well to methadone (Faupel, Horowitz, & Weaver, 2010; Mosher & Akins, 2014). However, the use of heroin-assisted treatments is not without significant controversy and misunderstanding from both politicians and the general public, particularly in Canada.

Another popular semi-synthetic opioid is oxycodone and its time-release version OxyContin. Synthesized from a small part of opium plant called thebaine, it is chemically similar to codeine but far more potent and thus able to produce more physical and psychological dependency (Faupel, Horowitz, & Weaver, 2010). Oxycodone was first manufactured in 1938 and is often used in the medical community as an oral medication for moderate to severe pain management (Csiernik, 2014a). It may be used alone, while in combination with aspirin it is known as Percodan, and in combination with acetaminophen as Percocet.

The controlled-release version of oxycodone, OxyContin, was introduced in 1995 (Faupel, Horowitz, & Weaver, 2010; Leukefeld & Stoops, 2009). It was initially believed that the slow-release properties of OxyContin would decrease its dependency potential compared to other opioids. However, this was not the case. Controlled-release properties can be eliminated when the substance is crushed and used intranasally or intravenously (Lankenau, 2009). After several years of legal battles, the creator of OxyContin, Purdue Pharma, was found guilty for misleading the public and doctors into believing that the substance was non-addictive and was forced to pay multi-million dollar fines. However, this did not prevent the family who owned Purdue Pharma from becoming among the richest families in America, ranking in the top 20 with a net worth of $14 billion (Morrell, 2015).

As a result of the problems with OxyContin, Purdue Pharma began the manufacture of another semi-synthetic opioid called OxyNEO. The creation of this new substance was intended to develop a tamper-proof version of OxyContin. Thus, Canada ceased using OxyContin in 2012 and OxyNEO was introduced as a replacement for pain relief. To make the substance tamper-proof, OxyNEO turns into a gel form when users try to breakdown or liquefy the substance. However, when users try to inject the substance, it poses significant health risks, as gel-like substances cannot be safely injected into a vein. Not surprisingly, OxyNEO is not without its limitations and, in fact, may be a more dangerous substance for those who use the substance to self-medicate or to recreationally obtain a sense of temporary euphoria (Levinthal, 2014). Thus, the supposed tamper-proof properties of OxyNEO may simply result in more health consequences and greater ingenuity amongst users trying to find a way to get the desired effects. The other unintended consequence of this fiasco was the increased use of heroin by those seeking alternative opioids, and the unintended surge in overdose deaths when expensive heroin began to be laced with far less expensive, but far more potent, synthetic fentanyl and carfentanil.

Synthetic Opioids

Synthetic opioids do not have any origin in the poppy plant. However, the effects and chemical structure are similar to semi-synthetic and natural opioids (Faupel, Horowitz, & Weaver, 2010). Even though there are many different opioids that have been created and synthesized in the past century, methadone, buprenorphine, and fentanyl are the most commonly known and used synthetic opioids.

Development of methadone began in Nazi Germany as a wartime analgesic alternative to morphine, though it was never deployed in the field. As part of wartime reparations, the patent was sold to an American pharmaceutical company but never became popular, as it does not produce euphoria like other opioids. Methadone remerged with a rather beneficial, albeit controversial, existence as a maintenance or substitution therapy in the medical community. During the 1960s, methadone was employed as a treatment for heroin addiction (Faupel, Horowitz, & Weaver, 2010), but it has since expanded to include many different forms of opioid dependence. Several communities across Canada offer methadone treatment for individuals with opioid dependence, while others only offer methadone maintenance. Unfortunately, there is significant resistance from some members of the public, who are often unaware of the differences between the two approaches. While some have incorrectly argued that methadone maintenance is the most effective treatment currently available (Ritter, 2011), others have accurately illustrated that methadone maintenance is a biopolitical attempt to control which substances are legitimate for consumption and which ones are not (Bourgois, 2000), serving as a means of social control of an undesirable population. Methadone maintenance, though widely accepted in the medical community as the most economically effective means of treating opioid dependence, is actually simply drug substitution, and without a counselling component the individual remains addicted to a psychoactive drug—only one with no euphoric effects. As long as it does not produce the pleasurable feelings that other opioids produce, the public and uninformed political leaders seem satisfied that this type of addiction is tolerable, though still not entirely acceptable; methadone is not entirely free from the stigma traditionally attached to substance use and misuse.

There are also economic issues related to methadone. A Canadian study reported that the average daily cost of methadone in 2010 was only $15.48/day, which comprised physician billing (9.8 percent), pharmacy costs (39.8 percent), and urine toxicology screens (46.7 percent), with the methadone itself costing merely $0.59/day. On average the annual cost is $5,651, or the equivalent of one three-week hospital stay every year (Zaric, Brennan, Varenbut, & Daiter, 2012). This is eight times less than the average health, social, and criminal costs associated with an untreated person using illicit opioids, which was estimated at $44,600/year (Health Canada, 2008). However, over the course of 35 years, with inflation, the cost of methadone maintenance will tally over $250,000 to keep each person legally addicted. This long-term cost could be substantially offset if, rather than only drug substitution, counselling was incorporated throughout the process to aid in moving individuals towards abstinence. Even if the process of methadone treatment were to take two or four years, which it often does, it is much shorter and much less costly both economically and personally than spending three-and-a-half decades regularly ingesting an addictive substance.

Fentanyl is used in medical communities for pain relief, but also used on the street because it is even more potent than heroin (Faupel, Horowitz, & Weaver, 2010). In fact, estimates suggest that fentanyl is upwards of 100 times stronger than morphine (Hart & Ksir, 2014; Sonne, 2009). Fentanyl can be used intra-venously, in a transdermal patch, and orally through a lozenge or a dissolving tablet. The unknown potency of illicit forms of fentanyl on the street dramati-cally increases the risk of health consequences and even death when it is smoked or placed inside the mouth. These same risks are not common in controlled or medically supervised environments.

There are many other synthetic analgesics that were developed for use in the medical community, such as Demerol (meperidine) and Talwin (pentazocine), that have found their way to the street (Stolberg, 2011). As has been the case with most opioids, the development of new formulations is usually based on the desire to find a less dependency-producing opioid. However, this has not been successful. In the case of Talwin, there have even been attempts to add naloxone, an opioid antagonist, to prevent the pleasurable effects that illicit substance users were trying to achieve (Csiernik, 2016).

Legal Classification and Penalties for Opioids

Most opioids, with only a few exceptions, are classified as Schedule I substances under Canada's Controlled Drugs and Substances Act (Government of Canada, 2015a) (Table 5.2). Depending on the offence, Schedule I penalties range from six months to life in prison. Minimum sentences ranging from one year to three years of incarceration are applied to special circumstances for trafficking, import-ing and exporting, and production offences. Possession offences can result in either a summary conviction or an indictment: the former is a less serious offence under the criminal code and does not result in a criminal record, and the latter is considered more serious and does result in a criminal record. As an indict-able offence, the maximum penalty for possession of opioids is seven years. As a summary offence, the penalty is six months in prison, a $1,000 fine, or both for a first-time offence. For subsequent offences, the penalty is one year in prison, a $2,000 fine, or both. Life imprisonment penalties are reserved for the most seri-ous trafficking, importing and exporting, and production offences.

Interestingly, two synthetic opioids, butorphanol and nalbuphine, are clas-sified as Schedule IV substances. The penalties associated with Schedule IV substances are significantly less than Schedule I. In fact, unlike Schedule I, Schedule IV does not regulate or control possession. Instead, seeking to obtain a substance listed under Schedule IV without authorization is punishable with up to 18 months in prison as an indictable offence, or 6 to 12 months as a summary offence. There is no rationale for why these two opioids would be classified under a different schedule with differing penalties.

Table 5.2: Legal Classifications of Psychoactive Drugs in Canada

CDSA Schedule I	
Types of Substances Included	
	Approximately 150 different substances, including opium and its derivatives, coca and its derivatives, amphetamines, methamphetamine, PCP, ketamine, MDMA, Rohypnol, and GHB
Offences and Penalties	
Possession	Indictable offence: max. 7 years in prison
	Summary offence: 6 months/$1,000 fine for first offence; 1 year/$2,000 fine for subsequent offences
Trafficking	Min. 1 year in prison if you commit the offence for a criminal organization; use or threaten violence in its commission; carry, use, or threaten to use a weapon in its commission; or within the previous 10 years you were convicted of a designated substance offence
	Min. 2 years if you commit the offence in or near a school or any other public place usually frequented by minors, at a prison, or with the assistance or involvement of a minor
	Maximum life imprisonment
Importing and Exporting	Up to 1kg. of heroin or cocaine: min. 1 year if you commit the offence for trafficking, if you abuse a position of trust or authority while committing the offence, or if you have access to an area that is restricted to authorized persons and use that access to commit the offence
	More than 1kg. of heroin or cocaine: min. 2 years in prison
	Maximum life imprisonment
Production	Min. 2 years in prison; 3 years if any of the following apply: (a) you use real property that belongs to a third party to commit the offence; (b) the production could endanger the security, health, or safety of minors at or close to the offence location; (c) the production constitutes a potential public safety hazard in a residential area; or (d) you set or place a trap, device, or other thing that is likely to cause death or bodily harm to another person in or close to the offence location, or permit such a trap, device, or other thing to remain or be placed in that location or area
	Maximum life imprisonment
CDSA Schedule II	
Types of Substances Included	
	All forms of cannabis preparations, derivatives, and synthetics, but excluding non-viable seeds, branches, and stalks (as long as there are no leaves, flowers, seeds, or branches on the stalk)

(continued)

Offences and Penalties	
Possession	Up to 30g of marijuana and/or 1g of hashish is a summary offence, max. 6 months in prison/$1,000 fine or both
	More than 30g of marijuana and/or 1g of hashish, the following applies:
	Indictable offence: max. 5 years less a day in prison
	Summary offence: 6 months/$1,000 fine or both for first offence; 1 year/$2,000 fine or both for subsequent offences
Trafficking	Min. 1 year in prison if you commit the offence for a criminal organization; use or threaten violence in its commission; carry, use, or threaten to use a weapon in its commission; or within the previous 10 years you were convicted of a designated substance offence
	Min. 2 years if you commit the offence in or near a school or any other public place usually frequented by minors, at a prison, or with the assistance or involvement of a minor
	Max. 5 years less a day for quantities up to 3kg
	Max. life imprisonment for more than 3kg
Importing and Exporting	Min. 1 year if you commit the offence for trafficking if you abuse a position of trust or authority while committing the offence, or if you have access to an area that is restricted to authorized persons and use that access to commit the offence
	Maximum life imprisonment
Production	Marijuana plant minimums:
	6 months if there are 6–200 plants
	9 months for 6–200 plants, and any of the following apply: (a) you use real property that belongs to a third party to commit the offence; (b) the production could endanger the security, health, or safety of minors at or close to the offence location; (c) the production constitutes a potential public safety hazard in a residential area; or (d) you set or place a trap, device, or other thing that is likely to cause death or bodily harm to another person in or close to the offence location, or permit such a trap, device, or other thing to remain or be placed in that location or area
	1 year for 201–500 plants
	18 months for 201–500 plants and any of the factors a through d, above
	2 years for more than 500 plants
	3 years for more than 500 plants and any of the factors a through d, above
CDSA Schedule III	
Types of Substances Included	
	31 different substances with varying effects, including some amphetamines, sedatives, hypnotics, hallucinogens, psychedelic stimulants, antidepressants, and stimulants for weight loss, euphoria, pain, and cough suppression; LSD, psilocybin, and methylphenidate

Offences and Penalties	
Possession	Indictable offence: max. 3 years in prison
	Summary offence: 6 months/$1,000 fine or both for first offence; 1 year/$2,000 fine or both for subsequent offences
Trafficking	Indictable offence: max. 10 years in prison
	Summary offence: max. 18 months in prison
Importing and Exporting	Indictable offence: max. 10 years in prison
	Summary offence: max. 18 months in prison
Production	Indictable offence: max. 10 years in prison
	Summary offence: max. 18 months in prison
CDSA Schedule IV	
Types of Substances Included	
	Approximately 130 different substances that are classified as barbiturates, benzodiazepines, anabolic steroids, non-steroidal hormones, appetite-suppressing stimulants, sedatives not classified as benzodiazepines or barbiturates, and a couple of synthetic opioids not in Schedule I
Offences and Penalties	
Possession	Possession not regulated under this schedule
	Seeking to obtain, indictable offence: max. 18 months in prison
	Seeking to obtain, summary offence: 6 months/$1,000 fine or both for first offence; 1 year/$2,000 fine or both for subsequent offences
Trafficking	Indictable offence: max. 3 years in prison
	Summary offence: max. 1 year in prison
Importing and Exporting	Indictable offence: max. 3 years in prison
	Summary offence: max. 1 year in prison
Production	Indictable offence: max. 3 years in prison
	Summary offence: max. 1 year in prison
CDSA Schedule V	
Types of Substances Included	
	The Minister of Health can add any substance to this schedule for a period of up to 1 year and can apply to have it listed for up to 2 years max., if it is in the interest of the public; the Minister of Health can also remove any substance from this schedule if it is in the interest of the public
	No substances were listed under this Schedule as of February 2018
Offences and Penalties	
Possession	N/A

(continued)

Trafficking	N/A
Importing and Exporting	Indictable offence: max. 3 years in prison
	Summary offence: max. 18 months in prison
Production	N/A
CDSA Schedule VI	
Types of Substances Included	
	Precursor substances
	Class A: chemical compounds used in the manufacture of clandestine substances
	Class B: solvents, acids, or bases that can potentially create a specific chemical reaction that is desired for the manufacture of some psychoactive substances
Offences and Penalties	
Possession	N/A
Trafficking	N/A
Importing and Exporting	Indictable offence: max. 10 years in prison
	Summary offence: max. 18 months in prison
Production	N/A
CDSA Schedule VII	
Types of Substances Included	
	Cannabis and cannabis resin in quantities >3kg
Offences and Penalties	
Possession	See Schedule II
Trafficking	See Schedule II
Importing and Exporting	See Schedule II
Production	See Schedule II
CDSA Schedule VIII	
Types of Substances Included	
	Cannabis >30g and cannabis resin >1g
Offences and Penalties	
Possession	See Schedule II
Trafficking	See Schedule II
Importing and Exporting	See Schedule II
Production	See Schedule II

CDSA Schedule IX	
Types of Substances Included	
	Designated devices used to compact or mould tablets or fill capsules
Offences and Penalties	
Possession	Indictable offence: fine of up to $5000, max. 3 years in prison or both
	Summary offence: fine of up to $1000, max. 6 months in prison or both
Trafficking	N/A
Importing and Exporting	Device must be registered for import or export otherwise it's prohibited
Production	N/A
Source: Government of Canada (2017)	

5.3: DEPRESSANTS

Depressants include a wide range of substances from culturally acceptable though quite dangerous substances like alcohol, to medically useful yet potentially dangerous preparations such as barbiturates and benzodiazepines, to inhalants and solvents that are used both in the medical community, industry, as well as recreationally. Like opioids, depressants slow down, CNS and peripheral nervous system processes. The respiratory system slows down, heart rate decreases, thought processes slow down, and reaction time decreases (Faupel, Horowitz, & Weaver, 2010). CNS depressants also produce euphoria, relaxation, and even some anaesthetic effect on the brain (Csiernik, 2014a).

Alcohol

The history of alcoholic beverages is believed to date as far back as 8000 BCE, when scholars have identified the first consumption of mead, a fermented form of honey (Levinthal, 2014). It is believed that beer and berry wine originated around 6400 BCE, and the more familiar grape wine emerged around 300 to 400 BCE. (Hart & Ksir, 2014). Evidently, alcohol has been consumed for a very long time, and its popularity in modern society is undisputable.

There are multiple forms of alcohol, though all alcoholic beverages that are consumed by humans involve the fermentation and sometimes the distillation of ethyl alcohol, also known as ethanol. There are three general classifications of alcoholic drinks: beer, wine, and spirits. Fermentation is used for beer and most wines, while distillation is used to create beverages, such as fortified wines and spirits, with alcohol content levels exceeding 12–15 percent (Hart & Ksir, 2014).

There are many misconceptions about the psychopharmacological effects of alcohol. Most believe that alcohol makes them happier, more sociable, and willing to do things they would not otherwise do when they are not drinking. This occurs due to alcohol's effects as a disinhibitor. While it is true that the substance lowers inhibitions and can have a stimulating effect, this depends on the social setting and the expectations of the user. However, when it comes to the actual properties of the substance and the effects on the CNS, alcohol actually works in the opposite way than most people believe: it is a depressant, not a stimulant (Hunt & Kilmer, 2009).

In general, alcohol has a high level of toxicity as it is a poison to human physiology, and there are many direct and indirect risks associated with alcohol consumption. The point at which alcohol becomes lethal for people is a mere 0.5 percent: this means that when the percentage of alcohol in one's blood reaches 0.5 percent there is significant risk of death. In addition to the potential loss of life caused directly from alcohol, every organ system in the human body can be affected over the long-term (Csiernik, 2016). Indirectly, alcohol consumption lowers inhibitions and reactions, leading to significant risk-taking and posing danger not only to oneself but also to others.

The potential dangers of alcohol cannot be overstated. In fact, even after the potential benefits of alcohol are taken into account, such as decreased heart disease at moderate levels of consumption, the total number of direct and indirect deaths attributed to alcohol in Canada is more than double the total number of deaths attributed to all illegal drugs (Rehm et al., 2006). Admittedly, there are far more people who consume alcohol in the population compared to those who consume illegal drugs (Health Canada, 2013a). However, it is the social acceptability of alcohol that makes it problematic and which contributes to it being responsible for 3.8 percent of all global deaths and 4.6 percent of global disability annually (Rehm et al., 2009).

A major risk associated with alcohol is its concurrent use with other psychoactive drugs. This is called a *pharmacodynamics effect*: when alcohol is consumed with many other drugs, rather than 1+1=2, the effect is 1+1=3 or in some cases 4. Being aware of the pharmacological and psychological effects of various substances is of utmost importance to understanding the potential risks associated with poly-substance use, or the practice of using more than one substance at the same time or during a short span of time. When different substances are combined, there are several potential problems depending on the substances being consumed. For instance, mixing alcohol with other depressants or opioids can intensify the risk of shutting down the respiratory system. Alternatively, if alcohol is mixed with stimulants, this confuses the body's CNA response and can lead to several physical complications, highlighted by cardiovascular collapse. When used in conjunction with cocaine, a new chemical is produced that is more toxic than either drug alone. The increasingly popular mixing of alcohol with energy drinks is another example, as is mixing MDMA with alcohol. Knowing the potential risks of mixing alcohol with other substances is rarely discussed, yet the consequences can produce a range of negative physical outcomes, including fatalities due to direct use or actions arising from impaired thinking.

Barbiturates

Barbiturates were originally developed at the beginning of the twentieth century to aid with inducing sleep and reducing anxiety (Csiernik, 2016). There are four major forms of barbiturates: ultra-short acting, short acting, intermediate acting, and long acting (Khanna, 2009). Ultra-short acting barbiturates have the shortest effect on the body, and when inhaled take effect in seconds and last only a few minutes, while short-acting barbiturates take effect after a few minutes and can last as long as eight hours. The intermediate and long-acting forms can take up to an hour to take effect when consumed orally, with the psychoactive effects lasting anywhere from six to twelve hours.

Over the short-term, and under careful medical supervision, barbiturates can be extremely effective in aiding with medical conditions such as epilepsy or injury from substantive physical trauma. However, physical and psychological dependence can develop within as little as two to four weeks of regular use. The withdrawal that results from barbiturate use is the most severe of any psychoactive drug and can include seizures, hallucinations, delirium tremens, high fevers, nausea, vomiting, agitation, and confusion (Baker, 2011). There is a high risk of fatality with immediate withdrawal and overdose from barbiturates (Faupel, Horowitz, & Weaver, 2010; Khanna, 2009). Barbiturates contributed to the deaths of celebrities such as Judy Garland and Marilyn Monroe. While the risk of barbiturates alone is problematic, adding other depressants, such as alcohol or opioids, to the equation can produce even greater risk of overdose, thus the recreational use of barbiturates is not common (Faupel, Horowitz, & Weaver, 2010; Khanna, 2009; Mosher & Akins, 2014).

Benzodiazepines

Once the potential dangers and noticeably addictive properties were identified with barbiturates, pharmaceutical companies developed an alternative that was marketed as being much safer and non-addictive (Hart & Ksir, 2014). The former was correct, the latter was not. This class of drugs, along with barbiturates, forms a subgroup of CNS depressants referred to as sedative-hypnotics. Sedatives help reduce agitation and anxiety, while hypnotics assist in producing sleep. Despite the original reasons that benzodiazepines were developed, many of the variations, while far less likely to produce an overdose than barbiturates, still produce physical and psychological dependency within as little as four weeks of regular use (Faupel, Horowitz, & Weaver, 2010).

Possessing sedative, hypnotic, and tranquilizing properties, like barbiturates, benzodiazepines became quite popular in the 1960s and 1970s for a variety of modern-day stresses and anxieties (Mosher & Akins, 2014). Aside from anxiety, benzodiazepines are used to treat insomnia in both the medical community and on the street. They are also mixed with methadone to produce a greater feeling of euphoria than when either drug is used alone. Additional misuse of benzodiazepines includes the infamous date-rape drug Rohypnol (flunitrazepam). When ingested in combination with alcohol, Rohypnol has the ability to induce anterograde amnesia, resulting in significant intoxication, temporary blackout, and memory impairment (Hart & Ksir, 2014).

Inhalants/Solvents

The last major group of CNS depressants to be aware of is inhalants or solvents. This group of substances are dispensed in vapour form and then inhaled by the user, producing a similar effect to alcohol or other depressants. There are two major groupings of inhalants based on their legal status: organics and anaesthetics (Faupel, Horowitz, & Weaver, 2010).

Organic inhalants refer to substances that are legally available but are not intended for human consumption. Many of these substances are common household products, such as gasoline, paints, lighter fluids, hairsprays, cleaning products, and glues. These products are easily accessible to children and youth who may not otherwise have ready access to other intoxicating substances (Hart & Ksir, 2014). Not surprisingly, young people are the most likely demographic to use organic inhalants for intoxication. This is confirmed by population-based surveys, where inhalant or solvent use is more common among younger students than older students (Boak, Hamilton, Adlaf, & Mann, 2013).

Anaesthetic inhalants are legally approved for use in the medical community, but are also used for recreational purposes to produce euphoria (Faupel, Horowitz, & Weaver, 2010). These include the former medical use of ether and chloroform and the current medical use of nitrous oxide, also known as laughing gas (Hart & Ksir, 2014). Another inhalant that made a brief appearance in some medical communities is γ-Hydroxybutyric acid (GHB). Originally believed to be an effective dietary supplement and growth hormone at low doses, GHB use became widespread in the 1980s (Hart & Ksir, 2014). However, there was never significant evidence to suggest that GHB was effective for these purposes. Nevertheless, its widespread availability for a period of time meant that there was greater experimentation with its potential uses as a CNS depressant, one such use being the adulteration of alcoholic beverages to induce a severe form of intoxication that includes temporary amnesia.

Both Rohypnol and GHB have become household names because of widespread media coverage of these substances. However, these two substances are not the only CNS depressants that pose dangers. In fact, large quantities of alcohol or opioids alone can produce similarly dangerous outcomes. It is the speed with which Rohypnol and GHB can produce impaired judgment and memory loss that sets them apart from these other substances and makes them more commonly used substances for date rape crimes (Hunter, 2009).

A major concern with inhalants is that they are available everywhere to virtually anyone who wants to try them. Young people wanting to alter their consciousness can find intoxicating substances in their homes. However, as with the other depressants described above, inhalants can be very dangerous for human consumption when they are not used for their intended purposes and are one of the few drugs that do actually produce permanent brain damage when misused (Filley, 2013; Kobayashi, 2014; Marulanda & Colegial, 2005).

Legal Classification and Penalties for Depressants

The legal penalties and classifications for depressants are rather complex. For instance, alcohol—the most widely used depressant—is not controlled or regulated under the Controlled Drugs and Substances Act (CDSA). However, there are several benzodiazepines, barbiturates, and a few sedatives and hypnotics not in those categories that are controlled and regulated under Schedules III and IV of the CDSA (Government of Canada, 2015a). Only a few different sedatives or hypnotics are listed under Schedule III, though the rationale for this classification is not clear. Why might some depressants lead to significant punishment for possession, while possessing a pharmacologically similar substance might not lead to punishment at all? For instance, some solvents that have a depressant effect are controlled under Schedule VI, as "precursor substances" that can also be used in the manufacture of clandestine substances; however, Schedule VI is only concerned with the importing and exporting—not possession and use—of these substances, making the use and misuse of many solvents and inhalants unregulated. Even more puzzling is the classification of GHB and Rohypnol. Rather than being classified Schedule IV, as most other sedatives or benzodiazepines are, they are actually classified under Schedule I. Though there is no explicit justification for classifying these two substances under Schedule I rather than Schedule IV, we can only assume that it is because of the misuse and abuse of these substances in sexual assaults that they are considered worthy of stricter penalties. While other drugs of this group have similar intoxicating potential, alcohol remains the drug most used against women in sexual assault situations, yet it is not controlled under the CDSA.

Schedule IV, where most of the depressants mentioned above are classified, carries some of the shortest and most lenient penalties under the CDSA. As mentioned, possession is not regulated for Schedule IV substances; however, seeking to obtain them without authorization or evidence to support one's need for such substances can result in six to eighteen months in prison, between $1,000 and $2,000 in fines, or both a fine and prison. Trafficking, importing and exporting, and production may result in a prison term ranging from one to three years.

5.4: STIMULANTS

Stimulants activate or excite the CNS, increasing mental awareness, motor coordination, and energy (Faupel, Horowitz, & Weaver, 2010). In a society that stresses success and achievement over everything else, it is not surprising that stimulants are among some of the most popular psychoactive substances available in North America, particularly in post-secondary settings. Used acutely, in low to moderate doses, stimulants do not usually pose a problem for users and tend to produce positive effects, such as a reduction in appetite and inhibition of sleep. However, some stimulants when used in excess over prolonged periods of time can produce detrimental and even fatal effects (Hanson, 2009).

Generally speaking, there are two categories of stimulants: major and minor. The more powerful the effects, the more likely a substance will be classified as being a major stimulant. Substances in this classification include cocaine and various forms of amphetamines, including methamphetamines and prescription stimulants such as Ritalin and Adderall. Caffeine and nicotine, on the other hand, are believed to produce less intense stimulating effects with less serious side effects, so they are considered minor stimulants (Hanson, 2009). A noteworthy point about the classification into major and minor stimulants relates to the legal and social status of these substances. Major stimulants tend to be illegal or restricted and socially disapproved, while minor stimulants are legal, widely available, and socially approved. While societal views of nicotine have certainly changed over the past few decades, nicotine products are still legal and available in many different forms.

Cocaine

Cocaine originates from the coca plant, which is primarily grown in the South American Andes. People in this region, including the Incas, chewed coca leaves for endurance and energy, medical remedies, as well as for religious and social reasons and continue to do so today (Johnson, 2011). It is believed that these original uses of the coca plant date back thousands of years to around 5000 BCE (Hart & Ksir, 2014). However, cocaine—the psychoactive ingredient in coca leaves—was not isolated until 1860. Soon after, cocaine became a commercial craze, and various products and elixirs were marketed for their beneficial effects, from antidepressant aids, to toothache remedies and cough drops, to prohibition beverages such as Coca-Cola (Levinthal, 2014).

Around the same time, pioneering psychoanalyst Sigmund Freud began using cocaine to treat his own mental health issues. For a few years, Freud advocated widely in both personal and professional circles for the use of cocaine to treat a variety of different ailments, including morphine dependence (Hart & Ksir, 2014). However, after watching his good friend experience increased dependence on cocaine and a drug-induced psychosis, Freud abruptly denounced the use of cocaine and other medicines to treat psychological disorders (Hart & Ksir, 2014), though it is not without small irony that his death was due in part to his cigar smoking.

Today, cocaine and its derivatives are strictly regulated under the Controlled Drugs and Substances Act. Although there are certainly medical uses for cocaine, such as its effectiveness as a local anaesthetic and a stimulant (Fischman, 2009), much of the use of cocaine is found in recreational settings. There are two different forms of cocaine that are available on the street: powder cocaine and crack cocaine. Powder cocaine is more accurately cocaine hydrochloride, which in an unadulterated form is a combination of 90 percent cocaine and 10 percent hydrochloric acid. However, being an illicit substance there is no quality control, and it is not unusual to find many additives in cocaine powder.

Although the common perception is that powder cocaine is less problematic than crack, they are virtually the same psychoactive substance ingested in different ways by different groups of people. The most substantive differences between crack cocaine and powder cocaine are the demographics most likely to use them, the routes of administration, and the penalties attached to the substances, particularly in the United States.

Powder cocaine is usually associated with higher status users, or people who can afford to purchase the powdered substance in larger quantities. Alternatively, crack cocaine is broken down by adding a weak base, such as water and baking soda, making it available for purchase at a significantly lower per-unit cost and in smaller quantities. Thus, crack cocaine has come to be associated with more impoverished and disadvantaged minority groups, though in a gram-to-gram analysis there is typically not much overall difference in price (Finegood, 2011).

As for the routes of administration, crack cocaine is usually heated and inhaled. The sound that the substance makes when it is heated is a crack or popping noise, which is why it is called crack. Powder cocaine is usually snorted, but can be injected or smoked if certain modifications are made to the powdered substance. However, in its usual state as a powder, it cannot be heated to produce a high (Calcagnetti, 2009).

Finally, and perhaps most controversially, there are significant differences in the penalties attached to powder cocaine and crack in some countries. In the United States, for instance, crack cocaine carries significantly more punitive penalties compared to powder cocaine. Although adjustments were made to federal legislation in 2010 under the Fair Sentencing Act, penalties for crack cocaine compared to powder cocaine are extremely unbalanced, with crack cocaine more severely punished (Mosher & Akins, 2014). Though most would like to believe that the differential penalties are connected to the relative harms associated with crack versus cocaine, this is not the case. The laws have a significant racial undertone when it comes to crack cocaine possession and use.

Amphetamines (Including Methamphetamine)

Amphetamines, including the very potent derivative methamphetamine, are synthetic substances that are chemically derived in laboratories, sometimes through clandestine operations. Originally, chemists were looking to create a drug that would mimic adrenaline (Faupel, Horowitz, & Weaver, 2010). For a period of time, not unlike many new psychoactive drug discoveries, amphetamines were believed to be miraculous non-addictive drugs and were widely used in many settings, including the military.

In the medical community, amphetamines are used for narcolepsy, weight loss, and attention deficit hyperactivity disorder (ADHD) (Bucossi & Stuart, 2009; Matuszak & Rajendren, 2011). For narcolepsy, a well-known but relatively rare condition, amphetamines are effective medications to increase alertness and wakefulness. In contrast, for weight loss, amphetamines are not an effective remedy (Bucossi & Stuart, 2009). Initially, activity levels increase and appetite is suppressed; however, tolerance quickly builds to these effects and the dose needs to continuously increase to produce the same level of activity and appetite suppression. Moreover, once the drug is no longer being taken, the weight loss is not maintained and withdrawal—the rebound effect of taking a drug when your body works to return to a homeostatic level—can lead to greater weight gain.

Prescription stimulants such as Adderall and Ritalin appear to have a paradoxical effect. When these drugs are given to children with excessive activity levels, like those with ADHD, these children slow down and are better able to focus on tasks. Though many believe that these medications help children and youth who have been diagnosed with ADHD to "behave" in the classroom, they are really only intended to treat the underlying symptoms of inattentiveness, distractibility, impulsivity, and hyperactivity, and not proper behaviour per se. Like all stimulants, they allow a person to focus better and stay on task. Historically, researchers were puzzled by the ability of a stimulant to have a calming effect on individuals diagnosed with ADHD, but recent findings suggest that these stimulants enhance focus by removing or at least minimizing background noise, as well as increasing motivation to complete tasks; this is true for anyone who uses them, not just those who have been diagnosed with ADHD (Levinthal, 2014).

These desirable properties of prescription stimulants have also resulted in the increased popularity of illicit use amongst university and college students (McCabe, Teter, & Boyd, 2006). In an attempt to meet the demands of higher education, an increasing number of post-secondary students use prescription stimulants to help them stay awake and focus on the many different tasks they are required to manage while in college or university, particularly during exam periods. Balancing the demands of work, school, parental pressures, and independence is challenging. For some, the illicit use of prescription stimulants can help them feel like they are able to meet all of these challenges. However, evidence suggests that the use of these prescription medications is not effective for increasing long-term or overall performance.

The widespread prescribing of amphetamines and other stimulants has not only led to a greater availability of these substances, but also to the increased use of other recently developed substances that are found primarily on the street. Methamphetamine is one such example of an amphetamine-like stimulant. It is a particularly attractive drug in recreational settings because it has a powerful rush and a sense of euphoria that lasts longer than cocaine (Faupel, Horowitz, & Weaver, 2010). As well, unlike cocaine, which needs to be imported from South America, methamphetamine can be made by almost anyone who can follow a recipe. However, methamphetamine can have detrimental and even fatal effects when taken regularly. Compulsive use of methamphetamine results in a lack of sleep, and possible psychotic episodes that can be accompanied by hallucinations (Irniger, Mutisya, & Harrison, 2009). Not only can this place the user at risk, but it may also place others around them in vulnerable situations. In addition, producing methamphetamine, while a comparatively simple chemical process, is also a toxic and dangerous one.

In addition to methamphetamine, other designer or club drugs have also emerged, and many of these substances have multiple psychoactive properties, including amphetamine-like effects. Most notable among these substances are bath salts, which are synthetic versions of a natural stimulant that grows around the Horn of Africa, khat. Bath salts are not the same as the traditional products one might bathe with, such as Epsom salts or sea salts. Instead, they are packaged to appear similar to these household remedies and typically contain warnings that they are not for human consumption. The packaging and warnings are only a guise to avoid detection by authorities. On the street, bath salts are used for their intense stimulating psychoactive effects, which are most often from mephedrone (4-methylmethcathinone) (Levinthal, 2014).

Nicotine

Nicotine, in combination with tobacco, is the leading cause of premature death of any psychoactive agent in Canada and the world, with doses as small as four milligrams producing severe illness. Nicotine is the psychoactive agent found in tobacco that makes its use a compulsive behaviour. When smoked, over 500 compounds are inhaled, including tar, ammonia, acetaldehyde, acetone, benzene, toluene, and carbon dioxide, which make the effects of smoking nicotine numerous and wide-ranging. The more recent development of electronic cigarettes now allows for the ingestion of nicotine without tobacco (Csiernik, 2014a).

Nicotine is a natural insecticide that, when ingested by humans, increases heart rate, pulse rate, and blood pressure. It depresses the spinal reflex, reduces muscle tone, decreases skin temperature, increases acid in the stomach, reduces urine formation, precipitates a loss of appetite, increases adrenaline production, and stimulates, then reduces, brain and nervous system activity. In non-smokers, small doses, even less than one cigarette, may produce an unpleasant reaction that includes coughing, nausea, vomiting, dizziness, abdominal discomfort, weakness, and flushing (Benowitz & Fredericks, 2009).

In addition to the harms of the individual user, nicotine crosses the placenta, and women who smoke during pregnancy tend to have smaller babies and are more likely to give birth prematurely. They also have a greater number of stillbirths and deaths among their newborn babies. Sudden infant death syndrome (SIDS) is also more common in the infants of smokers than those of non-smokers, as is the risk of having a child who develops ADHD (Thapar et al., 2003).

Nicotine also leads to the death of non-users through the inhalation of second-hand smoke. In addition to the many different, mostly negative, effects of nicotine, it also produces physical and psychological dependency. Nicotine has significant reinforcement properties, similar to other psychoactive substances such as heroin, cocaine, and alcohol, making quitting smoking a difficult task for many people (Lane, Graham, & Ovson, 2006; Zucker & Piasecki, 2009). Like alcohol, there are limited controls on the purchase and use of nicotine, which contributes to the global physical harm it produces.

Caffeine

In most instances, caffeine is usually related to the consumption of coffee, teas, and sodas, but it is also found in chocolate, pain medications, and energy drinks. It is often not considered a drug because of its widespread use and availability, but because of how it influences the human body and because of the potential for dependence and withdrawal, it is a psychoactive substance. Caffeine is the world's most-used psychoactive drug, with estimates of 120,000 tons consumed globally each year. Over 80 percent of Canadians consume caffeine on a regular basis, with an estimated 15 billion cups of coffee alone sold annually in Canada. Along with its ability to increase wakefulness, caffeine has a long list of therapeutic uses, including combatting migraine headaches, acting as a respiratory stimulant in babies who have had apnea episodes, and aiding fertility because of its ability to enhance sperm mobility (Csiernik 2016).

When used in small amounts, such as one or two cups of coffee, caffeine can produce stimulant effects on the CNS similar to those of small doses of amphetamines. These can include mild mood elevation, feelings of enhanced energy, an increased alertness, reduced performance deficit due to boredom or fatigue, postponement of feelings of fatigue and the need for sleep, and a decrease in hand steadiness, suggesting impaired fine motor performance. However, in excessive amounts of 1,000 milligrams per day, dependency can occur. Caffeine withdrawal consists of irritability, anxiety, restlessness, agitation, headache, light-headedness, rapid breathing, tremors, muscle twitches, increased sensitivity to sensory stimuli, light flashes, tinnitus, gastrointestinal upset, abnormally rapid and irregular heartbeat, and disrupted sleep. Chronic, long-term caffeine misuse has been linked to ulcers, persistent anxiety, increased cholesterol levels, and depression (Csiernik, 2014a).

Legal Classification and Penalties for Stimulants

Like depressants, the control and regulation of stimulants varies, with some substances widely available to everyone and others strictly controlled in Canada. Unlike the drug laws in the United States, the Controlled Drugs and Substances Act does not distinguish between powder cocaine and crack cocaine (Government of Canada, 2015a). Both substances are classified under Schedule I and carry the same standard penalties listed under that schedule. The disparities in how users are treated are more obvious when examining differential law enforcement practices. Crack cocaine users tend to be more visible and from more marginalized and oppressed backgrounds, which systematically disadvantages them both in their communities and through the criminal justice system.

Bath salts, along with many other amphetamines including methamphetamine, are also strictly controlled under Schedule I of the CDSA (Government of Canada, 2015a). However, this was not always the case. Many amphetamines, including methamphetamine, used to be classified as Schedule III substances. This is still the case for methylphenidate (Ritalin); however, since 2012, due to the perceived growth of amphetamine and other designer drug use, there have also been increases in the penalties attached to these substances, and a reclassification under the CDSA. Not only are the finished products controlled, but several precursor substances are now also controlled under Schedule VI. These precursors are contained in the CDSA to ensure that individuals do not have easy or illegitimate access to substances that are used in the creation of various designer drugs, including methamphetamine. Schedule VI, which names and classifies precursor substances, carries penalties ranging from 18 months to 10 years in prison for importing or exporting Class A or B precursors without proper authorization.

Nicotine and caffeine are two stimulants that are not controlled under the CDSA, but are still classified as having psychoactive properties. The sale and distribution of nicotine products is controlled and regulated, but not under criminal law. Caffeine, on the other hand, is completely unregulated. Anyone can purchase caffeine products in almost any convenience store or coffee shop. The wide availability and lack of criminal penalties attached to nicotine and caffeine are unrelated to the amount of harms produced by these substances.

5.5: HALLUCINOGENS

The health and social effects of hallucinogens have been widely debated. Some see these psychoactive drugs as dangerous because of the hallucinogenic or psychotic-like effects that can result, while others who use them argue that hallucinogens offer mind-expanding and even spiritual experiences. This has led them to be classified by various terms, including phantastica, psychotomimetics, psychedelics, and entheogens, each of which has implications concerning how the actions of each substance are conceptualized and thus how we relate to the changes in behaviour that they produce in each individual. Recently, more research has been undertaken exploring the effect of drugs such as MDMA (ecstasy) on post-traumatic stress syndrome (Mithoefer, Grob, & Brewerton, 2016) and ketamine (Special K) on depression (Newport et al., 2015). Whatever one's moral or sociological standpoint, biologically these drugs distort one's sensory perception, producing a disconnect between the physical world and the user's perception of the physical world. The context of use and the user's state of mind prior to consuming a hallucinogenic substance also can affect the nature, form, and intensity of the effects. These drugs do not produce physical dependency—with the exception of cannabis, which is sometimes classified as a hallucinogen. This is because a phenomenon known as tachyphylaxis, a rapid development of tolerance, occurs with regular hallucinogenic use. Since hallucinogens distort perception rather than create euphoria, they affect the brain in a unique manner compared to other drugs. After a few days of regular use, the brain no longer reacts to the drugs; in essence, total tolerance has developed to the drugs' effects. Nevertheless, psychological dependency is still possible.

Natural Hallucinogens

There are dozens of different plants that are naturally occurring hallucinogens (Table 5.3). Among the most prominent are peyote and its hallucinogenic component, mescaline. While historically used among Indigenous peoples of South America and the North American southwest, mescaline became popular along with other hallucinogens in the 1960s during the countercultural hippie and anti–Vietnam War movements. It was and remains preferred by many hallucinogen users over LSD because the effects are not as intense (Faupel, Horowitz, & Weaver, 2010).

Another prominent natural hallucinogen is psilocybin, typically referred to as magic mushrooms. Psilocybin is the active ingredient in the *Psilocybe mexicana* mushroom. Indigenous peoples in southern Mexico and the American southwest also used this drug in religious ceremonies. While chemically related to LSD, psilocybin is far less potent and has a shorter duration of action. The initial effects of this drug are felt approximately half an hour after ingestion and usually last several hours. Time and space perception are distorted and users are thought to be more suggestible and distracted. There is also evidence to suggest that psilocybin produces emotional extremes, where users can go from a feeling of euphoria to hilarity to deep depression. The short-term physical effects of psilocybin include an increase in blood pressure, heart rate, and body temperature, with some users initially experiencing nausea, vomiting, and intestinal cramping (Csiernik, 2014a).

Semi-Synthetic Hallucinogens

There is only one significant semi-synthetic hallucinogen, and that is LSD, which is derived from a fungus found on rye plants. LSD, the most potent of all known hallucinogens, is a colourless, tasteless, odourless chemical. When administered orally, initial effects are felt in less than an hour and generally last from 8 to 12 hours. Hearing and vision may be intensified or merged, and sense of time is often distorted. LSD is also associated with eliminating the perception of physical boundaries between the user and her or his surroundings. This can be a positive experience, though for some it can lead to panic as they lose a sense of themselves. As with other hallucinogenic drugs, LSD does not produce schizophrenia or other mental health issues; however, it can exacerbate existing issues and manifest latent biological neurochemical imbalances that might otherwise not have arisen if LSD had not been used. Chronic LSD use has been associated with amotivational syndrome, apathy, and disinterest in the environment and with social contacts, as well as a general passive attitude toward life. However, there are no known deaths directly attributable to the pharmacological effects of LSD, only fatalities through indirect actions when people were unable to distinguish between internal perceptions and what was occurring in the physical world around them (Csiernik, 2014a).

LSD has an interesting connection with Canada, as during the 1950s the leading facility conducting research on this drug was the Weyburn Mental Hospital in Saskatchewan where experiments on the drug were conducted on both staff and patients. Psychiatrists Humphrey Osmond and Abram Hoffer both used LSD themselves in an attempt to induce a personal state of psychosis, which they hoped would help them understand the chemical process, and encouraged other staff at the hospital to try LSD in order to better empathize with patients who suffered from schizophrenia (Dyck, 2010). They also began experiments to assess if LSD could be used as a treatment for alcohol addiction, something the Ontario Alcoholism and Drug Addiction Research Foundation would further examine (Smart & Storm, 1964). LSD was also experimentally provided to terminally ill individuals with hopes of separating their healthy mind from their pain-racked bodies (Grof, Goodman, Richards, & Kurland, 1972) and used in mind control experiments conducted by the Central Intelligence Agency of the United States, some of which were carried out at McGill University (Lee & Shlain, 1992). However, the use of LSD by the American counterculture (hippies) in the 1960s led to increasingly negative sensational publicity, which was created as part of President Nixon's "War on Drugs" to counter the momentum of the anti-Veitnam War movement in the United States. The result was the creation of mainstream public fear, leading to an end to research grants for studying LSD and other hallucinogens. The Canadian government enacted LSD prohibition in 1968, with research only recently resuming (Winkelman, 2014).

Synthetic Hallucinogens

Synthetics are prohibited based upon their chemical formula. As a result, there have been a variety of drugs synthesized in order to avoid legal prosecution. However, several synthetic hallucinogens were initially developed by pharmaceutical companies that were searching for legitimate medications. Many amphetamine-based drugs (MDA, MDMA, PMA, PMMA) were developed in an attempt to find more effective appetite suppressants for North American consumers.

Amphetamine-based synthetic hallucinogens produce both a separation of the senses from the environment along with a sense of heightened energy. This has made them particularly popular in clubs, bars, raves, and electric dance music festivals that emphasize loud music and extended opportunities to dance and socialize. While extensive or excessive use has been linked to memory impairment and cognitive impairment due to brain damage, the greater concern has been quality control. Due to the illicit nature of these drugs, most users have no idea what they are ingesting or the amount. It is this lack of quality control that most often leads to physical health complications and overdoses.

The other major group of synthetic hallucinogens are dissociative anaesthetics. The term *dissociative anaesthetic* refers to the state in which a person is aware of physical sensations such as touch, pressure, and pain, but the brain does not interpret the messages. These drugs were developed for use as anaesthetics; however, they produce a wide spectrum of unpredictable responses, making it difficult to know what type of experience a person will have from one usage to the next. The two prominent members of this subgroup are phencyclidine (PCP) and ketamine.

The pharmaceutical company Parke-Davis originally developed PCP in the 1950s as an experimental general intravenous anaesthetic. The makers called it Sernyl to reflect the idea of serenity it was hoped the drug would create. However, prior to active distribution, clinical trials found several undesirable side effects upon waking, including convulsions, delirium, confusion, visual disorientation, and hallucinations. PCP produces different effects at different dose levels, with as little as two milligrams producing a psychoactive reaction lasting from three to eighteen hours. At low doses, it can produce feelings of euphoria, relaxation, and sedation. Perceptual distortions of time, space, body image, and visual or auditory stimuli are also common. Impairment of attention, concentration, judgment, motor coordination, and speech can also occur. Higher doses of PCP can induce an acute toxic psychosis, including paranoia, confusion, disorientation, restlessness, anxiety, agitation, personal alienation, and violent behaviour, which has made it an unpopular drug of choice. Unfortunately, as it is comparatively easy to manufacture illicitly, it can be substituted for other drugs without the buyer's knowledge.

Ketamine is used primarily as a veterinary tranquilizer in North America, because it produces anaesthesia quickly; even low doses can produce delusions and mental confusion that can progress to hallucinations and degrees of dissociation bordering on a schizophrenic-like state and even psychosis. However, its low cost has made it the most commonly used anaesthetic in Africa. Ketamine

Table 5.3: Hallucinogen Classification

Natural Hallucinogens	Semi-Synthetic Hallucinogen	Synthetic Hallucinogens
Acacia spp.	d-Lysergic Acid Diethylamide (LSD)	Dimethyltryptamine (DMT)
Angel's Trumpet		Dimethoxyamphetamine (DOM/STP)
Arundo donax		Ketamine (Special K)
Ayahuasca		Methylenedioxyamphetamine (MDA)
Brugmansia		
Conocybe mushrooms		3,4Methylenedioxymeth-amphetamine (MDMA)
Delosperma		Paramethoxyamphetamine (PMA)
Hawaiian baby woodrose		Para-Methoxymethamphetamine (PMMA)
Hemerocallis		
Iboga/Ibogaine		Phencyclidine (PCP)
Morning Glory		Trimethoxyamphetamine (TMA)
Nutmeg		
Peruvian torch cactus		
Peyote		
Phalaris aquatica		
Psilocybe mexicana		
Psychotria viridis		
Salvia divinorum		
San Pedro cactus		
Syrian rue		
Source: Csiernik (2014a, 2016).		

is far less potent than PCP and when used recreationally is associated with the "K-hole" effect—a distinct feeling of mind-body separation that in severe circumstances can lead to stupor or unconsciousness, with a resulting feeling of confusion and loss of short-term memory. Chronic use, which is uncommon, can produce impaired memory and cognitive functions (Csiernik, 2014a).

Legal Classification and Penalties for Hallucinogens

Natural or semi-synthetic hallucinogens, including mescaline, psilocybin, and LSD, are all classified as Schedule III substances, while synthetic, multi-effect hallucinogens such as PCP, ketamine, and MDMA are classified as Schedule I substances (Government of Canada, 2015a). Schedule III of the

CDSA contains a wide variety of substances with varying effects beyond hallucinations, making generalizations difficult. Nevertheless, the possession, trafficking, importing and exporting, and production of many hallucinogens are less severely punished than the same offences for the synthetic or multi-effect hallucinogens classified under Schedule I. Hallucinogens that have been classified as Schedule I substances are punished in the same manner as cocaine and heroin.

5.6: CANNABIS (MARIJUANA)

There is likely no drug that is presently surrounded in more controversy than cannabis. It was banned in Canada in 1923 in the same legislation as heroin and cocaine as part of the first real attempt at drug prohibition laws, but will be legal again sometime in 2018. Due to a lack of empirical study regarding psychoactive drugs at the time, early drug laws were founded more in racial and cultural fears than scientific knowledge (Csiernik, Bhakari, & Koop-Watson, 2017). Cannabis is among the most consumed drugs globally and is the most used illicit drug in North America—though that is surprisingly changing in the United States and Canada as more jurisdictions are legalizing and taxing the substance. As well, there are a variety of medical uses for which this drug it touted; though again, only some of these have been empirically supported. Medical cannabis can be used to enhance appetite among those with HIV/AIDS and related disorders. It can ease the severe seizures some forms of epilepsy produce and helps manage the symptoms of multiple sclerosis (Health Canada, 2015).

Recreational users report a sense of well-being and euphoria as a result of smoking or eating cannabis, along with a distorted sense of time that is also associated with short-term memory loss and heightened physical and emotional sensitivity. Many have reported reduced anxiety and alternating periods from talkativeness and laughter to introspection and lethargy. However, these effects cannot be understood without taking into consideration the expectations and setting of the user. Ultimately, all psychoactive drugs alter the CNS of individuals in a unique way; thus, there is no such thing as a totally safe psychoactive drug—even those that have proven medical uses, such as cannabis (Arendt et al., 2008; Csiernik, 2016).

A major concern with cannabis is its affects upon brain development. We know that the most common group to use cannabis is youth between the ages of 15 and 24 (Health Canada, 2013a), yet it is also known that the human brain continues to develop until we are in our early twenties. Thus, the implications of early cannabis use, especially prior to the full development of the brain, can have unknown and potentially lifelong consequences. Researchers at Western University are only now beginning to disentangle the potential effects of cannabis on the developing adolescent brain. In experiments with rats, they have found early onset and chronic use of cannabis mimics a similar process in the brain as schizophrenia, and this process does not reverse itself in developing brains; however, cannabis use and even regular use among adults does not produce the same effects (Renard et al., 2017). Interestingly, the same team of researchers have also found that cannabidiol (CBD), another psychoactive chemical found in marijuana, may help treat the effects of schizophrenia, underscoring the paradoxical pharmacological effects of cannabis (Renard et al., 2016). Despite these findings, Canadian provinces will be able to set the legal age for purchase and use of cannabis products as low as 18.

Additionally, cannabis impairs short-term memory, logical thinking, and the ability to drive or operate machinery beause of its impairment of judgment and motor control (Asbridge, Hayden, & Cartwright, 2012; McClure, Lydiard, Goddard, & Gray, 2015; Solowij & Battisti, 2008). It also produces changes in the perception of time, distance, touch, sight, and hearing, affects balance, and produces amotivational syndrome (Rubino & Parolaro, 2008; Volkow et al., 2016).

Another popular concern or myth has been that cannabis is a gateway drug, and that regular use will eventually lead the user to move onto other "harder" substances to achieve the excitement and thrill they once got from cannabis. According to Faupel, Horowitz, and Weaver (2010), there are two fallacies associated with this notion: inevitability and causal fallacies. The inevitability fallacy suggests that all users of cannabis will eventually use harder drugs. However, the evidence does not support this. The problem with the inevitability fallacy is that we tend to look at drug use backwards: we start with heroin or cocaine users and then find that most of them have used cannabis before progressing to more potent substances. It is then concluded that people will inevitably use hard drugs if they begin using cannabis. However, when we look at cannabis users, we do not reach the same conclusions: many of them never progress to other illicit psychoactive substances and not all people who initiate cannabis use will continue their use for a prolonged period of time.

The second criticism that Faupel, Horowitz, and Weaver (2010) address is the causal fallacy. According to causal arguments, cannabis users progress to more potent drugs because they are no longer satisfied with the high that they get from cannabis alone; there is a direct link between cannabis and the desire for more potent or different kind of high. This is an argument that likely originates from the disease perspective on addiction. However, it is not necessarily a result of the limited effects of cannabis over the long-term. Instead, it could be that cannabis is the first illegal drug that users try, so progression to other illegal substances is easier once they have violated the law and used cannabis. Alternatively, it may be the subcultural involvements of an individual once they begin using cannabis that gives them greater access to other illicit psychoactive substances.

Legal Classification and Penalties for Cannabis

The controversy surrounding cannabis and its derivatives is partially fuelled by its legal status and the penalties in Canada. Under the CDSA, cannabis is regulated under three separate schedules (Government of Canada, 2015a). Schedules II, VII, and VIII are devoted exclusively to all forms of cannabis, with the exception of non-viable seeds and mature stalks and fibres as long as there are no leaves, flowers, seeds, or branches on the stalks. The main difference between each of the schedules dealing with cannabis is the quantities of the substance and the penalties associated with those quantities. Under the CDSA, the only substances that are controlled by quantities are heroin, cocaine, and cannabis. In the case of heroin and cocaine, however, there are not separate schedules that regulate differing quantities. Cannabis was the only substance under the CDSA that was covered by three schedules, a puzzling fact given that there are only eight schedules in total. Even more perplexing are the minimum sentences that were introduced in 2012 for cannabis. Trafficking, importing and exporting, and production of cannabis carry similar minimum penalties as Schedule I substances, in particular heroin and cocaine. As with most of the CDSA, there is no known evidence-informed justification for the harsh criminalization of cannabis, yet it continues to be classified as a distinct and threatening substance.

5.7: PSYCHOTHERAPEUTIC AGENTS AND PERFORMANCE-ENHANCING DRUGS

The drugs discussed thus far are used to slow down, speed up, or disrupt CNS and peripheral nervous system functioning. This final group of substances used to alter the mind or body does not necessarily follow the CNS classification scheme, but they are still important to consider. These substances can be organized into two distinct groups. The first are psychotherapeutic agents that balance rather than distort CNS functioning. The second, performance-enhancing drugs, include steroids and human growth hormones that, while altering physiology and at times behaviour, have no direct action on the CNS.

Psychotherapeutic Agents

Psychotherapeutic agents can also be referred to as mood-enhancing drugs. They are distinct from most other psychoactive substances discussed in this chapter in that their primary function is to move a user towards homeostasis rather than away from it. These drugs are intended for use with those with formally assessed and diagnosed mental health conditions. They are classified as psychoactive drugs because they also modify thought processes, mood, and emotional reactions to the environment. However, many substances within this family of drugs, particularly those that have been in use for longer periods of time, produce unpleasant side effects, including involuntary movements and tremors, a shuffling gait, nausea, dry mouth, insomnia, and constipation. As these psychoactive agents also tend to change mood slowly over a period of days or weeks, they are not generally subject to recreational use, and thus issues of abuse or addiction are limited.

Mood-enhancing drugs are classified into three categories: antipsychotics, antidepressants, and mood stabilizers (see Table 5.4). Antipsychotics are used to treat the underlying symptoms of various psychoses, including schizophrenia, by reducing behavioural and physiological responses to stimuli and producing drowsiness and emotional quieting. They work on positive symptoms, but have minimal impact on negative symptoms or cognitive deficits. Thus, antipsychotics are not effective in alleviating emotional flatness or social withdrawal, or increasing communication, but rather calm the user and minimize emotional and physical outbursts that can be harmful to the person or those around them.

Depression is a more complicated mental health issue, as there are biological and environmental factors, and interactions between the two, that lead to depressive states. Antidepressants taken over a period of time can alleviate depression that has a biological basis, but they are far less effective in resolving issues of daily living or trauma where counselling or the two in combination are a more effective response. Newer antidepressants that have emerged are SSRIs (selective serotonin reuptake inhibitors), NDRIs (norepinephrine-dopamine reuptake inhibitors), and SSNRIs (selective serotonin-norepinephrine reuptake inhibitors). Newer generation antidepressants produce far fewer side effects and can enhance mood even if depression is not an issue.

Bipolar disorder is a condition where a person moves from feelings of depression to those of mania, where the person has exaggerated perceptions of well-being or excessively positive views of themselves, their status, and/or their success. Persons suffering from bipolar mood disorder, formerly referred to as manic depression syndrome, may use lithium carbonate, carbamazepine, and valporic acid to help maintain personal functioning levels closer to homeostasis. Side effects can be unpleasant and include fatigue, dysphoria, vertigo, and slurred speech; thus, with this drug, as with many other psychotherapeutics, the concern is one of compliance rather than misuse or abuse (Csiernik, 2014a).

Performance-Enhancing Drugs

Performance-enhancing drugs do not have the same kind of effect on the CNS as opioids, depressants, stimulants, or hallucinogens, as they are not psychoactive. However, they are substances that can alter one's physical performance, can have negative consequences for society and the individual, and can be misused and abused. Their use is associated with the socialization of boys and young men into traditional masculine ideology, which leads to the pursuit of enhanced muscularity. There are three major types of performance-enhancing drugs that can readily and artificially produce this physique: proteins, anabolic androgenic steroids, and human growth hormones. Each of these substances is produced in our bodies naturally to varying extents; however, there are also artificial versions that mimic the same processes as the natural substances. When ingested it is believed that the substances will optimize performance, increase competitive edge, and improve body shape.

Proteins are an increasingly popular substance for both competitive and non-competitive athletes trying to get the most out of their fitness routines. Artificial proteins are contained in many different nutritional powders and shakes. Many of these are marketed in health stores for their potential benefits, and consumers endorse these substances for their ability to "pump them up" both in terms of energy and helping to build muscle. However, they are not unlike the more controlled and perhaps more stigmatized steroids: too much protein can have a negative effect on the body.

Like proteins, which are naturally occurring in humans, anabolic androgenic steroids are an artificial form of the naturally produced hormone called testosterone. Excessive amounts of testosterone can result in extreme irritability and aggressiveness, also known as "roid rage." Human growth hormones, which are typically used in the medical community for dwarfism, are also used

Table 5.4: Psychotherapeutic Drugs

i) Antidepressants by Pharmacological Category		
Type	**Drug**	**Brand Name**
Tricyclic antidepressants	amoxapine	Asendin
	imipramine	Tofranil
	amitriptyline	Elavil
	doxepin	Adapin, Sinequan
	desipramine	Norpramin, Pertofrane
	nortriptyline	Aventyl
	clomipramine	Anafranil
Monoamine oxidase Inhibitors	moclobemide	Manerix
	tranylcypromine	Parnate
	phenelzine	Nardil
Other cyclic antidepressants	*SSRIs*˙	
	fluoxetine	Prozac
	paroxetine	Paxil
	fluvoxamine	Luvox
	sertraline	Zoloft
	nefazodone	Serzone
	trazodone	Deseryl
	NDRIs˙	
	bupropion	Zyban
		Wellbutrin
	SNRIs˙	
	venlafaxine	Effexor
	duloxetine	Cymbalta
ii) Antipsychotic Agents by Pharmacological Category		
Type	**Drug**	**Brand Name**
Butyrophenones	haloperidol	Haldol
Phenothiazines	chlorpromazine	Largactil
		Thorazine
	trifluoperazine	Stelazine
	thioridazine	Mellaril
Rauwolfia Alkaloids	reserpine	Serpasil

(continued)

Thioxanthenes	chlorprothixene	Truxal
	thiothixene	Navane
	fluphenazine	Prolixi
New antipsychotics	clozapine	Clozaril
	loxapine	Loxitane
	risperidone	Risperdal
	olanzapine	Zyprexa
iii) Mood Stabilizers		
	Drug	**Brand Name**
	lithium carbonate	Eskalith, Lithane, Lithobid
	carbamazepine	Tegretol
	valproic acid	Depakene

*SSRI=selected serotonin reuptake inhibitors; NDRI=norepinephrine-dopamine reuptake inhibitors; SNRI=selective serotonin-norepinephrine reuptake inhibitors
Source: Virani, Bezchlibnyk-Butler, & Jeffies (2009).

for performance enhancement; however, there is no evidence to support the effectiveness of human growth hormones for these purposes (Faupel et al., 2010).

For sociologists, these performance-enhancing substances are of great interest for several reasons. They represent issues of competition, body image, economics, and the overwhelming desire for some people to be special and a select few to exceed their biology and genetics (Filiault & Drummond, 2010; Karazsia, Crowther, & Galioto, 2013). Use of these products has become a global issue: in a study of 508 male high school students from South Africa, 48 percent had used protein supplements or steroids to gain muscle mass, lose weight, or improve their appearance. "The pursuit of muscularity is no longer something relegated to a fringe bodybuilding subculture, but it is now an aspect of everyday life for adolescent boys" (Martin & Govender, 2011: 234).

Legal Classification and Penalties for Psychotherapeutic Agents and Performance-Enhancing Drugs

Given that most of these drugs are not typically abused and, in the case of many psychotherapeutic agents, compliance is more an issue than misuse, most are not included in the CDSA. A few antidepressants are included under Schedule III, but not all prescribed substances for moods are legally regulated (Government of Canada, 2015a). While there are over 40 different types of anabolic steroids listed in Schedule IV, protein-based substances are not controlled under the criminal law because they are considered a food. The central question is at what point, by whom, and based upon what evaluative criteria are substances regulated or penalties determined? What distinguishes a drug from a food? At what point is taking a substance an enhancement to promote your well-being and competitiveness and at what point does it become a criminal behaviour?

5.8: THE PROBLEM WITH DRUG EFFECTS AND LEGAL CLASSIFICATIONS

Aside from using crime control as a punitive means of dealing with drugs and drug users, for which there is no consistent justification, the most significant limitation of the CDSA is its lack of justification for classifying certain drugs under specific schedules, each of which carry different penalties. If or when new substances become listed on the CDSA we should be asking: Why this substance? Why now? Why this schedule? What are appropriate penalties? What are inappropriate penalties? And what's next? Too often, society accepts the regulations that are imposed under the CDSA, which are not always linked to a drug's effects. It is believed that the laws and penalties must be justified; otherwise, they would not exist. When it comes to psychoactive drugs, however, this is not the case. Psychoactive substances are far more complex than the law suggests.

In addition to biological and psychological properties, psychoactive substances are sociological phenomena. As Erich Goode contends "… any accurate and valid definition of drugs must include the social, cultural, and contextual dimension. The concept drug is in part a cultural artifact, a social fabrication, applied to certain types of substances in specific contexts or settings. *A drug is something that has been defined by certain segments of the society as a drug*" (as quoted in Faupel, Horowitz, & Weaver, 2010: 9; emphasis in original). In Canada, this is best represented through a critical examination of the known psychopharmacological properties of different substances and the Controlled Drugs and Substances Act. Such an examination suggests that the social lens of a governing political party can be far more influential in determining crime and punishment than the actual effects of a substance.

PARADOXES

1) The legal classification of psychoactive drugs is not congruent with their biological properties or the consequences of their use.

2) Psychoactive drugs themselves can appear to produce paradoxical affects. For example, stimulants can paradoxically calm individuals with ADHD, and benzodiazepine, a depressant, can actually create anxiety in some users.

3) Recent research on cannabis indicates that the mental health consequences of regular use may be detrimental to the developing brain, specifically prior to the age of 25. However, the proposed legalization of cannabis includes the option for provinces and territories to set the age limit on cannabis purchase and consumption as low as 18.

CRITICAL REFLECTIONS

1) Are drugs good or bad? Discuss the implications of asking this question from a sociological perspective.

2) The inclusion of protein and other performance-enhancing substances in this chapter underscores the issue of distinguishing between foods, supplements, and psychoactive drugs, all of which affect the mind and body in different ways. Proteins can be positive, but then so can opioids. Human growth hormone has legitimate therapeutic uses, but then so does cannabis. How is it determined that a substance has value and that it is a problem for society?

3) Does the presentation of a drug's psychopharmacological effects alongside its legal and punitive consequences implicitly affirm the "Just Say No" ideology?

4) A new, isolated society has been discovered that has never been exposed to or has never used any psychoactive substance. As a result of your ability to explain addiction you are made Minister of the Drug Secretariat. Prepare a list of psychoactive substances that you would allow and those you would ban and provide a rationale for which drugs you put in each category.

6 The Socially Constructed Problem of Drugs and Drug Users

Since the emergence of the concept of addiction as immoral, punitive punishment has been the primary response offered by society and the state. As with other moral panics, responses and punishment are targeted toward certain genders, races, ages, and classes (Bailey, 2005). In order to heavily punish these marginalized offenders, strong law enforcement and impractical drug policies are imposed (Cheung, 2000; Kellen, Powers, & Birnbaum, 2017). To justify these responses, the media plays an important role in publicizing and demonizing certain groups of people, so that the general public will support harsh punishments and policies (Boyd & Carter, 2014).

But why are substance users targeted more than some other social problems? As sociologists Goode and Ben-Yehuda (1994: 163) contend: "The public fears threats less according to their statistical likelihood than to the extent that they are seen as involuntary, uncontrollable, unknowable, unfamiliar, catastrophic, certain to be fatal, and delayed in their manifestation." Both today and historically, social sentiment indicates that the fear of addiction and substance use fit this explanation. According to Reinarman (2005: 314), media suggestions that addiction "can happen to anyone" defy the evidence that addiction, while complex, is predictable and less haphazard than popular belief suggests. Nevertheless, fear still remains in the collective conscience of society. The following are some examples of drug scares that have made headlines or have been presented in some way to the general public as a concerning issue in Canada. In each instance, it is evident that a particular type of drug or user is being targeted in an attempt to communicate to the public that there is evidence to not only be concerned about drugs and drug users but to be petrified of them.

6.1: BATH SALTS

One of the most recent drug scares presented in the Canadian media surrounded the use of "bath salts." This is the name given to a designer drug typically containing methylenedioxypyrovalerone (MDPV) or mephedrone, synthetic versions of the psychoactive drug khat, which became a prohibited substance in Canada in 1997 for social rather than pharmacological reasons. For a period of time, it seemed that people believed that these bath salts were the same product one might find in the beauty section in local stores; however, this is not the case. These amphetamine-type designer drugs do appear similar to regular bath salts, having a sugary or crystal-like appearance, and are often packaged with the name *bath salts* to avoid detection when imported and exported. Media claims have emphasized the erratic and violent nature of users found to be using these psychoactive drugs.

A *CBC News* headline from June 2012 read: "Calgary 'Bath Salts' Drug Incident Sends 2 to Hospital: User Overpowered Police in City's 1st Reported Incident of Drug's Use." Upon closer examination of the article, there is no evidence that the bath salts were what caused the user to be able to overpower the police. Perhaps the same man could have overpowered the police if he were intoxicated from alcohol. Only two days later, another headline in the *National Post* read: "'Bath Salts' Drug Believed to be Behind Violent Assault on Toronto Cops, Arrests in Calgary." Again, there is no confirmation that the bath salts were the actual source of the violent assault; it is merely suspicion. Perhaps the most dramatic example of suspected bath salt use was the US man who ate the face off of a homeless man (ABC News, 2012). This story made international headlines in 2012; however, a complete, evidence-informed, toxicological report by the medical examiner confirmed that the man was not impaired by bath salts or any other "exotic street drug" (CBS Miami, 2012).

Since this original, short-lived scare, and the making of "bath salts" illegal in Canada, there have been few cases reported in the media and even fewer cases of people self-reporting use. In fact, less than 0.5 percent of the student population in Ontario reported using bath salts in 2012 (Boak, Hamilton, Adlaf, & Mann, 2013).

6.2: ECSTASY

According the 2012 World Drug Report from the United Nations Office on Drugs and Crime (UNODC), Canada is the leading manufacturer and supplier of designer drugs, including ecstasy, a central nervous system (CNS) hallucinogen with secondary stimulant properties. In fact, the UNODC estimates that 60 percent of all seizures globally of 3,4-Methylenedioxyphenyl-2-Propanone, the precursor to ecstasy, were in Canada. However, a Public Safety Canada study found that Canada only produces between 0.6 and 4 percent of the world's supply of amphetamine-type stimulants, including MDMA (Bouchard et al., 2012). Thus, the media frenzy that Canada is one of the major suppliers of ecstasy appears to be vastly exaggerated, especially when only seizures are taken into account.

Another concern that has received heightened media attention recently is the questionable purity of drugs being sold under the guise of ecstasy. Media portrayals of ecstasy tend to focus on a younger demographic of middle-class partiers looking to have good time, without fear of the potentially fatal consequences of using other illicit substances. As one headline for *The Canadian Press* read in early 2012: "B.C. Ecstasy Deaths: Teen Overdose May Be Latest in String of Deaths" (Burgmann, 2012). Another *CBC News* headline from Calgary in 2012 proclaimed: '8 Alberta Deaths Linked to Ecstasy-Like Drug: Victims Think They Are Taking Ecstasy, but Actually Ingesting 'Dr. Death.'" What the British Columbia headline failed to communicate to readers is that the drug responsible for the death of the young teen may not have been MDMA; the second headline at least mentions that the drug responsible is not ecstasy. To the average reader, however, ecstasy may still be blamed for the deaths, as the headline mentions ecstasy and not the actual drug that caused the fatalities. A series of toxicology reports on previous deaths presumed to be from ecstasy actually show a different chemical present in the bodies at the times of death.

Paramethoxymethamphetamine (PMMA) is one of the substances being substituted to produce effects similar to ecstasy, as it is easier to produce and it is literally impossible to tell the difference between any of these illicit hallucinogens with stimulant properties. While PMMA mimics the effects of MDMA, it is much more toxic and takes longer to produce the hallucinogenic effects, so some people have overdosed on the drug because they are trying to produce the desired effects that they obtain from ecstasy. Similar accounts of PMMA have been found elsewhere, including Ireland (Mullally, 2014). This issue of purity is of major concern in Canada and other countries where psychoactive substances are criminalized. Under a prohibitionist regime, there is no way to regulate and control the potency or even the content of substances when they are being manufactured and distributed by criminal organizations and other individuals hoping to garner tax-free incomes.

6.3: CRYSTAL METH

Another drug that is a target of ongoing concern and regulation in Canada is crystal meth, the smokeable form of methamphetamine. Fear of the widespread use of methamphetamines is also closely linked to concerns about ecstasy, which is also an amphetamine derivate. Since the 1990s, drug education programs run by police officers enter public school classrooms and warn young people about the dangers of using crystal meth or similar substances. Using before and after images of crystal meth users supposedly showed the effects of accelerated aging and open sores that appear on the face after using these dangerous substances, as well as an inevitable involvement in crime to feed the addiction. For many young people, these images of meth users are forever embedded in their minds. Interestingly, the same three images of crystal meth users were featured in every major Canadian newspaper on multiple occasions, and are now readily accessible on the Internet, leading the critical reader to wonder if there were only ever three Canadians who experienced the negative effects of crystal meth. Interestingly, these images are not even Canadian.

More recently, scares concerning crystal meth and other synthetically produced stimulants have focused less on the users of crystal meth and more on the prevalence of meth labs that are supposedly popping up everywhere across the country. In 2006, the media and government focused on controlling various over-the-counter (OTC) cold remedies that contained ephedrine or pseudoephedrine. As one *CBC News* headline in April 2006 proclaimed: "Cold Remedies Removed over Crystal Meth Concerns." These efforts to control the sale of cold remedies containing traces of chemicals used to produce crystal meth were used to evoke concern and anxiety in the minds of citizens across Canada. The headlines confirmed that common household substances were now supposedly being abused in mass quantities or being purchased with the intention of manufacturing extremely addictive drugs, such as crystal meth.

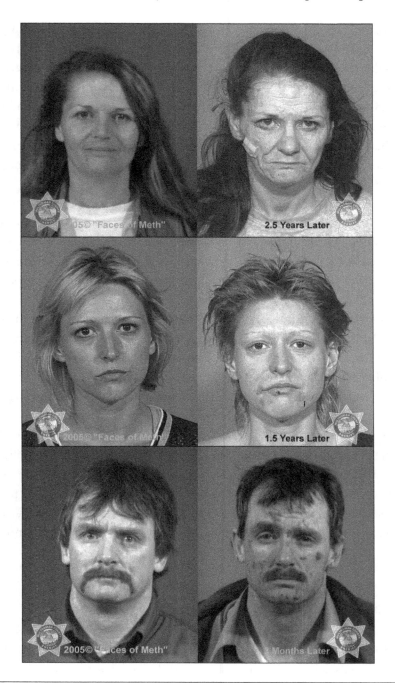

Figure 6.1: The Faces of Meth (Photos Appeared on the Front Page of the *London Free Press* on October 24, 2005)

Source: Images from the Faces of Meth V 1, 2005, CD© 300 dpi images F4, F18 and M36. Reproduced by permission of the Multnomah County Sheriff's Office.

To add to this fear campaign, media reports have focused on the unpredictability of meth labs and their locations; these concerns were further fuelled by the popular television series *Breaking Bad*. Some have noted the dangers associated with "cooking" meth, while others have emphasized the possibility that both rural and urban people may be making meth in their homes and even in the trunks of their cars. While these concerns have some legitimacy, and no one wants their home or family to be destroyed because of an explosion from a nearby crystal meth lab, the level of fear being produced by these reports is not proportionate to the actual number of labs discovered in Canada.

Relatively speaking, crystal meth is one of the least commonly used substances among Canadians. In Ontario, for instance, the 2013 Ontario Student Drug Use and Health Survey (OSDUHS) showed no evidence that the general population of youth in Ontario are using crystal meth or other methamphetamines; instead, there are indications of a decline in use. Less than 1 percent of the student population reported using methamphetamines in the past year (Boak, Hamilton, Adlaf, & Mann, 2013). Nationwide estimates have suggested that approximately 52,000 Canadians are methamphetamine users (Bouchard et al., 2012). In the same Public Safety Canada study, estimates for the number of amphetamine-type stimulant labs ranged from 560 to 1,400 across the entire country. Of course, these numbers may seem quite large; however, it is vital to consider how large Canada is geographically when assessing what the numbers represent. If the media delivers the message that meth labs are everywhere, the public begins to panic; yet, though certainly a public health concern, the problem is far less severe than the media and government have tried to convey, and there are even times when the market is oversupplied and prices for the drug decrease. This is not to suggest that we do not need to be concerned about the potential dangers associated with methamphetamine production, but rather to ask if the facts warrant the level of hysteria.

6.4: COCAINE

Similar to restrictions on traditional cold remedies to curb the production of crystal meth, a St. Louis, Missouri, legislator attempted to regulate the sale of baking soda to prevent individuals from being able to produce crack cocaine (White, 2007). If people had to provide identification when purchasing baking soda, the thought was that there would be fewer people purchasing the precursor substance and crack use would be curtailed. Similar attempts to ban or regulate these common household items did not happen in Canada, even though many of Canada's attempts to demonize cocaine have been borrowed from the United States.

The most notable attempt to create a cocaine scare in Canada was in the late 1980s, though early initiatives date back to the turn of the twentieth century. In 1986, when American President Ronald Reagan was re-energizing the War on Drugs in the United States—a "war" started by President Nixon during the Vietnam War to divert attention away from domestic political issues—public support for the then Conservative Canadian Prime Minister Brian Mulroney was rapidly declining. In an attempt to bolster his popularity and support, Mulroney decided to follow Regan's political strategy and wage a War on Drugs in Canada (Jensen & Gerber, 1993). Despite the fact that the general Canadian public did not support a War on Drugs, the legal apparatus and reports that followed attempted to portray drugs in Canada as a significant social ill. One example was in the 1989 proclamation that seizures of cocaine had increased 268 percent since 1985 (Erickson, 1992). However, as Erickson also insightfully highlights, this increase in seizures was largely the result of one massive confiscation of 500 kilograms of cocaine, and that the majority of the remaining seizures were small (less than one ounce) and intermediate (between one ounce and one kilogram) in size.

Most of the media frenzy surrounding cocaine and crack in Canada during the 1980s was directly borrowed from American media sources (Erickson, 1992). The targets of this media and criminal justice–based panic were largely African Americans, who were also disproportionately victimized by high unemployment, poverty, and an ever-increasing decline in social welfare supports (Reinarman & Levine, 1997); this lead to racially biased criminal justice responses (Albonetti, 1997).

Another notable element in the hysteria around crack in the 1980s was the widespread claim that crack use during pregnancy causes irreparable damage to infants. Researchers actually refute this claim (Avants et al., 2007; Kleiman, Caulkins, & Hawken, 2011; Peele, 1985a), suggesting that the direct causal connection between a mother's crack use and her infant's various physical and developmental concerns cannot be entirely separated from other aspects of their living conditions, including poor nutrition, lack of adequate housing, unsafe living conditions, and inadequate parenting that is often associated with many forms of substance dependence. Essentially, there is no definitive evidence to suggest that crack is the single and direct reason why children of crack-using mothers may experience greater difficulties in life. Thus, the term *crack babies* is misleading and stigmatizing to both mothers and children born into these circumstances.

The longitudinal work of Hallam Hurt and his research group underscores this conclusion. They followed a cohort of African-American children exposed to crack cocaine in utero living in inner-city Philadelphia. There were grave concerns over the long-term health and cognitive abilities of this group, which seemed justified when these children entered the school system and their academic performance was below national standards. However, their school performance, grade point average, reading level, and standardized reading and math scores were equivalent to those children in their community who had not been exposed to crack cocaine. Moreover, there were no significant differences in IQ, executive brain functioning, or general cognitive abilities. However, when examining the social context of both groups it was discovered that 81 percent of the children had seen someone arrested; 35 percent had seen someone shot; and 19 percent had seen a dead body in their neighbourhood by the age of seven. Those children who reported a high exposure to violence were also the most likely to have symptoms of depression and anxiety and to have lower self-esteem. Hallam's conclusion was that poverty was a far more powerful influence on the academic outcomes of inner-city African-American children than gestational exposure to crack, and that the underlying issue was one of the environmental surroundings imposed on particular racial groups rather than drugs (Avants et al., 2007; Farah et al., 2008; Hurt et al., 1997; Hurt et al., 2001; Hurt et al., 2005; Hurt et al., 2008).

More recently, crack cocaine resurfaced in the Canadian media in 2014 when it became known that the then mayor of Toronto, Rob Ford, had some experience with smoking crack. Originally denying the allegations, which included a video in which he was spotted smoking the illegal substance, Ford became the focus of media all over the world, especially when he eventually admitted six months later that he had smoked crack cocaine. After his admission, late night entertainment hosts made him a regular, including conducting in-person interviews. In a televised question-and-answer period, Ford told reporters: "Yes, I have smoked crack cocaine, but no, do I, am I an addict? No. Have I tried it? Probably in one of my drunken stupors, probably approximately about a year ago." It is puzzling to think that the mayor of the largest city in Canada, with a population greater than five of the nation's provinces, believes that he can use drunkenness as an excuse for crack use. Rather than any negative repercussions, his actions became a worldwide media event, including his aborted and then successful attempts to enter treatment. Critical to consider here are the media depictions of elite drug users versus marginalized substance users and the role of politics in the media.

6.5: PRESCRIPTION STIMULANTS: ATTENTION-ENHANCING PRESCRIPTION DRUGS

According to the 2014 World Drug Report released by the UNODC, among the countries that collect information on prescription stimulant misuse, Canada ranks fourth highest for rates of misuse of prescription stimulants primarily targeted at children, including Ritalin, Dexedrine, Concerta, and Adderall. To add to this, newspapers targeting children as the new drug dealers have fuelled heightened concern. As a 2001 *Globe and Mail* heading reads: "Children Trafficking in Ritalin, Dexedrine" (Walton, 2001), and the article continues: "they're trafficking in them and being bullied into giving them up in what has become a burgeoning school-yard drug trade." The overprescription of ADHD medications is certainly a public health concern; however, the media focus does not appear to be the overmedication of children, but rather fear regarding youth becoming drug dealers while at school. The reality is that the prevalence of self-reported non-medical use of ADHD among youths in Ontario is estimated to be about 1 percent in 2013, a rate that remained stable between 2007 and 2013. It seems that the data gathered by the UNODC and some newly published reports can be misleading. Moreover, the public portrayal of prescription stimulants in the media is inconsistent with the empirical findings of the most comprehensive set of data on young people and their drug use in Canada, the OSDUHS.

Another scare tactic used by the media is related to the potential side effects of ADHD medications. In 2012, the *Toronto Star* conducted an independent investigation of 600 adverse reaction reports by doctors, nurses, pharmacists, and parents (Bruser & Bailey, 2012). The main concerns highlighted in the news article included suicide, psychotic disorders, depression, convulsions, hallucinations, heart problems, overdoses, and strokes. A series of other potential side effects were also listed to heighten the concerns of the public about the utility of these drugs. The article also focused on the inadequate reporting of and lack of accountability for these adverse reactions. According to the *Toronto Star* investigation, pharmaceutical companies are left with the responsibility of recording and responding to any adverse reactions to these attention-enhancing drugs. Health Canada, on the other hand, takes no responsibility for monitoring or enforcing the reporting practices of doctors, nurses, and pharmacists. Thus, the real issue is not necessarily the drugs, but the lack of documentation to support their overall effectiveness and reveal whether we are using them as a mechanism of social control to deal with other issues, such as the under-funding of public schools. After reading this article, parents with children displaying ADHD characteristics may not want to treat their children, for fear that their child will experience one of the side effects. However, when used under proper supervision by a knowledgeable physician, prescription medications for ADHD can be effective and produce positive outcomes for otherwise distracted and struggling children (Tanner, 2009).

6.6: CANNABIS

The criminalization of cannabis has been dubbed "the solution without a problem" (Giffen, Endicott, & Lambert, 1991). The initial introduction of cannabis and its derivatives into Canadian public policy was when it was added to existing legislation in 1923 (Erickson & Hyshka, 2010) without any parliamentary debate. Both before and after this date, cannabis was not a significant social problem, despite what some political figures suggested. In fact, the first seizure of cannabis did not occur until 1937, over a decade after its original criminalization (Giffen, Endicott, & Lambert, 1991), but even then cannabis was not a significant problem. Today, cannabis is the most widely consumed illegal substance in the world. Thus, it is not surprising that there have been several crusades to demonize cannabis or marijuana and its derivatives.

Most recently, marijuana has been highlighted in political campaigning. In an attack of the Liberal Party's vow to legalize marijuana, Stephen Harper's Conservative government launched a series of advertisements aimed at inducing fear in the public about the potential consequences of legalizing marijuana. One particular ad reads: "Trudeau's Pot Plan: Trudeau wants marijuana in local stores, just like alcohol and cigarettes" (see Figure 6.2). The ad features a superimposed image of a youthful, bearded Trudeau looking and smiling at a young teen lighting a joint. For most parents, this image is disturbing; unfortunately, many people will view this image and believe what it says rather than question its legitimacy. As plans to legalize marijuana have been made public by the Liberal government, it is clear there is no intention of making marijuana widely available to youth. In fact, there will be significant penalties to distributors who sell to minors and to adults who attempt to purchase marijuana on behalf of any minor (Health Canada, 2016).

Additional concerns have been featured in the media in recent years, including problems with medicalized marijuana and supposed outbreaks of marijuana grow operations. In a recent study conducted by Boyd and Carter

(2014), they found that the media frequently reports inaccurate information or makes exaggerated claims about the size and scope of marijuana grow ops in Canada, including reporting on the dangers associated with the marijuana industry and the often assumed connection to organized crime. Many of the media reports are based on information gathered by the Royal Canadian Mounted Police (RCMP), who tend to present drug seizures at estimated street value, which, like drug potency, is not always consistent or accurate. Not surprisingly, some journalists do not question the legitimacy of the information they receive from the RCMP, so they deliver the message to the public with little regard for its accuracy.

Perhaps more problematic are the politicians who rely on this same distorted and demonizing information to make policy decisions and enact harsher laws. An example of this is the recent enactment of the Safe Streets and Communities Act in 2012, whereby more punitive penalties and mandatory minimum sentences were introduced for various drug-related offences (Government of Canada, 2012). Mandatory minimum sentences are particularly problematic, as they remove discretionary decision-making from judges and other criminal justice officials. This makes situational and environmental conditions obsolete in the criminal justice decision-making process, further reinforcing the notion that it is the drug and the drug user that are the problem, not their social environment or conditions.

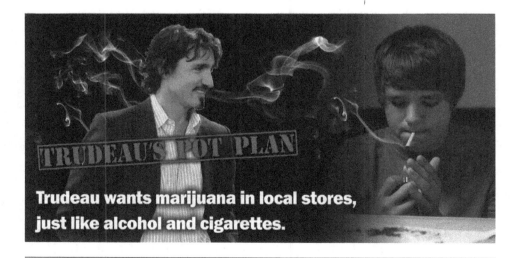

Figure 6.2: Conservative Government Federal Election Attack Ad, 2015

Source: Conservative Party of Canada, reproduced from the *Globe and Mail*, June 18, 2014 (Bryden, 2014).

6.7: SOLVENTS/INHALANTS

Concern about inhalant use is often targeted towards younger youth, as they are the most likely consumers of these intoxicants. In certain instances, the use of particular inhalants such as gas has also focused on marginalized Indigenous populations. Since the 1993 CBC documentary on the Davis Inlet, located in the north-eastern region of Newfoundland and Labrador, there has been heightened concern about the extent of gas sniffing and huffing in Indigenous communities across Canada (CBC, 1993). The media continues to frame the issue as a new and emergent problem. For instance, in a recent news article regarding gas sniffing and the Innu community that was moved from Davis Inlet, the reporter stated that "a recent escalation in gas sniffing involves children as young as seven" (Canadian Press, 2012). The report does not provide information on how much gas sniffing has escalated, and it fails to acknowledge that this particular community of Innu has had a longstanding problem with this particular practice. Moreover, it does not recognize the cause of the problem as being rooted in the official assimilation policies of successive federal governments both Liberal and Conservative. Finally, it ignores the impact of the centuries of trauma and economic exploitation that Indigenous groups have faced in Canada. Ironically, these peoples are among the few cultures on the planet never to have used drugs recreationally until introduced by an outside group.

Aside from targeting Indigenous groups as having a significant problem with inhalant use, the article also attempts to induce fear into the public about how young the users of inhalants can be. Of all the licit and illicit substances, inhalant use is most common among children and early adolescents, especially those who are marginalized. However, inhalant use, even among children and youth, is not widespread. In 2013, the Ontario Student Drug Use and Health Survey showed that less than 4 percent of youth had used any form of inhalant in the past year and less than 0.5 percent had used inhalants frequently (six or more times in the past year) (Boak, Hamilton, Adlaf, & Mann, 2013). This is the lowest inhalant use has been in over 15 years. Comparatively, the greatest recorded prevalence was in 1999, when almost 10 percent of Ontario youth reported using inhalants at least once in the past year.

Despite the empirical evidence showing a steady decline in inhalant use, in 2005 there was an additional scare referred to as "dusting." A June 16, 2005, headling from *CBC News* read: "Parents Warned of 'Dusting' Solvent Abuse." This inhalant practice involved the use of computer dusting cans to produce an intoxicating effect. The source of the problem, according to researcher

Colleen Dell from the Canadian Centre on Substance Abuse, is the lack of communication between parents and their teens, along with teens believing that dusting is harmless because it is just air from a can. However, this time the target of the scare was not marginalized groups; instead, it was predominantly middle-class youth with their own computers who were thought to be engaging in risky behaviour. In the same article, Dell admitted that there is no information being collected on this phenomenon in Canada, so there is no way to know how widespread the issue may be or even if anyone has died from dusting in Canada, though anecdotal from the United States indicates it is a rare occurrence (Alexander, 2005; ABC News, 2006).

6.8: PRESCRIPTION OPIOIDS

The use and misuse of prescription pain relievers or opioids has been in the head-lines of major newspapers across the country for several years now, highlighted by the banning of OxyContin, a longer-acting version of the established opioid oxycodone. The extent to which we can claim that a drug scare is being induced based on exaggerations or misrepresentations of this particular group of sub-stances would most likely appear to be insensitive to the objectively measured problems that exist as a result of these drugs. That is not our intent, as it has been widely expressed that opioid misuse is a growing public health issue (Canadian Press, 2016; Stack, 2016). What is worth highlighting here is how a significant social problem can be blown so far out of proportion and misrepresented that attempts to strictly control and regulate a particular drug epidemic may lead to adverse or unintended consequences.

In 2009, a *Globe and Mail* headline read: "Painkiller Deaths Double in Ontario." The article points to the 850 percent increase in the number of oxycodone prescriptions from 1991 to 2007 as the source of the problem (Mehler Papherny, 2009). People are dying because doctors are prescribing opioids without regard for the dependency issues known to be associated with these types of drugs. Admittedly, the focus of this article was not on the blameworthiness of the users or even the inherent dangerousness of the drug; rather, the focus was on the substantial overprescription of pain-masking agents by physicians. However, the zealous prescribing of OxyContin by physicians is partially attributable to the misrepresentation of the drug's potency and dependency liability by the manufacturer, in this case Purdue Pharma. In 2007, Purdue Pharma was fined $600 million, only a small percentage of the overall profits derived from their drug sales, for misleading physicians and the public about the dangers associated with OxyContin, namely promoting it as a non-addictive pain-masking agent (Spencer, 2007).

In a more recent headline from July 2014, it was claimed: "Opioid Use Increases after Oxycodone Crackdown" (Grant, 2014). These claims are based on findings from prescription-tracking firm IMS Brogan. Admittedly, the rates of psychoactive pharmaceutical abuse have increased significantly, though not to the extent that the media is trying to suggest. According to the 2012 CADUMS findings, approximately 1.5 percent of the Canadian population aged 15 or older reported abusing any form of psychoactive pharmaceutical, which includes stimulants and opioids (Health Canada, 2012). This number is significantly higher than the 2011 findings, where 0.7 percent reported abusing pharmaceuticals (Health Canada, 2011). Among youth, often the most likely to experiment and use substances, the CADUMS reported an increase in pharmaceutical use but not abuse, from 17.6 percent in 2011 to 24.7 percent in 2012. The problem with the CADUMS findings is that there is no distinction between the different kinds of pharmaceuticals. Comparatively, the 2013 OSDUHS indicated that the non-medical use of prescription opioid pain relievers was at an all-time low since 2007. The rates of use have steadily declined from 20.6 percent in 2007 to 12.4 percent in 2013. Despite these declines in use, the non-medical use of prescription opioid pain relievers is the third most common among youth, with cannabis ranking second and alcohol first.

However, what must also be considered is the broad therapeutic use of opioids, including the short-term use of codeine or Tylenol 3 after minor injury or surgery and the humane use of drugs such as morphine and Dilaudid among palliative patients in hospitals, nursing homes, and hospices across Canada (Pergolizzi et al., 2008; Strassels, McNicol, & Suleman, 2008; Wigmore, & Farquhar-Smith, 2016). The vast majority of users do not develop any addiction issues. In fact, of all the pharmacological categories of drugs, opioids have the least serious physical side effects when used as prescribed.

6.9: HEROIN

The most recent heroin scare in Canada is directly linked to the recent crackdown on prescription opioids referred to in the above section. In a 2014 *Vancouver Sun* headline, journalist Denise Ryan proclaims: "Heroin Addiction on the Rise among Young Drug Users." The story behind this headline suggests that as the government tries to place greater controls and regulations on prescription opioids, drug users are turning to heroin instead. While it may be the case that the unavailability of legitimate prescriptions is forcing people to seek relief from their withdrawal symptoms through heroin, it is certainly not the case that heroin use has increased dramatically among young drug users. From a population standpoint, heroin is one of the least used drugs among youth (Boak et al., 2013), even among high-risk populations such as street youth (Public Health Agency of Canada, 2007).

The focus on heroin, however, has been increasing due to increasing reported overdoses and a lack of treatment response. *CTV News* broadcasted a disturbing headline related to heroin in July 2014; the caption read: "'Killer Heroin' Prompts Warning for Montreal Drug Users." Between January and August 2016 there were on average over 60 illicit drug deaths per month in British Columbia, while Ontario Health Minister Eric Hoskins stated that six to seven Canadians die daily from an opioid overdose. None of these deaths should occur, as there are pharmacological interventions (Narcan), treatment options (heroin replacement therapy), and facilities (supervised injection sites) that have all been empirically demonstrated to address opioid overdose (Csiernik, Rowe, & Watkin, 2017). However, when substances are illegal, there are no regulations on the purity or content, so users have no idea what they are buying and using, which can lead to potentially fatal outcomes.

6.10: HALLUCINOGENS

There is a long history of hallucinogen use around the world, as these substances are derived from a broad variety of plants. However, whether a particular hallucinogenic substance is deemed licit or illicit remains somewhat random, and when they are banned it is typically for political rather than biological reasons. Hallucinogens such as kava, jimson weed, morning glory seeds, peyote, psilocybin, and *Salvia divinorum* are all used in religious ceremonies and to promote or enhance spiritual transcendence (Jeeves & Brown, 2009; McKenna & Riba, 2015). Hallucinogen use has also influenced human art, dance, fashion, film, literature, and music, and has played a distinct role in the creation of subcultures such as Rastafarianism and the North American hippie movement of the 1960s.

An example of the paradoxes surrounding this family of drugs can be seen with ayahuasca. Ayahuasca is a hallucinogenic tea derived from two plants native to the Amazon, with dimethyltryptamine (DMT) being the primary psychoactive component. It has been used for generations by Indigenous peoples living in Brazil, Ecuador, and Peru in a specific ritualistic manner for medicinal, cultural, and spiritual purposes. However, in the latter half of the twentieth century, ayahuasca's psychoactive properties gained increasing notoriety—increasing global demand changed who was using it, even producing a drug-related tourism industry in parts of South America (Grunwell, 1998; Holman, 2011). Ayahuasca became a commodified drug, used in cross-cultural Indigenous-style healing rituals conducted primarily for non-Indigenous participants by non-Indigenous healers. In Canada, possessing or selling plants used to make ayahuasca is not a criminal act, but possessing a preparation made from them can still lead to criminal charges, which led to a protracted legal case in Quebec (Tupper, 2008c, 2009).

In May 1996, Céu do Montréal, a chapter of the Brazilian Eclectic Centre of the Flowing Universal Light, was opened in Montreal. Céu do Montréal is related to the Santo Daime religion, which uses ayahuasca in a tea form during its religious rituals. From 1996 to 2000 the Céu do Montréal imported ayahuasca into Canada with approved Brazilian agricultural export documents to use as part of their faith-based practices. In September 2000, the Canada Customs and Revenue Agency intercepted a shipment of the tea and requested that the Royal Canadian Mounted Police (RCMP) conduct a chemical analysis. The outcome of the analysis led RCMP officials to notify Céu do Montréal representatives that the tea contained both DMT and harmala alkaloids, and therefore possessing or distributing their sacrament was an offence under the Criminal Code of Canada. No charges were laid at the time, but the church was told that any additional importation or distribution could lead to members being charged with trafficking a controlled substance. However, the church was also informed that they could apply to Health Canada's Office of Controlled Substances for a legal exemption. In 2006, the Director General of Health Canada's Drug Strategy and Controlled Substances Programme wrote that risks of issuing an exemption for the religious use of the tea were lower than the risks associated with refusing the request. While Céu do Montréal adherents could use this substance, the ruling indicated that those using the substance in a manner unrelated to their faith were at risk. As such, anyone outside the designated group could still be charged for distributing or trafficking a controlled substance under the Criminal Code (Tupper, 2011).

6.11: BRINGING TOGETHER THE OBJECTIVE AND SUBJECTIVE REALITIES

The preceding sections have illustrated the ways in which the government and the media help to create moral panics when it comes to drugs and drug users in Canada. These representations quickly become embedded in the minds of the general public, as they believe that the media and government are truthfully representing the safety and interests of society. Instead of being educated by these sources of information, there is a reinforcement of the underlying fear-based perceptions most people have of the drugs they themselves do not use. As illustrated, the reports are often exaggerated and misrepresentative of the objective reality of drugs and drug users. Admittedly, psychoactive drugs do cause real harm to a minority of users and to society as a whole, and it is critically important to address these concerns. However, the questions remain as to the extent and manner in which we should address them. To what extent are people's lives being ruined by drugs and drug use, and to what extent should we be publicly addressing these concerns? Does our response continue to follow a criminalization model? How do we respond to the facts and view this as a health and social issue, not one of criminality? What are some of the current policies and practices that are effective, and are they responding to the actual needs of individuals, including structural issues, or are they responding to the hysteria of a phantom threat? Equally important to ask is what policies and practices are producing more harm than good and how these policies and practices are reflected in our institutions. Finally, we need to ask who benefits from this type of misinformation.

PARADOXES

1) The state, as a primary social influencer, uses this influence to create images of fear and panic when promoting drugs. They do this to justify a criminal justice approach, despite other government employees promoting a public health model based on knowledge.

2) The media has a significant influence on societal beliefs about drugs and drug users, yet the information provided to the public is not always factual or given appropriate context. Thus, beliefs about drugs and drug users are not necessarily founded in facts, yet these beliefs help to shape who is valued and what is feared in society.

3)   Used therapeutically, a substance can have great value; used excessively, the same substance can create the need for therapeutic intervention.

CRITICAL REFLECTIONS

1)   Why are psychoactive drugs, and thus substance users as a group, more targeted by the criminal justice system than some other social issues?
2)   What do the psychoactive substances examined in this chapter have in common?
3)   What factors led cannabis to be prohibited from 1923 to 2018? What factors led to the rescinding of this prohibition?
4)   What value is there in creating a moral panic surrounding psychoactive drugs? Who benefits from this?

7 Studying Substance Use

Given the complex nature of substance use and misuse, there are several different ways in which information is gathered. Three prominent methods exist for gathering information about substance use and substance users: population-based, field-based, and clinical population studies. In addition to these traditional methods, and given the growing concern with substance use amongst certain populations, Indigenous methodologies are also becoming an important area of focus in social science research. Each approach has different strengths and weaknesses, depending on the objectives of the research. Regardless of the method used, we also need to ascertain what is being asked, why, and by whom.

7.1: POPULATION-BASED STUDIES

Population-based studies are typically composed of a sample or randomly selected group from a previously identified population. It is far too expensive and sometimes logistically impossible for researchers to reach out to every single person in a given population. Thus, probability sampling allows for a more cost-effective and time-efficient means of gathering information from a given group.

The intention with sampling is to draw a smaller proportion of cases from the much larger population that will serve as a representation of the population. Ideally, samples that are drawn from a population should mirror the characteristics of the group, so that certain known facts such as the proportion of men and women, racial and ethnic groups, regional location, and age are similarly reflected in the sample. There are a variety of distinct sampling techniques and strategies that can be used for population-based studies.[1]

Large-scale population-based studies on drugs and drug use come in many different forms. For sociologists interested in drug research, the most important sources of population-based information can come from international, national, or provincial studies.

International Studies

Two significant international studies that examine substance use are the World Drug Report, formerly called Global Illicit Drug Trends, and the Health Behaviour in School-Aged Children (HBSC). The World Drug Report is an annual overview of illicit drug use and illicit drug markets compiled by the United Nations Office on Drugs and Crime (UNODC). The objective of the World Drug Report is to collect international information to better understand the global impacts of drugs and drug use, and to develop strategies for combatting illicit drug use and drug markets. Unlike most other sources of information, the World Drug Report is not founded solely upon independent survey research that is conducted by the UNODC. Instead, it is a compilation of responses from the UNODC annual questionnaire, combined with results from national surveys from each of the member states. Each year, the World Drug Report examines trends in drug use and the illicit drug market, while also devoting special attention to emergent drug issues ranging from controlling illicit drug markets to addressing illicit drug use. Examining both the supply and demand sides of illicit drugs from several different countries, the World Drug Report offers the most comprehensive global picture of illegal drugs in society.

In 2012, the UNODC World Drug Report highlighted prevalence rates, age, gender, and regional variations, reporting that approximately 5.2 percent of the world's population had used an illicit substance in the past year. North America had the largest illicit drug market; however, illegal drug markets exist worldwide and in some nations they are vital to the economy and survival of the state. At the individual user level, the findings suggest that drug use is particularly prominent among young people between the ages of 18 and 25, and that illicit drug use, like many other forms of risky behaviour, is most prevalent among young men (UNODC, 2012). The most common substances used at least once among people aged 15 to 64 years old include cannabis, opioids, cocaine, and amphetamine-type stimulants, not including ecstasy (UNODC, 2014).

Shifting the focus to more specific drug market and manufacturing issues, the 2013 World Drug Report focused on "new" psychoactive substances such as synthetic cannabinoids, synthetic cathinones (bath salts), *Salvia divinorum*, and khat, among multiple other substances whose increasing use had brought them to the attention of governmental authorities (UNODC, 2013). More recently, the 2014 World Drug Report examined precursor substances used in the manufacture of synthetic and semi-synthetic drugs (UNODC, 2014). In Canada, several different precursor substances are regulated and penalized under Schedule VI of the Controlled Drugs and Substances Act (Government of Canada, 2015a). This international examination of precursor substances reveals that the United Nations believes that strict control efforts by member states are able to decrease supplies for clandestine operations for some psychoactive substances. However, there are two key challenges for the current situation with precursor substances: maintaining a balance between legitimate use and illegal use of precursors is difficult, and so too is trying to control an ever-expanding number of substances that can be used as replacements for traditional precursors.

A second important international study that includes issues surrounding substance use is the World Health Organization's collaborative cross-national survey on Health Behaviour in School-Aged Children (HBSC). Every four years, the HBSC surveys youth 11, 13, and 15 years old. Given that substance use is typically initiated during adolescence, the HBSC is an important starting point for understanding the factors that influence the decision to begin using a psychoactive substance. However, beyond this rudimentary information, there are distinct limitations in using the HBSC as an international source of information regarding substance use. The first is the cross-sectional nature of the survey. Several significant influences may be identified in any given year, but when a second group does not show the same results, it is difficult to ascertain if this is because of differences in the individuals surveyed or some other unknown factor. A second limitation is the group being studied. While substance use may begin for some youth between the ages of 11 and 15, there are many others who may wait to initiate substance use later in adolescence or upon becoming independent from their parents in early adulthood. These people are not captured because of the narrow age focus of this study; those not attending school are also not taken into consideration.

National Studies

International studies are important for generating a global picture of social issues to better understand the differences and dynamics between countries. However, it is also crucial to have a clear understanding of social issues from within a nation. Admittedly, the national studies on illicit drugs in Canada are rather disconnected and incomplete. Ideally, to monitor drug trends and the various issues related to drug use and drug markets, a constant body of data and knowledge should be developed and consistently pursued. As with most drug-related activities in Canada, government-led national surveys are inadequate in both their scope and their consistency. Searching the Health Canada and Statistics Canada archives over the past few decades, it is apparent that there is no single source or benchmark survey that Canadians can consult for information regarding trends pertaining to psychoactive substances. There is neither a comprehensive source of information, nor a guaranteed annual survey regularly conducted at the national level. Thus, the majority of Canadian information regarding substance use and illicit drug markets comes from multiple distinct sources and surveys, making year-over-year comparisons limited and difficult.

In 1989 the source for Canadian drug trends was the National Alcohol and Drug Survey. Canada's Alcohol and Other Drugs Survey followed in 1994, which was followed in turn by the Canadian Addiction Survey (CAS) in 2004. The CAS was a significant departure from previous survey research, as it was not solely sponsored by Health Canada or Statistics Canada. Instead, it was conducted through a collaborative initiative with several different groups across the country, but due to funding issues, this survey was only conducted once (Adlaf, Begin, & Sawka, 2005). In 2008, Statistics Canada introduced the Canadian Alcohol and Drug Use Monitoring Survey (CADUMS), which only lasted four years. In 2013, the CADUMS and the Canadian Tobacco Use Monitoring Survey (CTUMS) were replaced by the biennial national survey referred to as the Canadian Tobacco, Alcohol and Drugs Survey (CTADS). The longevity of this survey is yet to be determined.

In addition to these substance use–specific surveys, there are several other national surveys that, while not focused specifically on psychoactive drugs, do include questions regarding substances and substance use. These more general surveys allow researchers an opportunity to examine drug use within a different context. The Canadian Campus Survey, which was conducted in 2004, is one such example. The main focus was on drinking, drugs, mental health, and gambling behaviours among undergraduates attending universities across Canada (Adlaf, Demers & Gliksman, 2005). Another national study that draws from the general population, rather than one specific demographic, is the Canadian Community Health Survey (CCHS), which began collecting information biennially in 2001 and then annually in 2007. This is one survey that still remains active today (Statistics Canada, 2014). The CCHS survey aims to better understand diseases and health conditions, lifestyle and social conditions, and includes some questions on drugs and alcohol.

Although each of these studies provides important data, there is limited or virtually non-existent information regarding families, peers, and general community-based measures, all of which are important in developing a fuller understanding of substance use. Moreover, all of the national surveys discussed above are cross-sectional in their approach. This means that the data collected, even if it is collected on an annual basis, is being collected from different samples of people each time. There is no way to make causal inferences about certain findings, as there is no guarantee that the newly sampled people are the same as the previously sampled people.

Longitudinal studies are much more expensive and time-consuming, though they offer the advantage of being able to monitor people and outcomes over time, which also allows for researchers to make causal conclusions. One source of longitudinal information focusing on young people, including their substance use, families, schools, and peers, was the National Longitudinal Survey of Children and Youth (NLSCY). The NLSCY began collecting information on children and youth in 1995 and continued until 2009 (Statistics Canada, 2010). It was limited in its coverage of substance use, as that was not the primary focus of the survey. However, a significant strength was that there were often two sources of information: the youths themselves and the person most knowledgeable (PMK) about the youth, which was most often the mother. Unfortunately, since the discontinuation of NLSCY, there have not been any alternative nationwide longitudinal studies that include information about individuals and their substance use. Thus, the sources of national information about substance use and substance users are limited to basic descriptive details, such as the prevalence rates, age, and gender, contained in the CTADS. Beyond this, there is no national data that is a comprehensive source of information about psychoactive substances and the multitude of factors related to use and misuse, which if it existed could be used in program and policy development on a national level.

Provincial/Regional Studies

Given the limitations of the national reports, even those that are focused ex-clusively on psychoactive substances, it is not surprising that many researchers turn to provincial studies to better understand substance use in Canada. Several provincial studies across the country have captured information concerning sub-stance use among youth. At one time or another, most of the provinces have con-ducted surveys of youth ranging from grades 7 to 12, with Saskatchewan being the major exception. Ontario has the longest-running cross-sectional survey of students in Canada. Beginning in 1977, the Ontario Student Drug Use Survey (OSDUS) has collected information about student drug use every two years. The survey is now called the Ontario Student Drug Use and Health Survey (OSDUHS), as the biennial survey has expanded to include other health behav-iours, including risk-taking and physical and mental health.

Since there is no federal requirement to collect information about sub-stance use, there is significant inconsistency in the surveys that are used and the scheduling of these surveys. Moreover, the limited scope of national surveys has made it imperative for the provinces to collect information about substance use. However, since each province collects different information and uses dif-ferent sampling methods, provincial comparisons can be difficult or inaccurate. In 2011, the Student Drug Use Surveys Working Group, with representatives from each provincial survey and in collaboration with the Canadian Centre on Substance Abuse, released the first-ever report on inter-provincial comparisons of student alcohol and drug use (Young et al., 2011). This report serves as a start-ing point from which researchers can better understand national and provincial prevalence rates of substance use among youth. However, there are no com-parable provincial studies of the adult population beyond the national surveys discussed above.

Advantages and Disadvantages of Population-Based Studies

There are two notable strengths of population-based studies that use survey de-signs. The first advantage is the generalizability of the findings. If the group being studied has been carefully selected to best represent the population of in-terest, researchers are able to generalize their findings from their sample to the entire population. Large-scale comparisons and descriptions of populations are important strengths for drug research. Moreover, the advancement in statisti-cal techniques in recent years increases the generalizability and further enables drug researchers to better understand the complexities of drug use and misuse. The second advantage is the standardization that is required for survey-based research (Babbie, 2016). Unlike other methods, surveys ensure that everyone is asked the same question in the same manner. This is particularly helpful in trying to make generalized statements about a population. Moreover, it is helpful to researchers when there is a standard or accepted method of measuring a given concept, as there is less ambiguity in the meaning that each concept represents.

Some of the strengths of population-based survey research are also the foundation for some of its weaknesses. Depending on its objectives, survey research can be limited by sampling issues and the quality of responses (Babbie, 2016). Some sampling issues might include non-response from various participants and inaccurate estimation of the population characteristics. Moreover, the quality of the responses may be limited by the standardization of survey questions or the truthfulness of the respondents (Goode, 2008). Standardization of survey questions is helpful for general characteristics, but it can at times be difficult to capture social complexities and individual characteristics with survey-based questions. Truthfulness is also difficult to guarantee with most forms of social research, especially anonymous or confidential surveys and studies of marginalized populations (Harrison, 1997). However, some argue that truthfulness is not as problematic as we might think, especially when making comparisons over time, as there is a consistently small number of respondents who misrepresent themselves (Goode, 2008). As well, when examining these types of studies we cannot forget to ask what is being asked, why, and by whom.

One of the sampling issues with population-based studies is that they often exclude hard-to-reach populations such as street youth, homeless people, early school leavers, and other marginalized groups, such as those living in the lightly populated northern regions of Canada, on reserves, or in institutions. Technically, these groups belong to the general population of Canada, and thus should be included in any samples of the population. However, it is difficult, for practical and political reasons, to ensure that all people are captured in representative numbers in a given study.

A major issue with population-based studies is that samples originate from a list of all possible respondents in a given population. Usually, these lists are derived from existing sources such as home addresses, telephone lists, or class lists for school-based surveys. However, those who do not have a home or a phone are automatically excluded, as is the case with those who leave school early. Indigenous Canadians living in the northern regions, as well as those living on reserves, are also difficult to survey because of past exploitative research practices, research ethics regarding information ownership, and location; thus, they are typically excluded from the selection process.

For some types of population-based survey research, these sampling issues do not pose much concern. However, for drug researchers, these hard to reach populations are some of the most vulnerable groups in society and are at a greater risk of using and misusing substances. Thus, we must also use methods that allow us to capture the experiences of hard-to-reach populations. One approach is to use field studies where researchers seek out a specific setting or group that meets the characteristics of the study objectives.

7.2: FIELD-BASED STUDIES

Traditionally, in sociology, field-based studies refer to various qualitative research methods. Though quantifying drug use and drug patterns is important, there are still many questions left unanswered by population-based studies. Sometimes studying certain topics, such as drugs and drug use, requires a more personalized approach. Psychoactive substances are a sensitive topic to examine because there are many different meanings attached to certain substances and substance users, with issues of stigma, oppression, and criminality still surrounding the field. Moreover, marginalized groups are difficult to reach in a typical survey sample, yet we know from field research that these groups are also more likely to be using or misusing substances. Thus, researchers attempt to connect with them in their natural settings or public spaces where they are known to frequent. Three different types of field studies used to collect qualitative information include in-depth interviews, focus groups, and observational or ethnographic methods.

In-Depth Interviews

In-depth qualitative interviews are similar to conversations, where researchers may engage in unstructured, semi-structured, or structured discussions with participants (Ireland, Berg, & Mutchnick, 2010). Unstructured interviewing can be useful in the beginning stages of research when there is minimal information about a topic. However, semi-structured and structured interviewing techniques are more useful when researchers are attempting to derive themes and generate theories from the data that is collected. Semi-structured and structured interviewing techniques begin with a set of predetermined ideas or questions that the researcher will ask individual participants. The main difference between semi-structured and structured techniques is flexibility. In structured interviewing, interviewers guide participants through a series of predetermined open-ended questions. Although the answers to the questions are not controlled, the pace and structure of the interview is generally more rigid than in semi-structured interviews. In semi-structured interviews, there is greater opportunity for participants and interviewers to discuss topics that were not originally part of the predetermined questions.

For example, Small and colleagues (2011) conducted 50 in-depth open-ended interviews with Insite clients to examine the barriers associated with accessing North America's first supervised injection facility located in Vancouver, British Columbia. The interviews began with a set of predefined or a priori themes and subsequent interviews continuously built upon the themes as new ones emerged. This research illustrated how semi-structured, in-depth interviews can help inform future interviews by uncovering topics that the researchers may not have considered in the beginning phases of the research. While open-ended semi-structured interviewing is useful for identifying themes that the investigator may not have considered, there remain limitations with this approach. One of the most significant is that not all participants will be exposed to the same set of questions or topics. Thus, it is difficult to determine if the interviews with earlier participants might have produced different findings.

Focus Groups

Focus groups are similar to in-depth interviews except that they are conducted in small group settings where multiple participants are interviewed or engage in a discussion at the same time (Babbie, 2016). In this type of research setting, the interviewer acts more as a facilitator than an interviewer, managing the discussion in a way that allows all participants an opportunity to have their views heard, while at the same time managing any temptation to influence or control input from participants.

Focus groups are an efficient way of gathering information from multiple people in a short period of time in terms of both time and cost. Since focus groups are composed of different people, each of them has something unique to offer, and the group process can produce insights that individual interviews would not uncover. When one participant raises an idea or discusses an experience, this may trigger another participant to refute or build on that idea. Thus, focus groups offer a significant amount of flexibility for the researcher to garner new insights and perhaps adapt new topics for future focus groups. However, this also means that the researcher facilitating the focus groups must be well trained and be comfortable managing group dynamics with inherent dominant and passive participants, and with issues ranging from conflict to silence.

Fischer and colleagues' (2002) study of attitudes towards methadone treatment used focus groups as the method of data collection. Using a multi-site approach, 47 opiate users in Toronto (N=24), Vancouver (N=12), and Montreal (N=11) were divided into focus groups ranging in size from five to eight participants. In total, seven focus groups were held over the course of five months. In addition to a facilitator for each focus group, there was also a recorder present to take notes. This approach is beneficial for this type of research as it is difficult for a facilitator to both take accurate notes and keep the discussion on track. Moreover, body language and group dynamics cannot be captured with audio recordings, so the person acting as the recorder can incorporate these important features of the focus group into her or his notes.

As with most forms of qualitative field research, focus groups are generally exploratory. Fischer and colleagues (2002) sought to better understand the attitudes of opioid users towards methadone and other forms of treatment for opioid dependence. Some of the themes identified through the focus groups included: the relationships users have with their substance of choice; the significance of the route of administration; the strict rules imposed on users through methadone treatment; the benefits of methadone treatment; opinions about the ideal opioid treatment program; and attitudes towards heroin treatment programs. Although it is impossible to generalize the findings from 47 opioid users to all users, the themes that emerged from this work can inform future research.

Ethnographies

Ethnographic research methods are perhaps some of the most time-consuming and detailed forms of field research. This approach involves immersing oneself in a particular social setting and observing the environment and individuals that the researcher is most interested in better understanding. In contrast with most research methods examined, ethnographies require a significant amount of flexibility and openness from both the researcher and the participants. When observing people in their natural environments, there are many details for the researcher to interpret and reinterpret. In survey research and interviews, researchers pose a question and the participants respond. However, with observational research, participants may behave in ways that are complex and contradictory, leaving the researcher to subjectively interpret the phenomenon being investigated. Similar to interviewing, ethnographic researchers are generally concerned about exploring the unknown. They enter the field with minimal assumptions about the subject they are investigating, while hoping their observations will help them to better understand the setting and the people with whom they are interacting and/or observing.

A recent Canadian example of ethnographic research examined the use of an unsanctioned safer smoking room (SSR) by current crack cocaine users in Vancouver (McNeil, Kerr, Lampkin, & Small, 2015). The researchers spent 50 hours in the field observing crack cocaine users from within the SSR over the course of four months. To supplement their observational data, they also conducted 23 in-depth interviews with crack cocaine smokers. Currently, there are no government-sanctioned safe smoking rooms for crack cocaine users in Canada; however, there are a few SSRs operating in Europe. The existing data on the effectiveness of SSRs is rather limited, making ethnographic research a viable and methodologically prudent starting point for better understanding how this type of environmental intervention may or may not be an effective strategy. Similar to existing research on safe-injection facilities for opioid users, the researchers concluded that the SSRs are effective at reducing the health and social harms associated with smoking crack cocaine.

Another notable example of Canadian-based ethnography is Philippe Bourgois and Julie Bruneau's (2000) examination of intravenous drug users in Montreal along with Bourgois's (2000) account of methadone maintenance programs in both Montreal and East Harlem. This work challenges the empirical claim that harm reduction programs, including both needle exchange and methadone maintenance programs, are effective at reducing use and stabilizing people's lives. Drawing on personal accounts and observations from the field, the authors contend that harm reduction programs, though more widely accepted today and celebrated by governments as being effective, are actually a means for the state to control individual bodies and populations of users. This ethnographic work helps to illustrate how survey data and population-based studies, which are founded on the quantification of outcomes, are not showing the complexities of substance use. Missing from survey representations is the lived experience of users, yet quantified studies are often the basis of policy and program decisions.

Advantages and Disadvantages of Field-Based Studies

In general, field studies can generate a wealth of information that cannot be captured adequately with typical, predefined, closed-ended survey questions. Rather than valuing only outcomes generated by quantified studies, field studies provide more comprehensive and nuanced understandings of individuals, relationships, and social settings. Rich descriptions of social reality often increase validity, which is analogous to accuracy, though at the potential expense of reliability (Babbie, 2016). Observations that are considered valid are thought to truthfully capture what the researcher intends to measure. Reliability, on the other hand, refers to the consistency with which individuals or the social phenomenon of interest produces the same results each time they are measured. In field research, reliability is difficult to achieve. Everyone behaves in unique ways, even when exposed to the same social conditions. Adding to this complexity, people describe social experiences differently. Thus, the meaning attached to one particular phenomenon may have many different connotations, making reliable or consistent observations a challenge for researchers; this also speaks to the complexity of the addiction field of study.

Nevertheless, the abundance of valid, detailed data collected from field studies is often used to provide insight into hard-to-reach populations, develop theories, and direct future research. The theories that can be generated from field studies are founded upon the assumption that researchers should allow their observations to tell the stories and patterns that are derived from fieldwork. It is rare for a good qualitative researcher to enter a field of study with preconceived notions of what to expect. Instead, the researcher should be open to any and all possibilities that present themselves in the course of field research.

While theory building and theory generation are distinct advantages of field research, reaching a point of theoretical saturation, when there appears to be no more unique findings or observations, can be time-consuming and unpredictable. It can also be difficult for a researcher to determine the point at which theoretical saturation has been achieved. Unlike a survey, field research is dynamic and ever changing. This fact can produce unique insights into a phenomenon, but may also be frustrating when dealing with a social reality where people inevitably change, as do their social circumstances.

Ethically, conducting field research can be challenging in most social science research; however, there are some unique challenges when dealing with drugs and drug users. One such challenge is the fact that drugs and drug use, in many cases, are violations of the law and many of the related activities of drug users may pose risks to themselves or others. Researchers must balance confidentiality, the pursuit of knowledge, and the preservation of participants' safety. Amidst drug-using subcultures there is a risk that researchers may have to report people being harmed or posing harm to others. This compromises the ability of researchers to be fully involved in any participatory manner. Another ethical challenge when conducting research with drug users is the capacity for informed consent. Intoxication undermines the capacity to consent to involvement in any research. If the object of study is individual drug use, it is difficult to navigate boundaries surrounding informed consent, as individuals may not be fully aware of what they are consenting to when they are intoxicated (Bell & Salmon, 2012; Csiernik & Birnbaum, 2017; Olsen & Mooney-Somers, 2014).

7.3: CLINICAL POPULATION STUDIES

Clinical population studies, though not an official methods classification, include two important populations that are often excluded from survey and field methods: individuals being treated for addiction issues and correctional populations. There is significant variation in how studies are conducted with these populations. Some use experimental designs, others use survey designs or risk assessment tools, and others might use unobtrusive methods, involving case histories and other existing documentation. In some instances, multiple methods of data collection and analysis are used to develop a more comprehensive understanding of substance use and the substance user. This is often referred to as a mixed-methods approach. As the name suggests, mixed-method studies combine elements of more than one type of research method. In some instances this might include using survey data to complement fieldwork, or vice versa; it can also entail combining multiple forms of field methods into one study, as was the case in the above example of crack cocaine smokers and SSRs. Whichever approach is selected, the information gathered from treatment and correctional populations is an important part of understanding substance use and substance users, especially among higher-risk groups.

Treatment Studies

There is wide variation in the methods used in examining specific populations receiving treatment for their addiction issue. Part of this variation is a result of the lack of national treatment standards. Substance treatment is a multidisciplinary field with no agreed upon national guidelines and only some agreed-upon best practice principles. As discussed earlier, there are no continuous national studies measuring even the prevalence of substance use; thus, it should come as no surprise that there are no national practices in place, nor are there any national treatment studies that have ever been conducted in Canada.

With a lack of acknowledged standards for treatment practices and no agreed upon certification standards, Canada's treatment research is fragmented. On the one side, there is the recovery movement. This is led by agencies and counsellors, who themselves had issues with psychoactive drug dependency, working on the front line with people who experience similar types of substance use problems that their counsellors have overcome. Their orientation is typically based on experience, founded in their own path to recovery from addiction. On the other end, there are those with no direct personal history but who have extensive formal education, often at the graduate level, and are practicing based upon evidence-informed principles. Between these two poles there are outreach workers and harm reduction agencies, whose primary goal is to decrease use rather than be concerned about abstinence-based outcomes. Each group provides a different lens for social research, explaining in part the significant variation in the types of research being conducted across the country.

One landmark example of a treatment study was a Canadian-based harm reduction initiative, known as the North American Opiate Medication Initiative (NAOMI). This was an important comparative study, as there is widespread criticism by the public, mostly fuelled by the media, that heroin-assisted treatments should not be available in Canada; however, these claims made by the public are not founded in empirical evidence. Accordingly, the NAOMI set out to determine, with evidence, what the most effective forms of pharmacological treatment were for a known group of opioid users (Lasnier, Brochu, Boyd, & Fischer, 2010; Nosyk et al., 2012; Oviedo-Joekes et al., 2009; Schechter & Kendall, 2011).

This mixed-methods study began with a randomized controlled trial of the effectiveness of injectable diacetylmorphine (DAM or heroin) or hydromorphone (HDM) compared to traditional oral methadone maintenance treatments (Oviedo-Joekes et al., 2008). Participants were recruited from Montreal and Vancouver between 2005 and 2008, resulting in a final sample of 251 long-term opioid users. The objective of this study was to replicate other controlled trials being conducted in Europe, while also developing a Canadian profile of effective treatment for people dependent on opioids. The study results essentially indicated that different users require different modes of treatment, and that heroin-assisted treatments are an effective alternative for those who are not responsive to other treatments, such as methadone maintenance.

A second sub-study or follow-up was conducted in 2008 using qualitative interviewing with a stratified probability sample of participants who had completed a full 12 months of the trial treatment (Oviedo-Joekes et al., 2014). The objective of this qualitative component was to better understand the experiences and perceptions of the study participants from the randomized controlled trial. Taken together, NAOMI offers a multi-faceted understanding of opioid treatments from both the user's perspective and the overall effectiveness of the randomized controlled trial findings, which is not a standard practice among most clinical population studies.

The most well-known form of helping in the addiction field, Alcoholics Anonymous (AA), was developed using the personal experiences of two men in the 1930s, though it was primarily structured around the thinking of Bill Wilson, a businessman with repeated failed attempts at maintaining his sobriety. In 1935, when he began to develop the 12 steps and 12 traditions of Alcoholics Anonymous with the support of Dr. Bob Smith, not only was the stigma significant around addiction—hence the need for anonymity—but empirical social science studies were also minimal. Since its inception, the anonymous nature of AA has limited the types of research that can be conducted with participants. However, the historic lack of empirical success of AA among its adherents has not been a barrier to membership, as there are over two million active members worldwide (Alcoholics Anonymous, 2015). In 2011, AA members from Canada and the United States were asked to complete an anonymous survey. Over 8,000 responses were obtained; only basic demographic data was collected, but this did provide an overview of the basic membership of this organization, which still very much reflects its origins. The majority of those who belonged to AA, when the survey was conducted, were white males between the ages of 31 and 60. In terms of the length of sobriety, existing members tended to belong to two groups: those who had been sober for more than 11 years and those who had been sober for less than a year (Alcoholics Anonymous, 2012).

Smaller studies of actual therapeutic utility have also been conducted, but again the anonymous nature of AA makes anything other than one group pre-post tests difficult to conduct (Csiernik, 2010). Despite this limit, Humphreys and Moos (1996) were able to conduct a larger comparative study. They followed 200 individuals dependent on alcohol in San Francisco for a three-year period. One hundred and thirty-five of the study's participants attended AA, while 65 attended professional outpatient aftercare counselling. Despite the cohort using AA having lower incomes, less education, and more severe drinking experiences than the comparison group, at both one- and three-year follow-ups, the AA-attending group had lower health care costs than those who only attended professional aftercare groups.

Perhaps the most rigorous and expensive national treatment study ever conducted was an American study called Project MATCH (Glaser, 1999). With 1,726 patients participating in a multi-site controlled trial of psychotherapies, Project MATCH sought out to determine which form of treatment was most effective for different types of patients with alcohol dependence. Patients were randomly assigned to one of three dominant treatments: cognitive behavioural therapy (CBT), motivational enhancement therapy (MET), or Alcoholics Anonymous (AA). However, the results of Project MATCH were not as promising as the investigators had hoped. Despite the scientific rigor and the admirable amount of funding that went into this project, there was a significant amount of skepticism surrounding the study design and findings.

One significant limitation to the study design was that all of the participants included in the study were voluntarily seeking treatment. Thus, it can be argued that they exhibited a motivation to change that is not likely to be evident among people with alcohol dependency who were not seeking treatment, let alone those using illicit substances (Ball, Carroll, Canning-Ball, & Rounsaville, 2006; Howatt, 2003; Prochaska, Norcross, & DiClimente, 1994). In addition, there was no control group in this study, so there is no way to ascertain if the treatment offered would be significantly different from those who did not receive treatment (Walters, 2002). Finally, the project set out to test the significance of 16 different hypotheses concerning the matching of patients to certain types of treatment, of which only one was statistically significant: 12-step programs are more effective than CBT for patients with lower psychiatric scores—a finding that numerous experts have criticized. Undoubtedly, many expected the results of Project MATCH to be more fruitful. Though it may not have produced the intended outcomes, it still made a significant contribution to treatment and science. The national scale on which this study was founded is unparalleled by any other study.

Correctional Populations

National estimates indicate that 70 percent of offenders in the federal prison system had some form of substance use problem in the year prior to imprisonment (Kellen, Powers, & Birnbaum, 2017; Weekes, Thomas, & Graves, 2004). However, federal estimates are problematic when appraising substance use problems, as many drug infractions are classified as summary offences. In contrast with indictable offences, which are dealt with at the federal level, summary offences fall under the domain of the provinces and territories. Thus, federal estimates do not accurately represent the extent of substance use problems in correctional populations. Moreover, provincial and territorial estimates are difficult to ascertain in Canada, as different jurisdictions use different methods of assessment. Federally, the Computerized Assessment of Substance Abuse (CASA) is used to identify the severity of substance use problems upon entry into the correctional system (Kunic, 2006). Despite having been tested for efficiency and accuracy, the CASA has yet to be implemented across provinces and territories. This leaves most substance users in the provincial and territorial systems to deal with a variety of challenges, including disconnected services and a lack of evidence-based clinical practice.

Research on correctional populations and substance use generally supports the view that substance use and criminality intersect with one another. There is further evidence to suggest that the same risk factors associated with criminal offending are also associated with substance use problems. The work of Plourde, Gendron, and Brunelle (2012) is a recent example of Canadian research that illustrates these overlapping risk factors. In a multi-site study of federally incarcerated women, a subsample of 39 Indigenous women completed in-depth semi-structured interviews on psychoactive substance use. A significant proportion of the women interviewed reported having alcohol and/or drug use problems at some point prior to incarceration, approximately 77 percent and 82 percent, respectively. In addition to their substance use, a large proportion of the women reported psychological problems. The qualitative themes derived from this study indicated that many of the women began using substances for experimental and social reasons, but that substance use eventually evolved into a coping strategy for the difficulties they faced, whether it was escaping current problems, dealing with past trauma, issues of oppression, or self-medicating for mental health reasons. Although the findings from this are not necessarily generalizable to the total population of incarcerated individuals and certainly not the general population of all substance users, there does appear to be preliminary evidence to suggest that incarcerated Indigenous women are at significant risk of having substance use histories, along with traumatic and difficult lives prior to incarceration. By extension, the researchers suggest that integrated intervention programs are necessary both within correctional settings and in the communities where the women will reside upon release, to help them develop new, culturally sensitive strategies for adapting to adversity.

Advantages and Disadvantages of Clinical Population Studies

Clinical population studies focus on a specific subgroup of the population. While large-scale population-based studies fail to capture some groups in society, these targeted studies allow researchers to seek out high-risk groups in treatment, corrections, or even those who are accessing services from the street. Though the samples may not be fully representative of the entire population of high-risk people, research with these groups still provides comprehensive knowledge about some of the most problematic and vulnerable cases.

While there is substantial research and debate concerning treatment and correctional populations, there is also a lack of implementation of evidence-informed practices and laws at the program and policy levels. Generating knowledge among treatment and correctional populations does not necessarily translate into practice. The silencing of scientists and a lack of consistent federal funding for nationwide studies are two significant barriers to evidence-informed practice and policies. The social sciences suffered significantly under the Harper-led Conservative majority. Research was stifled because it did not meet the ideological objectives of the political party in power, and social science research was deemed unnecessary or unimportant.

In addition to these barriers, most studies of vulnerable or high-risk groups are narrowly focused on a particular group in a specific location. These studies leave out a significant proportion of the general population. Without a matched sub-sample from the general population, it is impossible to determine if the findings from clinical population studies are significant enough to support widespread program and policy changes. Beyond individual differences in high-risk samples and the general population, location-specific sampling can limit the potential outcomes of a study. Solutions identified for one particular location may not be effective or feasible in an alternate location. These limitations are further confounded by the structure of health care and criminal justice in Canada. While both health care and criminal justice are federally mandated, it is mostly up to the provinces to deal with substance use, yet across provinces there are significant variations in how criminal justice and health care providers deal with the issue.

7.4: INDIGENOUS METHODOLOGICAL APPROACHES

Another emerging area in substance use research is Indigenous methodological approaches. In Canada, we have a limited empirical base for understanding substance use patterns amongst Indigenous populations. A prominent reason for this lack of information is that we simply do not routinely collect ethnic background information in our population-based studies. Moreover, survey collection methods tend to exclude Indigenous people living on reserves. Perhaps more importantly, even the research that has been historically conducted with Indigenous populations is not necessarily reflective of Indigenous social and cultural practices. As Champagne states, "Western academic scientific theory and social interpretations are positivistic, materialistic, reductionist, objectivist, and focused on compartmentalizing knowledge into specialties" (2015: 58). Indeed, the methodologies and resultant research presented in this chapter would be characterized by most as being exclusively Western.

Even more problematic is that historically research involving Indigenous peoples in Canada has been defined and carried out primarily by non-Indigenous researchers. The approaches have not generally reflected Indigenous world views, and the research has not necessarily benefited those of First Nations, Inuit, Innu, and Métis heritage or their communities. As a result, Indigenous peoples continue to regard research, particularly research originating outside their communities, with a certain amount of apprehension and mistrust. However, Indigenous methodologies can offer great insight into culturally relative issues and solutions that typical methodologies do not fully appreciate.

In a comprehensive review of the effectiveness of different types of cultural practices used with Indigenous people experiencing substance dependence, researchers have found a variety of different practices and treatment solutions unique to Indigenous peoples. Among the studies examined, treatment facilities for Indigenous peoples included ceremonial practices such as sweat lodges and talking circles; traditional teachings led by elders using the medicine wheel; cultural activities including drumming, singing, storytelling, and land-based activities; and the use of natural foods, medicines, and fasting to support the recovery process (Rowan et al., 2014). Many of the interventions reviewed in this study were offered in tandem with Western modalities of treatment and, in most cases, a range of cultural interventions were offered within different treatment programs. This suggests that there is a need to be flexible and sensitive to the population being treated, as there is no panacea that will lead to the most beneficial outcome. However, for Western-trained researchers, this poses a distinct problem: How do we compare and generalize our findings from different studies if no two methods or approaches are alike? Do we need to have identical or even similar approaches to be able to measure effectiveness?

Rowan and colleagues (2014) responded by suggesting that it is our frame of reference for approaches that needs to change. Rather than identifying each distinct intervention, such as sweat lodges, talking circles, or traditional elder-led teaching, it may be useful to examine the interventions in terms of the functions they are intended to serve, such as developing a cultural identity, establishing relationships with others, or connecting with lost language and spirituality.

Social researchers have begun to develop more distinct and culturally sensitive approaches to conducting research with Indigenous groups that will no doubt continue to evolve as Indigenous voices and researchers become more widely represented and appreciated. Champagne (2015) further suggests that Indigenous methodologies do not have to follow the same rigid systematic standards set out in social science research. Instead, alternative perspectives and paradigms that are rooted in the cultural practices of Indigenous populations should be developed and welcomed as meaningful contributions to our understanding of substance use from a cultural perspective.

In addition, ethical standards of practice in research must be properly developed and followed (Champagne, 2015). This issue takes on even greater importance when working with Indigenous peoples, given the historic exploitation that has occurred. Codes of research practice with First Nations, Inuit, Innu, and Métis peoples need to go beyond the scope of ethical protections for individual participants and extend to the interconnection between humans and the natural world. This includes the obligation to maintain, and pass on to future generations, knowledge received from ancestors as well as that developed in ongoing research initiatives. Concern for welfare must include the consideration of participants and prospective participants in their physical, social, economic, and cultural environments, along with the community to which participants belong. This acknowledges the important role of Indigenous peoples in promoting their collective rights, interests, and responsibilities, rather than only considering the welfare of individual research participants. In the past, abuses stemming from research have included the misappropriation of sacred songs, stories, and artifacts; the devaluing of Indigenous knowledge as primitive or superstitious; the violation of community norms regarding the use of human tissue and remains; the failure to share data and resulting benefits; and the presentation of information that has misrepresented or stigmatized entire communities (Csiernik & Birnbaum, 2017).

7.5: CONCLUSION

There is a significant amount of knowledge generated from social science research on substance use and substance users. Unfortunately, Canada has yet to develop a consistent and comprehensive nationwide study that addresses the complexities of substance use amongst Canadians. Much of the national information we have pertaining to substance use and substance users is either lacking in empirical rigour or is derived from other nations, such as the United States, which has a very different orientation to the field. However, this does not mean that Canadian researchers have not continued to work diligently to better understand substance use and substance users. Rather, it means that the government has not adequately supported or funded nationwide studies. Instead, the state of Canadian substance use research is composed of a myriad of differently funded studies, leading to a classic case of researchers doing the best they can with what they have.

This chapter focused on Canadian research, to the extent that it exists. The main objective was to highlight what we can and cannot learn from different methods of inquiry. Consistent with the overarching theme of this book, studying substance use and substance users is paradoxical: knowledge does not always translate into practice. Based on the knowledge we have acquired through various studies, we should expect policies and practices to reflect these research advancements. This is not the case. There are no consistent, evidence-based practices in Canada, nor are there standards for counsellor certification. We continue to treat substance users and substance use as criminal or as having a lifelong disease with no cure. At worst, substance use is a lifetime of condemnation through the criminal justice system. At best, substance users can receive treatment without having to travel outside their home community, but there is no agreed standard or assurance that what is offered is actually going to work. Our health care and criminal justice responses to substance use are not based on solid, longstanding evidence. This leaves us with some important questions to ask: Why is it that, while we know far more than we did only a few decades ago, our policies and practices are regressing? Why, when we know the cost effectiveness of offering treatment and early intervention, do we continue with more expensive, less effective options? Why in the twenty-first century are substance abusers still oppressed, and the dominant form of assistance still requires anonymity? These questions demonstrate why Canada is in dire need of a national strategy that addresses the health care and criminal justice aspects of substance use in a consistent and evidenced-based manner (Weekes, Thomas, & Graves, 2004).

NOTE

1.   For an in-depth examination of population-based research and survey designs refer to Babbie (2016) and Miller and Salkind (2002).

PARADOXES

1) Drug use is a major societal issue in terms of health, criminal justice, and economics, yet no systematic data collection method exists at a national or provincial level.

2) The government-funded treatment protocols that exist provincially and nationally have been established without reliance on any empirical database.

3) Substance abuse is a prominent social and media issue that is regularly discussed and reported upon, yet the prominent form of assistance, Alcoholics Anonymous, is based upon anonymity.

4) Knowledge does not consistently translate into practice in this field.

CRITICAL REFLECTIONS

1) What types of knowledge do the different methods for gathering information about substance use and substance users provide us? What is the inherent value and limit of each?

2) If you were asked to advise the government in developing a national data collection protocol, what would you recommend and why?

8 Demographic Correlates of Substance Use in Canada

Sociologists attempt to better understand substance use and substance users by examining the patterns of relationships or associations that exist within a population. These are often referred to as correlates. Correlations do not confirm causation; however, they do help us recognize the various influences that may contribute to an increased risk of substance use and misuse. It is important to recognize that substance use patterns do not exist in isolation; rather, there are many different factors that are related to substance use and misuse. Some of the most common demographic correlates include age, sex,[1] ethnicity, race, socioeconomic status, and geographic location. Of course, these are not the only factors with which sociologists are concerned, and the next chapter will consider several relational correlates, such as peers, partners, and families. Demographics are simply a starting point; they allow us to gain insight into substance use patterns in the general population by identifying shared characteristics.

As the previous chapter demonstrated, there is a lack of consistently funded national studies on substance use in Canada and there are virtually no longitudinal studies that have been conducted on substance use in particular. This makes it difficult to determine changes over time and the changes in individual substance use patterns. It also leaves us with a series of disconnected and ever-changing sources of information; however, we can begin by examining the data that does exist, despite its inherent limits. Fortunately, we can derive some sense of the patterns and correlates of substance use among particular demographics in Canada from cross-sectional national and provincial studies measuring substance use.

8.1: GENERAL PREVALENCE RATES OF SUBSTANCE USE IN CANADA

Before examining the correlates of substance use, we should first consider the prevalence of use for various psychoactive substances. This allows us to establish a baseline understanding of the occurrence of different types of substance use in the general population. Not surprisingly, tobacco, alcohol, and cannabis are the three most commonly used psychoactive substances amongst Canadians that are officially measured. According to the 2013 Canadian Tobacco, Alcohol and Drugs Survey (CTADS), where 14,565 Canadians were surveyed, alcohol is by far the most commonly consumed psychoactive substance in Canada (Figure 8.1). When examining lifetime use, roughly 90 percent of Canadians report having ever drank alcohol, with almost 76 percent reporting that they have used alcohol in the past year. The second most commonly used substance is tobacco: 14.6 percent of Canadians report being current smokers, while 25.9 percent report being former smokers; 59.5 percent of the population has never smoked. Cannabis is the most commonly used illicit substance, ranking third overall of the most commonly used psychoactive substances. Estimates suggest that approximately 33.7 percent of Canadians have at least tried cannabis in their lifetime, but only 10.6 percent of Canadians report having used cannabis in the past year—though it will be most interesting to monitor how this changes with the drug's changed legal status.

Caffeine use is also common amongst Canadians, but it is not measured in the CTADS or any other comparable national substance use–specific survey.[2] In 2004, as part of the nutrition section of the Canadian Community Health Survey (CCHS), Canadians aged 19 and older were asked about their beverage consumption, including water, coffee, caffeine, tea, soft drinks, alcoholic beverages, milk, and fruit juice. Garriguet (2008) examined patterns of beverage consumption and found that coffee was the second most consumed beverage amongst Canadians. Furthermore, approximately 20 percent of men and 15 percent of women aged 31 to 70 drink more than the recommended daily limit of 400 milligrams of caffeine each day, which is the equivalent of three 8-ounce cups. Coffee is not the only source of caffeine that Canadians ingest: many teas and soft drinks and, of course, energy drinks contain caffeine. However, coffee is comparatively the main source of caffeine consumed through beverages. Approximately 81 percent of caffeine is consumed through coffee, while 12 percent is through teas and about 6 percent is from soft drinks. Though these estimates are important starting points for understanding caffeine consumption, there is no accounting for caffeine contained in other substances that we consume, including chocolate, medications, and energy drinks.

Past-year illicit drug use patterns, excluding cannabis, are relatively low, with less than 1 percent of the Canadian population reporting use. This pattern of illicit drug use has been consistent across time, as less than 1 percent of Canadians reported the use of cocaine, heroin, or LSD in the 1990s as well (Single et al., 1995). However, lifetime illicit drug use patterns are quite different (Figure 8.1). Approximately 7 percent of Canadians have ever tried cocaine or crack, about 3 percent have used amphetamines, 11 percent have used hallucinogens, 4 percent have used ecstasy, roughly 2 percent have used *Salvia divinorum*, and less than 1 percent report ever using heroin. Lifetime use estimates are important indicators of the number of people in the population who may have used a substance but did not necessarily progress to frequent or habitual use. Indeed, one of the

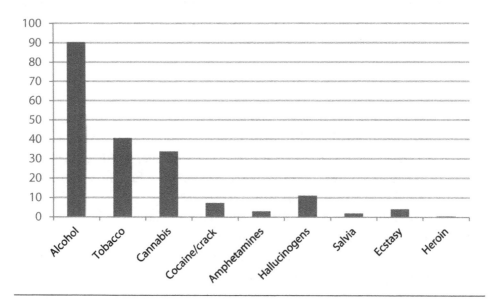

Figure 8.1: Percentage of Canadians Reporting Lifetime Use of Psychoactive Substances

Source: Canadian Tobacco, Alcohol and Drugs Survey (Health Canada, 2013a).

complexities of studying substance use is trying to understand different patterns of use at different stages in the life-course. Why is it that few people report past-year use of most illicit substances, while a much larger proportion have used these substances at some point? If substance use is something that is all-consuming and leads inevitably to addiction, why do the differences in past-year use and lifetime prevalence suggest otherwise?

8.2: DEMOGRAPHIC CORRELATES

The five demographic correlates consistently examined in substance use research are age, sex, ethnicity and race, socioeconomic status, and geographic location. In some instances, there is a well-established pattern of association between certain demographics and various substance use patterns; however, in other instances, the patterns we might expect do not exist at all, are spurious, or change over time. It is important to consider demographic correlates of substance use and misuse not only to understand broader population patterns, but also to better inform us about which groups in society are most vulnerable to substance-related problems and which groups are least vulnerable. Understanding demographic patterns of substance use and misuse informs future research, allows us to better target prevention programs, and allows us to dispel myths about what groups are most likely to use certain types of substances.

Age

It is a well-established social fact that young people are the most likely to use and misuse substances (Canadian Centre on Substance Abuse, 2007). National studies confirm that substance use generally increases with age, peaking in late teens and early twenties and then declining or stabilizing once full-time employment is secured and/or families are launched.

The national estimates of tobacco, alcohol, and cannabis from the 2013 CTADS illustrate the well-established connection between age and substance use (Figure 8.2). For all three substances, people aged 20 to 24 are the most likely to report past-year use. Some have suggested that availability and legal restrictions help to explain why a smaller proportion of 15 to 19 year olds report having used tobacco, alcohol, and cannabis (Csiernik, 2016). But how might we explain why those who are 25 and older also have a lower proportion of people reporting use? Surely availability and legal restrictions cannot the

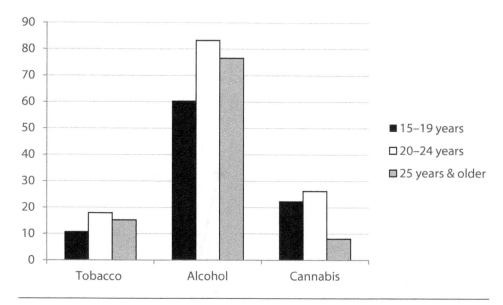

Figure 8.2: Percentage of Canadians Reporting Past-Year Use of Tobacco, Alcohol, and Cannabis by Age Group

Source: Canadian Tobacco, Alcohol and Drugs Survey (Health Canada, 2013a).

explanation. Instead, it has been argued that social bonds and obligations, such as employment and families, lead to lower numbers of people using substances (Antone & Csiernik, 2017).

With the exception of cannabis, the percentage of people reporting past-year use of illicit substances by age group is difficult to estimate because the percentage of people reporting use is quite low. This results in the actual estimate derived from the sample being suppressed or excluded from national reports. The 2004 Canadian Addiction Survey, however, measured lifetime use of several illicit substances across different age groups (Figure 8.3). Again, the general conclusion from this survey was that young people aged 20 to 24 are the most likely consumers of most illegal substances, with a few exceptions. Cocaine and crack use, injection drug use, and steroid use tend to follow a slightly different pattern, with older groups being the most likely users.

There are a few more significant exceptions to the age correlation. Inhalant use is more common among younger groups and declines with age (Boak, Hamilton, Adlaf, & Mann, 2013). For several years, the Ontario Student Drug Use and Health Survey (OSDUHS) has shown that students in grade 7 and 8 are the most likely to report inhalant use in the past year. Similar to one of

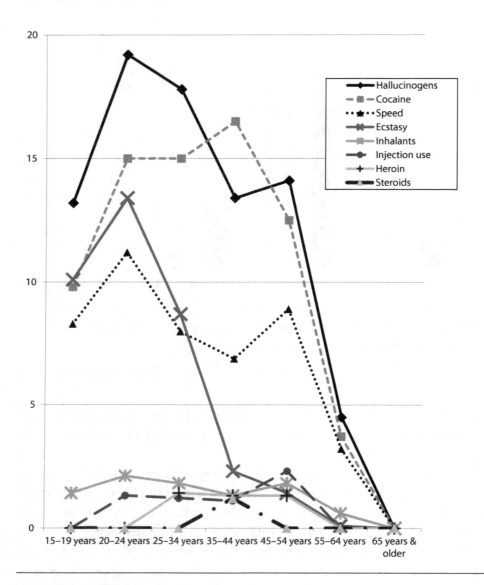

Figure 8.3: Percentage of Canadians Reporting Ever Used Select Illicit Drugs by Age Group, 15 Years and Older

*There is no available data on past-year use by age group in the 2004 CAS. There is only life-time use by age group.
Source: Canadian Addiction Survey (Adlaf, Begin, & Sawka, 2005).

the above arguments concerning tobacco, alcohol, and cannabis use, inhalant use is more common among younger populations because it is widely available. Many households have various chemical substances, including paints, cleaners, and even food-based products such as compressed whipping cream, that young people can use to inhale and get high when they do not have the economic resources to access less toxic substances.

Another exception to the age correlation is the use of benzodiazepines and psychotherapeutic drugs, primarily antidepressants, by the elderly. In a comparative population-based study, Kassam (2005) found that Canadians over the age of 65 were among the most at-risk group for using benzodiazepines and related sedative-hypnotic drugs. A study of people aged 65 or older in Quebec found that approximately 32 percent of the older population living at home in Quebec uses benzodiazepines. Compared to the 9 percent of users in the general population, this is significant. The study further found that roughly 17 percent of older people were using antidepressants. Perhaps most striking in this study was the finding that the overprescription of antidepressants or benzodiazepines to treat mood or anxiety disorders in older populations is likely ineffective, as many users did not experience recovery or even partial remission (Préville et al., 2011). Even more problematic is the off-label use of antipsychotics to physically and emotionally control seniors in long-term care facilities and nursing homes (Zagaria, 2008).

Sociological explanations for the connection between substance use and age emphasize social control, subcultural involvements, and social learning. Young people and the elderly, the two groups noted above, are at greater risk of substance use and misuse because of their relative lack of social control. Young people, as compared to children and older adults, are exposed to greater freedom and independence, have less parental supervision, and are not yet settled into their adult roles in work and family life (Link & Smith, 2014). From a social control perspective, these factors can increase the likelihood that a person will use and potentially misuse substances. From a subcultural standpoint, greater freedom and fewer obligations, including economic responsibilities, means there is more time for leisure activities. If one's peers are involved in substance use, then it is more likely that leisure time will be spent engaging in activities involving substance use. Similarly, social learning explanations suggest that young people learn what substances to use and how to use them from the people they associate with most often. If young people frequently hang out with others who are using substances, they are more likely to engage in it themselves.

On the other hand, seniors have slightly different substance use experiences that are most often a reflection of social control or social bonds, mostly due to loss and isolation. Many have transitioned out of the workplace, no longer have their children to look after, and they may have experienced the loss of their spouse, friends, and in some cases children (Link & Smith, 2014). Significantly, they have more time to engage in substance use and there are fewer people involved in their lives that would notice or attempt to control their substance use patterns. Emotionally, they may use substances as a means to cope with a lack of social connection or the significant trauma associated with losing loved ones.

Sex

Another demographic that is consistently related to different types of substance use and misuse is sex, or one's identification as being either male or female. National studies consistently show that males are more likely than females to use most illicit psychoactive substances, while males and females tend to have more similar rates of use when it comes to legal substances (Figure 8.4). For alcohol, 93 percent of males and approximately 88 percent of females report having used alcohol at some point in their lives. In 2013, lifetime tobacco use was much lower with approximately 16 percent of males and 13 percent of females reporting use. Even the use of cannabis is higher than tobacco, with roughly 41 percent of males and 27 percent of females stating that they had used. Almost 10 percent of males and approximately 5 percent of females reported using cocaine or crack, while a much smaller percentage of males (about 4 percent) and females (about 2 percent) reported using other amphetamines such as methamphetamine or crystal meth. Hallucinogens are the second most commonly used illicit substance, with 14 percent of males and 8 percent of females having ever used them. *Salvia divinorum* lifetime use is significantly lower than other hallucinogens for both males and females, at approximately 3 percent and 1 percent, respectively. Ecstasy, though thought to be widespread, has only been used by about 5 percent of males and 3 percent of females. Finally, heroin use has been reported by less than 1 percent of the males and females in the Canadian population, making comparison by gender difficult.

Though males are generally more likely to use most substances, pharmaceutical use is the exception (Figure 8.5), as women are far more likely to be given a mental health diagnosis and label than men (Forchuk et al., 2011). In 2013, the past-year use of any type of psychoactive pharmaceutical was about 19 percent for males and almost 26 percent for females (Health Canada, 2013a). A larger percentage of both males and females report using opioid pain relievers than stimulants or depressants; however, the gender differences in past-year opioid use are slight, with 14 percent of males and roughly 16 percent

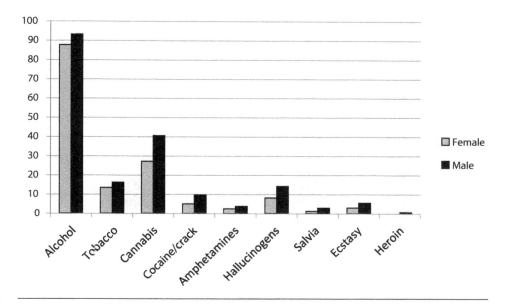

Figure 8.4: Gender Differences in Lifetime Substance Use Patterns

Source: Canadian Tobacco, Alcohol and Drugs Survey (Health Canada, 2013a).

of females reporting use. Only about 1 percent of Canadians, both male and female, report having used stimulant medications. The stark gender differences in pharmaceutical use are driven almost exclusively by the use of sedative medications, which are often used to mask anxiety and serve as a temporary sleep aid. Over 13 percent of females but only about 7 percent of males report using sedatives in the past year. Of course, these estimates include those who are using the substances for medical reasons and those who have admitted to abusing the substances. Of those who reported using sedatives in the past year, approximately 3 percent of males and 2 percent of females reported they had used the substance for the experience (i.e., to get high) or for reasons other than the intended prescription by a medical professional.

Ensminger and Everett (2001) outline two important sociological explanations for why differences by sex exist. The first is based on the notion that there are different norms or rules of conduct that males and females are expected to follow in society. For males, acting out and risk-taking are common, whereas for females, conformity and internalization of problems is considered appropriate behaviour. According to these explanations, males have a greater propensity to engage in drinking and drug use because it is externalized behaviour. On the other hand, women have lower rates of drinking and drug use because it does

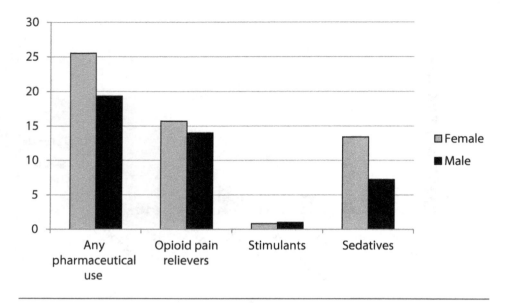

Figure 8.5: Gender Differences in Past-Year Pharmaceutical Use

Source: Canadian Tobacco, Alcohol and Drugs Survey (Health Canada, 2013a).

not fit with the gendered norms. However, women are more likely to seek help for internalized conflicts, thus making them more likely to be prescribed pharmaceutical drugs.

Another related explanation is based on social control theory (Ensminger & Everett, 2001). Males and females are socialized in different ways and experience different forms of social control, meaning they are monitored and regulated in different ways. Males are monitored less and are even celebrated for their recreational substance use (Svensson, 2003). Females, on the other hand, are viewed as being more vulnerable and are told not to engage in such risky activities. It is also argued from a social control perspective that women have closer ties to society, whether it is family, school, work, or even a more abstract respect for the law (Ensminger & Everett, 2001). When social bonds and connections are strong, people are less likely to use substances because they do not want to compromise these relationships. Thus, from this perspective, being a woman is somewhat of a protective factor. An extension of this argument is based on the idea that women are also more likely to uphold the law, making illicit drug use harder or more inappropriate for many women. Pharmaceuticals that are prescribed by a medical professional, however, are deemed as legitimate and necessary forms of substance use for women.

Ethnicity and Race

In studies of substance use and misuse, ethnicity and race are the most controversial and misunderstood demographic correlates. Ethnic and racial identification have long been interconnected with substance use patterns. Canada's early drug laws and treatment of Asian populations in the late nineteenth and early twentieth centuries is a notable historical example. A contemporary example is our treatment, or lack of compassionate treatment, of our First Nations, Inuit, Innu, and Métis populations in Canada. For Csiernik and Rowe (2017), society oppresses certain groups of people because they are not like the rest. Addiction is oppression, much like belonging to a racial or ethnic minority group, which places people in a marginalized and feared category. Can you imagine the oppression felt by ethnic and racial minorities who also have substance use problems? What about those groups that are believed to have substance use problems but actually do not? Under the guise of trying to avoid racism and discriminatory treatment towards minority groups, the Canadian tradition has been to ignore or intentionally exclude ethnicity and race in social research. This has enormous consequences for individuals and society alike.

Canadian researchers at the Centre for Addiction and Mental Health are aware of this problem and have recently started to examine ethnic and racial identification as it relates to health and health care outcomes (Agic & McKenzie, 2013). Though there are Canadian studies on minority groups and their substance use patterns (Homma, Chen, Poon, & Saewyc, 2012; Walls, Sittner Hartstorn, & Whitbeck, 2013), there is no population-based nationwide study that allows for comparisons between ethnic and racial minority groups and the general population. The conclusions from non-comparative studies can be misleading, as there is no way to determine if the group in the study is actually different from the general population. Thus, we rely on findings from American research, where substance use research has been far more comprehensive and diligent in examining ethnic and racial connections with substance use and misuse. The results from these studies are illuminating, as they challenge many preconceived notions about minority groups, while at the same time they tend to support the idea that social science research has long advocated—that opportunities matter.

The War on Drugs in the United States and the mass incarceration of African Americans and Hispanics has led many to believe that these groups are more likely to use and misuse substances than other groups. However, this is not always true. There is greater complexity and variation in substance use patterns than many people assume. Mosher and Akins (2014) summarize the differences in substance use patterns among whites, African Americans, Hispanics, Asians, and Indigenous groups in the United States, noting several interesting age patterns and concluding that racial and ethnic differences in substance use are not constant. The differences change depending on the age group being examined. Amongst adolescents, Asians are the least like to use illicit drugs, while Indigenous adolescents are significantly more likely to use illicit drugs than any other group. African American adolescents are actually less likely to use illicit drugs than whites, Hispanics, and Indigenous people. Finally, adolescent Hispanics are quite similar to whites in their patterns of illegal drug use. However, these patterns change as young people transition into adulthood, with African Americans showing a clear trend towards greater use and whites and Hispanics decreasing in their use. Compared to all of the other groups, Indigenous people remain the most likely to use illegal drugs after the age of 26. Within group comparisons show that African Americans have the greatest proportion of users after age 26, when the group rates begin to resemble the rates of whites and Hispanics. These crude estimates of ethnic and racial variations in illicit drug use help to illustrate the complexities of substance use patterns. Age is connected to substance use in different ways for different groups.

Admittedly, studying ethnic and racial identities is far more complex than simply checking a box on a survey. People self-identify in many different ways depending on several different factors, such as their national origin, amount of exposure to the country in which they are currently residing, socioeconomic status, and language (Khanna, 2012). Given the wide range of responses when people are asked to identify their ethnicity or race, it can be difficult for researchers to ascertain the connection between any one group of individuals and substance use patterns. Moreover, the simplification of ethnicity and race into a relatively small number of groups, as is often the case with most studies, may be misrepresentative. This does not mean that ethnicity and race are too complex, not important, or inherently misleading for researchers; however, it does suggest that any research that examines these demographic attributes must be interpreted with caution, and researchers need to be mindful of other factors that may contribute to substance use and misuse. One such factor that is often intertwined with ethnicity and race is socioeconomic status.

Socioeconomic Status (SES)

Socioeconomic status or social class is an important indicator of social behaviours and outcomes. Income and education level are some of the most commonly used proxies for socioeconomic status. Estimating household income is some-times difficult, as research participants are often reluctant to disclose this information (Wray et al., 2013). Thus, we often use education level as an alternative or additional measure to estimate where someone is positioned in the social class hierarchy. As with most demographics, socioeconomic status is related to substance use in different ways for different substances. The most recent estimates of socioeconomic status and substance use in Canada are derived from the 2004 CAS (Adlaf, Begin, & Sawka, 2005). Thus, it must be recognized that much has changed in the Canadian economy since 2004, including the greatest economic upheaval since the 1930s.

The 2004 CAS included measures for both education level and income adequacy, which was based on combining the total household income with the total number of people in the household. When examining income adequacy and alcohol use, those with higher incomes are more likely to have had alcohol in the past year; they also drank more frequently and exceeded the low-risk drinking guidelines, a finding that has been reiterated in more recent studies in both the United Kingdom and the United States (Iparraguirre, 2015; Jones, 2015). Despite these increased likelihoods, Canadians with high income adequacy rankings were no more likely to be considered heavy drinkers, measured as more than five drinks on a single occasion, than lower income groups (Adlaf, Begin, & Sawka, 2005).

Level of education and alcohol use indicated similar findings, with a few exceptions. Education was not related to exceeding low-risk drinking guidelines, but when measuring heavy drinking, people with a university degree were less likely to drink heavily than those with less formal education (Adlaf, Begin, & Sawka, 2005); however, binge drinking is most closely associated with those attending a post-secondary institution (Arbour-Nicitopoulos et al., 2010; Carlson, Johnson, & Jacobs, 2010). Quantity of alcohol consumed decreased with higher levels of education after the completion of studies.

Compared to many other demographic characteristics, income adequacy and education level are not strongly associated with illicit drug use, and most of the significant associations are linked to cannabis, not other illicit substances (Adlaf, Begin, & Sawka, 2005). There were some differences in illicit drug use patterns by income and education, but often not in the direction that most would expect. Interestingly, past-year cannabis use was not associated with income adequacy or education. However, lifetime cannabis use was higher amongst higher income groups. The association with level of education was non-linear, showing that the lowest lifetime use of cannabis was amongst those who had not completed high school, followed by those with a university degree; the group with the highest percentage of lifetime users of cannabis was those with some post-secondary education. Part of this is likely based on the age of the users, and part may be explained by the experiences of being in post-secondary education. Moreover, lifetime use reporting is always subject to recall biases, with individuals possibly misrepresenting their use histories, not intentionally but from a lack of memory.

Geographic Location

The areas where people live and the connections these locations have with substance use patterns is an important sociological consideration. There are multiple ways in which geographic locations are examined in national and provincial studies. The 2013 CTADS compared substance use rates across provinces, while the 2004 CAS examined urban and rural differences using postal codes. The annual OSDUHS also makes regional comparisons based on the location of various school boards in the province. Each of these geographic comparisons offers a different understating of substance use patterns.

According to the 2013 CTADS findings, there are few provincial differences in substance use patterns for tobacco, alcohol, and cannabis (Health Canada, 2013a) (Table 8.1). For Canadians aged 15 or older, the current rate of tobacco smoking is about 15 percent, with British Columbia having the lowest rate of current smokers at 11 percent and New Brunswick with the highest at 20 percent. The remaining provinces are not significantly different from the national average. The percentage of Canadians reporting past-year alcohol use is about 76 percent, with Ontario and Newfoundland and Labrador having the lowest rates of past-year alcohol consumption at around 73 percent. Quebec has the highest rate across the country, with approximately 83 percent reporting use of alcohol in the past year. Not surprisingly, the most commonly used illicit substance across all of the provinces was cannabis, with approximately 11 percent of Canadians aged 15 and older reporting past-year use. Saskatchewan has the lowest rate of past-year use at 8 percent, while British Columbia, perhaps not surprisingly based on its comparatively liberal stance on marijuana, has the highest rate of cannabis use at 13 percent.

Unfortunately, provincial comparisons for past-year use of all other illicit substances lack stable estimates due to high sampling variability and the low percentage of users included in the survey. The good news is that this means these substances are not as widespread as tobacco, alcohol, and cannabis. However, it is somewhat discouraging that we lack provincial data on variations in the use of illicit substances.

Table 8.1: Percentage of Canadians Aged 15 and Older Who Reported Using Tobacco, Alcohol, and Cannabis by Province

Province*	Substance		
	Tobacco (Current)	Alcohol (Past year)	Cannabis (Past year)
Canada	14.6	75.9	10.6
Newfoundland and Labrador	19.5	**72.5**	9.6
Prince Edward Island	17.3	74.6	10.9
Nova Scotia	19.4	76.2	12.5
New Brunswick	**19.6**	73.9	10.1
Quebec	17.1	**82.8**	10.7
Ontario	12.6	**72.7**	10.3
Manitoba	17.4	74.8	10.2
Saskatchewan	17.6	75.5	**8.1**
Alberta	16.0	74.5	9.1
British Columbia	**11.4**	75.3	**13.3**

*Percentages in bold are significantly different from the remaining nine provinces and the country as a whole.
Source: Canadian Tobacco, Alcohol and Drugs Survey (Health Canada, 2013a).

Similar to the CTADS, the results from the 2004 CAS show a few notable differences between people living in urban versus rural locations (Adlaf, Begin, & Sawka, 2005). For all measures of alcohol use, including prevalence, frequency, and quantity, there are no significant differences between rural and non-rural use patterns. Moreover, there appear to be no significant differences in the percentage of people experiencing alcohol problems or the harms associated with using alcohol. However, differences emerge with illicit substances. For lifetime use of cannabis, there are no significant differences between those living in rural areas and those living in urban areas; in fact, the urban and rural differences for lifetime use of any illicit substance are generally quite small. Differences between rural and urban places do appear to be significant, however, only when considering past-year use. Those living in rural locations are less likely to report using illicit substances in the past year compared to those living in urban locations. Urban dwellers are about one-and-a-half times more likely to report using cannabis compared to rural dwellers. The differences in the percentage reporting past-year use of cocaine, speed, ecstasy, hallucinogens, and heroin are much smaller but still significant. Approximately 3 percent of Canadians living in urban areas reported using one of these five substances in the past year, compared to 2 percent of people living in rural areas.

There are two convincing arguments for why there are some significant differences amongst urban and rural populations. Mosher and Akins (2014) suggest that availability of illicit substances is more restricted in rural locations. There are few drug dealers in these areas, so gaining access to illicit substances is more difficult, leading to fewer users. A second argument is that people who are most likely to use illicit substances gravitate to more urbanized areas. Part of this may be in pursuit of a particular lifestyle, or it may be driven by the desire to have access to illicit substances.

While there is no population study of substance use and misuse that accounts for the entire population of Canada, we cannot talk about geography in Canada and not talk about the territories, given that we know there is more alcohol problems and solvent use in these areas. In a revenue-versus-cost analysis of alcohol in Canada, Senior Research and Policy Analyst at the Canadian Centre for Substance Abuse Gerald Thomas (2012) illustrates the stark differences between the provinces and territories. In 2002, the per-capita surpluses and deficits associated with alcohol prevention, research, and transfer payment programs are rather negligible for most of the provinces, ranging from a surplus of $26.99 in Prince Edward Island to a deficit of $55.57 in New Brunswick after revenues are taken into account. The remaining provinces fall somewhere in between this range. However, when examining the per-capita deficits and surpluses in the territories, all three have significant deficits, with the Northwest Territories having a deficit of $134.19, the Yukon Territory at $228.15, and most significantly Nunavut at $563.25. This represents a per-capita deficit that is ten times higher than the costliest province. Surely this indicates a reason to be concerned about alcohol use in Canada's three territories.

Per-capita estimates of alcohol problems across Canada are not collected and reported. However, by taking population estimates and estimates of heavy drinking collected by Statistics Canada from each of the provinces and territories, we can compare rates of heavy drinking in the territories relative to the provinces (Statistics Canada, 2015a; Statistics Canada, 2015c). Likewise, similar estimates can be derived for smokers by combining estimates (Statistics Canada, 2015b; Statistics Canada, 2015c). Table 8.2 summarizes these estimates in percentages by country, province, and territory. Comparatively, the Northwest Territories has the highest percentage of heavy drinkers, with one

Table 8.2: Heavy Drinkers* and Smokers in Canada by Province and Territory, 2012

	Total Heavy Drinkers, 2012	Total Smokers, 2012	Total Population, 2012	% Heavy Drinkers	% Smokers
Canada	5,042,829	5,933,095	34,751,476	15	17
Newfoundlanc and Labrador	118,862	115,412	526,895	23	22
Prince Edward Island	24,903	27,401	145,259	17	19
Nova Scotia	179,721	190,986	944,835	19	20
New Brunswick	126,003	152,124	756,836	17	20
Quebec	1,268,559	1,626,375	8,084,768	16	20
Ontario	1,737,737	2,161,957	13,409,558	13	16
Manitoba	195,035	201,163	1,250,406	16	16
Saskatchewan	151,017	168,557	1,087,223	14	16
Alberta	594,025	689,302	3,888,552	15	18
British Columbia	625,452	568,961	4,542,578	14	13
Yukon	6,791	8,882	36,189	19	25
Northwest Territories	10,899	12,498	43,648	25	29
Nunavut	3,825	9,477	34,729	11	27

*People agec 12 and over who reported having five or more drinks, on one occasion, at least once a montᏂ in the past 12 months.
Source: Compiled from Statistics Canada (2015a, b, c), CANSIM, tables 105-0501 and 051-0001.

quarter of the entire population fitting into this category, defined as those aged 12 and over reporting that they have had 5 or more drinks on one occasion each month for the past year. Newfoundland and Labrador has the second highest percentage of heavy drinking with 23 percent of the population. Nova Scotia and the Yukon Territories have similar percentages of heavy drinkers at almost one fifth, or 19 percent. Interestingly, the current estimates suggest that Nunavut has the lowest percentage of heavy drinkers in the population—yet in Thomas's (2012) cost analysis, Nunavut had the greatest deficit related to alcohol. It is unclear why such a discrepancy exists, though issues of data collection due to geographic isolation and self-reporting, especially in supposedly dry communities, must be considered.

As for smoking, there is a clear pattern of significantly higher rates of smoking in the territories relative to the provinces. Almost one third of the population of Northwest Territories, or 29 percent, are smokers, followed by 27 percent in Nunavut and 25 percent in the Yukon. Newfoundland and Labrador has the highest percentage of smokers among the 10 provinces at 22 percent. British Columbia has the lowest percentage of tobacco smokers at 13 percent, while the remaining eight provinces have between 16 and 20 percent of the population who smokes.

8.3: CONCLUSION

There are several demographic characteristics that are important to consider with substance use. These correlates have important implications for how we view and treat substance use and misuse. However, the greatest impediment to our knowledge is the simple fact that we do not routinely collect all of the necessary demographic information when conducting research on substance use. This is particularly true for racial and ethnic groups, as Canadian population data is significantly limited.

As this chapter has shown, age, sex, ethnicity and race, socioeconomic status, and geographic location help us to better understand patterns of substance use. These factors are also often overlapping, which further illustrates the complexities of understanding substance use patterns. There is not one single factor that can explain substance use and substance misuse. The individual, as well as the social context, must be taken into consideration. Accordingly, the next chapter examines relational correlates, including peers, romantic partners, and families.

NOTES

1. The manner in which questions have been historically posed in survey research is through a closed-ended binary male-female categorization. While we use the terms *sex, female,* and *male* here, we do recognize that individuals are more fluid in their actual self-identification and that there is a distinction in the biological and social constructions of self. Our language used here is influenced by what is currently available in the survey research conducted to date, not individual realities of alternate forms of identification.

2. Caffeine is actually the most used substance not only in Canada but globally; however, most survey research does not include caffeine as a psychoactive substance.

PARADOXES

1) The Canadian government does not collect all of the necessary demographic information when conducting research on substance use to assess outcome effectiveness.
2) Illicit drugs are the substances we hear the most about in terms of the risks associated with use, yet the prevalence rates of use are relatively low compared to other legal substances we know produce harm when used excessively.
3) Even without proper data and well-defined estimates, the government still establishes policies and allocates funding to prevention and treatment programs that are not necessarily the most effective means of dealing with drugs and drug use.

CRITICAL REFLECTIONS

1) What is the value of having the various correlates discussed in this chapter when developing a sociological understanding of psychoactive drug use?
2) Which correlate(s) provide the greatest insight into understanding substance use in Canada?
3) What are the strengths of using demographics when attempting to understand drug use and addiction in Canada?
4) What are the limits of relying only upon demographic characteristics when trying to understand drug use and addiction in Canada?

9 Relational Correlates of Substance Use in Canada: Peers and Families

While demographic characteristics enable social science researchers to identify patterns of behaviour among particular groups of people, these factors tell us little about the influence of interpersonal relationships on substance use patterns and the potential development of substance dependence. Many sociologists are interested in the interactive nature of social life. Unlike psychologists, who are more interested in individual behaviours, sociologists are interested in examining broad patterns of individual behaviours and outcomes that are a product of social relations and social environments.

Pro-social relationships with peers, intimate partners, and family members can have protective effects (Barnes, Reifman, Farrell, & Dintcheff, 2000; Bègue & Roché, 2009); however, negative relationships can also increase the risk of substance use initiation and substance using patterns, including dependence (Barnes et al., 2007; Butters, 2002, 2005; Erickson, Crosnoe, & Dornbusch, 2000). Moreover, interpersonal relationships in certain social contexts can have both positive and negative influences (Alaggia & Csiernik, 2017; Francis, Alaggia, & Csiernik, 2010; Fleming, White, & Catalano, 2010). Thus, when attempting to understand substance use patterns, we also need to examine the many risk and protective factors involved in interpersonal relationships and social environments.

9.1: PEERS

A longstanding assumption regarding substance use initiation and continuation is that peers have a significant impact. While substantial evidence supports the connection between peers and substance use (Bahr, Hawks & Wang, 1993; Bahr, Hoffman & Yang, 2005; Clark & Lohéac, 2007; Duncan, Duncan, & Stryker, 2006; Elliott, Huizinga, & Ageton, 1985; Marcos, Bahr, & Johnson, 1986), the relationship is rather complex, as not all people are equally affected by their peer relationships (Allen et al., 2012). Many parents fear the overwhelming potential of "peer pressure," believing that their children will be forced or lured into substance use or misuse by the people they hang out with either at school or in their free time. The problem with this notion of peers pressuring individuals to use or misuse substances is its inaccuracy: the reality is far more complex than friends forcing or encouraging one another to use substances. Instead, the relationship between peers and individual substance use is more accurately described as "peer influence." This conceptualization recognizes that peers can have a significant and enduring effect on substance use patterns while also acknowledging that the individual and other social factors can play a role in substance use and dependence.

Indeed, several studies on youth substance use have examined the impact of peer influence, with relatively consistent findings: peers play a significant role in explaining patterns of substance use (Clark & Lohéac, 2007; Duncan, Duncan, & Strycker, 2006; Elliott, Huizinga, & Ageton, 1985; Korotkikh, 2008; Martino et al., 2006; Tang & Orwin 2009). While most studies find that peers increase the risk of substance use, there is evidence to suggest that the influence of peers is not necessarily the same for all types of substances (Clark & Lohéac, 2007; Kiuru et al., 2010), nor does the influence of peers have the same effect for all age groups (Tang & Orwin, 2009). Moreover, the influence of peers is not always direct (Fleming, White, & Catalano 2010). There are several individual and social factors that can modify or even amplify the influence that peers may have on substance use and dependence. Three areas of research that examine the multi-faceted nature of peer influence include (1) perceptions of peer substance use versus actual peer substance use, (2) the types of social activities that individuals are involved in with their peers, and (3) the selection of peers.

Perceived Peer Use Versus Actual Peer Use

Social influences in an individual's immediate environment can influence individual perceptions or beliefs about substances and substance use (Martino et al., 2006). While the decision to use a particular substance may be a matter of individual choice, social influences can still impact individual perceptions about drugs and alcohol, leading to the indirect influence of others on the decision to indulge or refrain. Research has generally supported the notion that beliefs and attitudes about substances are important predictors of substance use. In general, the findings indicate that those who believe that substance use is not risky or harmful and those who generally approve of using substances are more likely to use both alcohol and cannabis (Flanagan, Stout, & Gallay, 2008; Johnston, O'Malley, Bachman, & Schulenberg, 2006).

Peer attitudes towards substance use show a consistent connection with individual substance use patterns, but this relationship may be conditional upon ethnicity, race, and sex, with white females more influenced by their peers' attitudes than males and other ethnic and racial comparison groups (Mason et al., 2014).

Some researchers have further argued that individuals are more likely to use certain substances if they believe that their peers are also using those substances (Aseltine, 1995; Urberg, Luo, Pilgrim, & Degirmencioglu, 2003). According to this argument, it does not matter if peers are actually using substances; instead, if an individual simply thinks they have used, this can impact their decision to use substances themselves. Deutsch, Chernyavskiy, Steinley, and Slutske (2015) systematically compared perceptions of friends' substance use versus their actual substance use. In general, perceived substance use among one's friends has a greater effect on one's substance use than a friend's actual use of substances. These effects of perceived use also seem to depend on the type of substance and type of use, whereby different substances and amounts of use are more influenced by perceptions than other substances.

Social Activities and Peers

It has long been argued that social activities that involve hanging out with peers results in more cannabis and alcohol consumption (Hundleby, 1987). Osgood and colleagues (1996) further argue that unstructured, unsupervised, peer-dominated activities are conducive to a range of deviant behaviours, including substance use, while Thorlindsson and Bernburg (2006) examined how different types of leisure activities and peers can influence the likelihood of substance use. They found that the connection between peers and substance use partially depends on the types of activities in which individuals are routinely engaged. If young people are more often involved in partying and socially defined delinquent activities, then peers can influence the likelihood of substance use. On the other hand, if individuals are involved in structured and supervised activities with their peers than the likelihood of substance use is diminished.

In a recent Canadian study of adolescent alcohol and cannabis use, Gallupe and Bouchard (2013) extended these peer-based situational explanations by examining the connection between specific partying situations and peer substance use. They found that the more friends drank or used cannabis the more likely individuals are to use themselves. They also found that, as peers drink more at each subsequent party, there is a significant increase in individual use patterns. Finally, they found that alcohol and cannabis use is more likely to occur in smaller groups.

When examining the potential sex differences in substance use patterns and situational explanations, some research indicates there are no significant differences in the effects of unstructured, unsupervised activities on substance use in general (Bears Augustyn & McGloin 2013). However, others have found that there are some specific substance use differences. Positive or protective peer groups are especially important for young men's tobacco and marijuana use, in that young men are less likely to be influenced by risky situational activities that may involve tobacco or marijuana if they have a good group of positive and protective friends rather than negative or risky friends. However, there appears to be no effect of peer groups and risky situations on young women's substance use (Mason et al., 2015).

Selection of Peers

While peer relations can certainly have a dominant influence on the substance use patterns of young people, the influence of peers does not exist in isolation from social bonds to the family. Research concerning peers and substance use has generally supported the argument that close relations with substance-using peers often counteracts the effect of positive or close relations with families: close friendships, especially with those who are engaged in substance use themselves, tend to increase the risk of substance use (Bahr, Hawks, & Wang, 1993; Bahr, Hoffmann, & Yang, 2005; Clark and Lohéac, 2007; Elliott, Huizinga, & Ageton, 1985). However, there is also evidence to suggest that family experiences can have an impact on the selection of peers and, by extension, the influence that peers can have on a person's substance use (Liebregts et al., 2013).

In a longitudinal study examining the shift from early adolescence into early adulthood, family influences changed in importance as children aged (Van Ryzin, Fosco, & Dishion, 2012). While parental monitoring is important in early adolescence, the quality of family relationships becomes more important in the transition to high school and throughout adolescence. Family relationships and parental monitoring also had a significant indirect connection to substance use and peer influence, in that there appears to be an important role for the family in the choice of friends earlier in the life-course.

Intimate Partners

Another important emerging area in the research on peers focuses on intimate partner influences on substance use. There are two major foci of research on intimate or romantic partners: the basic connection between an individuals substance use and their partner's; and the effect of the nature, seriousness, or status of romantic relationships on substance use. Depending on the population being studied, most studies have suggested that partner effects are complex and differ based on individual characteristics, the ways in which romantic or intimate partners are being studied, and the substance being used (Catalano et al., 2010; Fleming, White, & Catalano, 2010; Gudonis-Miller et al., 2012; Kim et al., 2013; Kreager, Haynie, & Hopfer, 2012).

In a longitudinal analysis of young women and men from the National Longitudinal Study of Adolescent to Adult Health, formerly known as the National Longitudinal Study of Adolescent Health, Gudonis-Miller and colleagues (2012) found significant evidence that partners influence alcohol and tobacco use: having a partner who uses these substances increases individual use. For marijuana use, however, they found that as the seriousness of the relationship increased, marijuana use decreased.

Kim and colleagues (2013) conducted a longitudinal study of high-risk young men in their early-to-late twenties and found that even high-risk groups of young men generally decrease their use of alcohol as they progress into their later twenties. However, having a romantic partner who used alcohol and being in a new relationship were both associated with young men using alcohol to a greater extent in their late twenties than would be the case if their partner did not use alcohol and they were in a longer-term relationship. These findings suggest that being in a relationship is not necessarily protective for high-risk young men.

Catalano and colleagues' (2010) study of a larger sample of both men and women aged 18 to 20 years old found that relationship status changes, such as getting into a new relationship or getting more serious in the relationship, did not result in decreased use patterns. However, breaking up or getting into a new relationship within six months of ending a previous relationship were connected to specific substance use increases: dissolution of a relationship and starting a new relationship shortly thereafter was significantly related to increased use of tobacco and marijuana. The ending of a relationship was also significantly connected to heavy drinking, which was partially explained by experiencing depression and being more exposed to other substance-using peers when relationships dissolve or are newly formed. Liebregts and colleagues (2013), in a three-year qualitative longitudinal study, examined the role of social relationships in cannabis use and found that cannabis dependence could be explained by cohabitation and, for females especially, a new partnership.

However, as in the case of peer interactions, romantic partnerships do not exist in isolation from other peer influences, both direct and indirect. Taking a networking approach to peer and partner connections by examining direct peer influence, partner influence, and partner's peer influence, Kreager, Haynie, and Hopfer (2012) found that a partner's friends, a more distant measure of peers, influence drinking but not smoking. Individual smoking behaviour, however, is more associated with partner's smoking and direct peer associations. Thus, smoking is more closely related to direct peer associations, whereas drinking can be influenced by more distant connections.

9.2: FAMILIES

Though romantic dyads are important for understanding substance use patterns, and can rightfully be considered family-based measures, there is a separate area in substance use literature that focuses on the influence of the family. There are several different ways in which the family can have an influence on individual substance use and dependence. In fact, there is perhaps no other area of research or known correlate for substance use and dependence that highlights the necessity of a biopsychosocial approach. While several biological and psychological studies were considered in Chapter 3 (see Agrawal & Lynskey, 2008; Ball, 2007; Jessor & Jessor, 1977; Kaplan, 1975), there are many social aspects of the family that are worthy of consideration. These social aspects can be categorized broadly into sibling influence, non-substance-related parental influences, and substance-using parental influences.

Sibling Influence

Similar to research on peers, siblings are known to have a significant impact on the decision to use substances. According to Bahr, Hoffman, and Yang's (2005) study, not only do siblings have a direct influence on individual alcohol and cannabis use, but this influence also remains after taking into consideration peer influences. Massey and Krohn (1986) also found a significant influence of siblings on individual cigarette use. In fact, a sibling's use of cigarettes was actually more important than parental use of cigarettes.

Research tends to support the notion that older siblings have an impact on younger siblings' substance use (Boyle et al., 2001; Kothari, Sorenson, Bank, & Snyder, 2014). Boyle and colleagues (2001) similarly found that parental influence is not as important as older siblings for tobacco, alcohol, and marijuana use. Moreover, there appear to be stronger similarities in families when the siblings are all male and are two years or less apart in age. The similarities are also stronger among older siblings aged 19 to 24.

The expanding research on sibling influence on substance use in recent years provides a more detailed understanding of the potential role of interpersonal sibling relationships, as well as the role of a peer group in connection to sibling influences. With respect to sibling relationships, Samek and Rueter (2011) found that close bonds with an older sibling protects against substance use, but they did not find support for a social learning effect in siblings. According to this research, it is the emotional aspects of the sibling relationship that matter, not the assumed imitation or modelling of sibling substance use.

In contrast, other research has found that the combination of having shared peers and modelling the substance use behaviour of one's sibling has a significant impact on substance use behaviours (Whiteman, Jensen, & Maggs, 2013). These researchers further found that an individual's alcohol use is more strongly associated with an older sibling's use when they share the same friends; however, these conditional or amplifying effects were not supported with other substance use patterns beyond alcohol. Thus, patterns of sibling substance use are an important factor in attempting to understand individual use patterns.

Parental Influences

In comparison to sibling influences, much greater attention has been paid to various parental influences for explaining substance use patterns. Interestingly, there is no substantive literature directly examining the social influence of parental substance use on that of their children. Rather, the focus is divided along two distinct lines: one area focuses on parents with substance use or dependence in their histories, while the other area focuses on ways in which parents can influence substance use patterns regardless of whether they use themselves. While distinct, these two areas are not mutually exclusive. From both perspectives, the role of parents in explaining substance use patterns typically focuses on three distinct influences: structural, instrumental, and emotional. Structural influences include the gender of the parent and family composition as it relates to the presence of parents in the lives of children and youth. Not entirely unrelated to the more structural aspects of parenting, instrumental influences on substance use patterns typically focus on supervision and monitoring, while the emotional influences emphasize elements of attachment, parenting styles, and levels of family conflict. The following focuses broadly on these various parental influences, where the substance use of parents is not explicitly considered.

Comparing the relative impact of family structure and family attachment on adolescent alcohol and drug use, Barfield-Cottledge (2015) found that family attachment is more important than family structure in explaining substance use patterns. Specific parenting styles are also connected to substance use amongst adolescents, as authoritarian parents, defined as being strict and controlling, increase the risk of adolescent smoking, whereas permissive parents, who are usually more lenient and tolerant, decrease the risk of drinking (Loke & Mak, 2013).

In contrast with some attachment and parenting style findings, Jones, Ehrlich, Lejuez, and Cassidy (2015) examined 203 adolescents from two-parent families and found that attachments styles were not directly related to adolescent alcohol and marijuana use; instead, insecure attachments negatively influence the knowledge that parents have about their adolescent's involvement in activities, as well as their general knowledge about where their adolescent is when she or he is away from home. Moreover, the more parents know about their adolescents' whereabouts and activities, the less likely youth are to engage in alcohol and marijuana use.

Several researchers have examined the role of parental monitoring or supervision on the substance use patterns of adolescents (Barnes, Reifman, Farrell, & Dintcheff, 2000; Clark, Shamblen, Ringwalt, & Hanley, 2012; Fulkerson, Pasch, Perry, & Komro, 2008; Kim, 2004; Parsai, Marsiglia, & Kulis 2010; Tang & Orwin, 2009). Bahr, Hawkes, and Wang (1993) examined the competing roles of peers and families and found that parental monitoring has a strong and direct inverse effect on adolescent substance abuse, meaning the more parents monitor their adolescents, the less likely adolescents will abuse substances. These researchers also found that parental monitoring is indirectly related to substance abuse through peer drug use. Thus, parents need to not only monitor their adolescent's behaviour but also the behaviour of his or her peers in order to effectively control or prevent their adolescent from becoming a substance abuser.

Kim (2004) found similar direct and indirect effects of parental monitoring on adolescent alcohol use.

However, among younger adolescents aged 11 to 15, parental monitoring may not influence tobacco, alcohol, and cannabis use unless there is a direct consequence attached to the behaviour as a result of parental monitoring (Parsai, Marsiglia, & Kulis, 2010). Parental monitoring of marijuana initiation appears to be more effective in preventing use in early adolescence, but diminishes in strength in later adolescence (Tang & Orwin, 2009). However, Clark, Shamblen, Ringwalt, and Hanley (2012) claim that effective parental monitoring is a significant protective factor at all ages, even among high-risk youth.

In addition to supervision, spending time with parents can be protective. Compared to teens who have frequent family dinners (five to seven per week), those who have infrequent family dinners (fewer than three per week) are twice as likely to have used tobacco or marijuana, and more than one-and-a-half times more likely to have used alcohol. Of course, this is a finding of correlation and not causation, for the actual factor decreasing risk of use is family engagement—being together is what decreases risk (National Centre on Addiction and Substance Abuse, 2009, 2012). From this research, we can conclude that attachment between parents and youths may indirectly influence substance use through parental knowledge and supervision of their adolescents' activities.

In contrast, family conflict, a measure of interpersonal relations within the family, has shown relatively consistent connections with various forms of substance use (Butters, 2002, 2005; Branstetter, Furman, & Cottrell, 2009; Loke & Mak, 2013) and recovery from substance misuse (Best & Wilson, 2014). In general, family conflict increases the likelihood of substance use and reduces the likelihood of improved functioning even after formal treatment has been initiated. The importance of this area of research is that it does not just consider the parent-child relationship, but can also include conflicts between other family members such as parents in conflict with one another, siblings in conflict with parents, and siblings in conflict with one another.

Parental Substance Use

One area of research that is gaining attention from sociologists is the multigenerational transmission of substance use and related behaviours. As some previous research has illustrated, parental substance use is not regularly considered and thus not always measured. There are inevitably some people who engage in substance use and misuse as a consequence of structural or emotional aspects of the family, even without researchers knowing the substance use behaviours of the parents (Alaggia & Csiernik, 2017). However, substance use amongst parents is not mutually exclusive from structural and emotional factors in the family. It is difficult to estimate precisely how many children are affected by parental substance use (Kroll, 2004). However, research indicates that each person with an addiction seriously influences the lives of four to six other people (Abbott, 2000). Grant's (2000) study found that one in four children in the United States lived in a family with a history of alcohol abuse, while an Australian study reported that 22 percent of all Australian children were estimated to be affected by their parents or caregivers using alcohol, including more than 10,000 who were involved in the child welfare system (Laslett et al., 2015). Many current estimates are based on cases that have come to the attention of authorities, including counselling agencies, courts, and child protection agencies. Nevertheless, such evidence should indicate that the number of children and youth affected by parental substance use is far greater than we are currently aware.

There are many adverse outcomes that can result from parental substance use and dependence, including weakened or broken attachments, poor family dynamics or functioning, impaired relationships (Kroll, 2004), and behavioural problems (Raj, Kumar, Sinha, & Dogra, 2012). A Canadian study found that children exposed to parental addiction were 69 percent more likely to develop depression in adulthood compared to their peers with non-addicted parents (Fuller-Thomson et al., 2013). Abusive use of substances is also strongly correlated with violence in the family (Murphy & Ting, 2010). Healthy attachments, and the physical and emotional well-being of the child, are all compromised in these homes, which can also impact a child's ability to cope with adverse circumstances and adapt to adulthood in a healthy manner.

An important debate in the study of the familial transmission of substance use and dependence centres on the "nature versus nurture" argument. Is substance use and related problems a product of genes or environment? Knop, Goodwin, Jensen, and Penick (1993) address the nature/nurture question with results from a 30-year follow-up cohort study of the sons of alcohol-dependent fathers in Denmark. This study used a multidisciplinary approach to alcohol dependence by combining biological, psychopathological, and psychosocial measures. During pregnancy and at birth there were no significant differences between sons of alcohol-dependent fathers, defined as high risk, and sons of non-alcohol-dependent fathers, defined as low risk. However, by the time the boys were one year old, the high-risk group were significantly less likely to be living in suitable housing. Upon entry into school, the problems had grown: the high-risk boys scored significantly higher on the impulsivity and restlessness scale, had significantly more language and learning disorders, and had more frequent referrals to the school psychologist. When the boys were followed up with at 19 and 20 years old, the high-risk group reported more stressful life events, such as severe financial problems, marital breakdown between their parents, and continued problems with an alcohol-dependent parent. At the 30-year follow-up, the young men who had grown up with an alcohol-dependent father were significantly more likely to be dependent on alcohol or cannabis themselves. On all other measures of psychopathology, there were no significant differences.

Arguably, the familial transmission of substance dependence is not a straightforward process with guaranteed predictability. Different studies produce different results, depending on the measures and objectives of the studies. Kosten, Rounsaville, and Kleber (1985) surveyed 638 people who were dependent on opioids and compared those who had alcohol-dependent parents with those who did not. The people with at least one alcohol-dependent parent were more likely to be alcohol dependent in addition to their opioid dependence, and were more likely to report major depression and/or antisocial personality disorders. Moreover, they experienced more traumatic childhoods, with alcohol-dependent mothers being particularly damaging. Similarly, Taplin, Saddichha, and Krausz (2014) found that mothers who used substances were more likely to have children who experienced multiple forms of trauma, including sexual and emotional abuse, as well as physical neglect. Fathers who used substances, on the other hand, had a higher risk of their children experiencing physical abuse in childhood. These experiences of trauma directly increased the risk of earlier initiation into injection drug use amongst offspring.

Miller, Downs, Gondoli, and Keil (1987) compared 45 alcohol-dependent women and 40 non-alcohol-dependent women. They found that the former group was significantly more likely to have a parent who had alcohol problems and more likely to have experienced sexual abuse. While the alcohol-dependent parents did not perpetrate most incidences of sexual abuse, environmental and psychological factors such as supervision and parental mental health issues were believed to influence the occurrence of sexual abuse in alcohol-dependent homes.

Among high-risk youth, Mylant, Ide, Cuevas, and Meehan (2002) found that children of alcohol-dependent parents were at greater risk of negative outcomes than youth who did not have a parent with a substance use problem. Youth who admitted to having a parent with a substance use problem had significantly lower resiliency, as indicated by family and personal strengths, and lower school bonding. Additionally, children with substance-misusing parents scored significantly higher on at-risk temperament, feelings, thoughts, and behaviour measures.

In an attempt to understand parent–child interactions, Moser and Jacob (1997) found that alcohol-dependent families exhibited more impaired parent–child interactions, with significantly more negativity and less positivity than non-alcohol-dependent families. Unexpectedly, dual alcohol-dependent families (both mother and father)[1] had the highest levels of congeniality. According to the researchers, this counterintuitive finding may suggest that characteristics such as likability and friendliness may not be helpful indicators of problematic family dynamics when both parents are alcohol-dependent. Alcohol-dependent mothers had the largest impact on parent–child interactions. Fathers from alcohol-dependent families were more likely to be authoritarian in their parenting style, whereby they try to control their children using discipline and very little nurturing. Indeed, alcohol-dependent families can lead to substantial negative psychological and behavioural outcomes, particularly when the alcohol-dependent parent is the mother. Despite these negative findings, Moser and Jacob (1997) also found that non-alcohol-dependent mothers in these homes could moderate the negative impact of the father's parenting style by providing the child with positive interaction.

Moreover, maternal history of drug use can have an indirect impact on marital disruption and, ultimately, family structure. Research shows that mothers who are divorced or never married had children with greater negative outcomes (Kandel, Rosenbaum, & Chen, 1994). The negative effects of family structure may be more pronounced for children born to adolescent mothers when compared with older mothers, and the impact and range of negative substance use outcomes appears to be more significant for female children when compared to male children.

While most studies of children living with substance-dependent parents focus on the negative outcomes or possible risks, Hussong and colleagues (2005) examined resiliency, in particular social competence, among children of alcohol-dependent parents. Using a comparative cohort study of alcohol-dependent families and non-alcohol-dependent families living in the same community, results indicate that the effect of parental alcohol dependence on social competence varies over time, is more pronounced for girls, and depends on who is reporting on the measure—the teacher, parent, or child.

Tweed and Ryff (1991) state that not all outcomes for children of alcohol-dependent parents are negative. Instead, they argue, there is substantial variability in the experiences of living with an alcohol-dependent parent. Findings from their non-clinical comparative study of adult children of alcohol-dependent parents and adult children from non-alcohol-dependent families support the contention that adult children of alcohol-dependent parents do not live wholly miserable lives. When compared to adults whose parents were not dependent on alcohol, adult children of alcohol-dependent parents experienced similar levels of psychological well-being, personality characteristics, and personal development. Differences did emerge, however, when they were compared on measures of anxiety and depression: children from non-alcohol-dependent homes were less likely to experience such distress.

Harter (2000) examined controlled studies of the psychosocial adjustment of adult children of alcoholics (ACoAs) between 1988 and 1999. The population was at increased risk for substance abuse, antisocial behaviours, depressive symptoms, anxiety disorders, low self-esteem, difficulties in family relationships, and generalized distress and maladjustment. However, none of these outcomes were uniformly observed. Thus, while living with an alcohol-dependent parent can have negative effects, successful adjustment into adulthood is not impossible.

One obstacle to increasing social support is the social acceptance of children and family members of people who are substance dependent. Many people hold negative opinions about substance users, especially those that are identifiably substance dependent. Perhaps more surprising, however, are the negative attitudes society holds about family members or significant others who are associated with the substance-dependent person. In a population-based study, Corrigan, Watson, and Miller (2006) examined public attitudes towards family members of physically ill, mentally ill, and/or drug-dependent persons. The findings revealed that the general public endorses discriminatory behaviour towards those who have a family member who is drug dependent. More specifically, parents and spouses are blamed for the onset and relapse of a person's substance-use problem. Even worse, children of drug-dependent parents are perceived as being the most contaminated when compared to the other illness groups. This contamination belief is perpetuated by biological and genetic assumptions about addiction or substance dependence as a disease, though the lasting impact of the moral model remains evident.

The view that children of substance-dependent parents are somehow contaminated is particularly troubling, for the experiences of many children living in homes with substance dependence require compassion on behalf of the public. By stigmatizing vulnerable children and youth, we are further ignoring their needs and treating them as though they are unworthy, or worse, invisible, creating a sense of oppression that can surround them for their entire lives.

9.3: CONCLUSION

Research and development in the area of relational correlates and substance use is expanding. Though the precise mechanisms by which peers, partners, siblings, and parents may influence individual substance use is not fully understood or explored, there is substantial evidence to suggest that these sociologically relevant relationships are important. The extent to which each relationship affects a person depends on several different factors, including but not limited to individual characteristics, social circumstances, close relationships, and societal perception.

NOTE

1. In many family studies, there is an assumption that dual-parent households contain a mother and a father; this, of course, is not always the case. We recognize that this is a flaw in the existing research and the generalizations that we are making. We are reporting the results as they appear in the current literature, not suggesting that dual-parent families must include a mother and father.

PARADOXES

1) The belief that one's peers are using drugs is a greater influencer on teen drug use than actual peer drug use.

2) Peers are thought to be one of the strongest correlates of substance use, yet it is not the peers that necessarily pressure individuals in the conventional way that we are taught to think about "peer pressure"—social context and type of peer associations increases or decreases substance use and addiction risk.

3) Though many people reduce family patterns of substance use and dependence to biological and psychological explanations, there are distinct and often ignored sociological factors that influence use patterns.

4) Children and youth are stigmatized for coming from a family with substance dependence, yet many of them are resilient against the familial effects of substance use.

5) Belonging to a family with a history of addiction often results in significant stigmatization of children and youth. We do not see the same sorts of stigmatization for children and youth with parents or family members who have other illnesses, yet the dominant contemporary belief is that addiction is a disease that the individual cannot control.

CRITICAL REFLECTIONS

1) Through what mechanisms do peers, partners, siblings, and parents influence individual substance use?

2) Of your various social relations, who has influenced you the most in making choices around drug use and who is currently your most significant influencer?

3) What are the strengths of using relational correlates in attempting to understand drug use and addiction in Canada?

4) What are the limits of relying only on relational correlates in attempting to understand drug use and addiction in Canada?

10 Prevention Strategies for Drugs and Potential Drug Users in Education

There are many ways in which substance use can, in theory, be prevented. As some of the topics in previous chapters have suggested, structural and environmental conditions significantly impact the likelihood of engaging in substance use and potentially experiencing problems or risks as a result of substance use. There are several conceivable structural and environmental solutions that can mediate substance use and the potential development of substance dependence. These include:

- greater opportunities for employment that pays a living wage;
- alternative education opportunities;
- affordable housing;
- community solutions for people experiencing poverty;
- universal child care; and
- financial support for extracurricular activities.

These are only a few of the potential solutions that could help prevent substance, or at least reduce the risk of substance dependence amongst higher-risk groups.

While there are programs and policies currently in place that attempt to address some of these issues, there is no guarantee that these programs will continue, nor is there any assurance that everyone will have equal access to such opportunities. Perhaps more puzzling is that despite our awareness that structural and environmental conditions increase the risk of some people becoming dependent on substances, improving these conditions is not the primary method we use to prevent drug use and its problems. Instead, the main method of prevention is drug education, which fails to directly address structural or environmental stresses. Despite being implemented institutionally via schools, the core focus of drug education is on the individual, holding them accountable for drug-using decisions and outcomes.

Aside from the significant limitations of problematizing and individualizing drug use, there is substantial debate about the effectiveness of drug education in preventing or reducing drug use and related problems. Hawthorne (2001) argues that the paradox of drug education as a prevention strategy is the disjunction between political and public ideas about effective drug education and actual evaluations of the programs being offered. He illustrates that exaggerated, ideological anti-drug messages are needed to obtain funding, yet these approaches have not produced effective drug education outcomes. As sociologist Robin Room (2003: 1) once proclaimed: "Popular approaches are ineffective, effective approaches are politically impossible."

The following chapter examines the types or levels of prevention education; various delivery methods; a few examples of promising school-based programs; the limitations of the most popular approaches; and an illustrative example of drug education programs offered in schools in Ontario.

10.1: TYPES OF PREVENTION IN EDUCATION

Educational programs focused on preventing drug use and related problems can have different goals depending on the targeted group (Figure 10.1). Prevention is typically divided into three categories: universal, selective, and indicated. These categories are sometimes used synonymously with primary, secondary, and tertiary prevention (Coggans, Evans, & O'Connor, 1999; Evans, 1999).

Universal Prevention

Universal prevention is an effort that is directed towards entire populations without consideration of the levels of risk for particular individuals (Evans, 1999). This might include all students in grade 6, or all students in general.

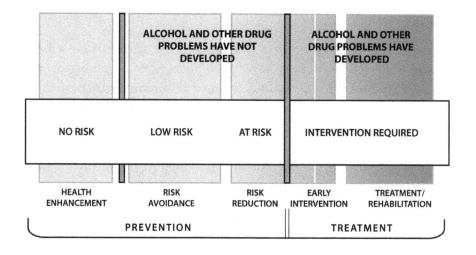

Figure 10.1: The Risk Continuum

Source: British Columbia Ministry of Children and Family Services (1998).

Depending on the intended aims of the prevention effort, the population can vary. Prevention efforts aimed at entire populations ensure that everyone has an equal chance of being exposed to programming that is intended to help build resilience, promote healthy living, and reduce the risk of using or misusing substances—or at the very least delaying the onset of use. While universal prevention efforts are beneficial for many, there are some higher-risk groups that will need additional supports and prevention programming that universal programs do not provide (Csiernik, 2016).

Selective Prevention

Selective prevention efforts are targeted at groups that have been identified as being at a higher risk for substance use and related problems (Evans, 1999). These groups have not yet initiated substance use, nor have they experienced problems as a result of substance use. Thus, selective prevention efforts attempt to address known risk factors and establish greater protective factors to potentially mitigate future substance use. The focus of selective prevention is on providing longer and more intense programming in smaller group sessions to at-risk individuals who can be easily identified based on their individual, academic, familial, demographic, and peer backgrounds (Csiernik, 2016).

Indicated Prevention

Indicated prevention is aimed at individuals who are already using substances and those who may be showing early warning signs of becoming dependent (Evans, 1999). This type of prevention is aimed at minimizing risks without the requirement of complete abstinence. Unlike universal and selective prevention strategies, indicated prevention may include treatment and maintenance programming that can be combined with family-based counselling (Csiernik, 2016). Indicated programming provides individualized support and treatment, if necessary, so that individuals do not progress in their use patterns.

10.2: DRUG EDUCATION IN SCHOOLS

The first method of formal drug prevention education that individuals usually encounter is through the school system. However, it is important to recognize from the outset that drug education occupies a rather marginal status in terms of its importance in society. Unlike the standardized education curriculum, usually determined by individual provinces, there is no consistent mandate that schools must offer comprehensive drug education, and there are no regulations concerning the type of drug education delivered. Thus, many students never receive any form of drug-related education. Those who do obtain drug education are likely exposed to ineffective programming and delivery methods (Csiernik, 2016).

The most popular school-based drug education programs have long been a subject of controversy in academic discourse, as there is significant evidence that many of these programs are either ineffective or counterproductive (Berberian, Gross, Lovejoy, & Paparella, 1976). The most widely evaluated and criticized program has been DARE, or Drug Abuse Resistance Education. During the 1990s, in particular, the DARE program underwent many formal evaluations to determine its effectiveness. Several researchers found that there were no significant changes in substance use behaviours, though the program did seem to have a positive effect on awareness, attitudes, assertiveness, and perceptions of media (Ringwalt, Ennett, & Holt, 1991; Sigler & Talley, 1995). In a meta-analysis, Ennett, Tobler, Ringwalt, and Flewelling (1994) found that DARE typically had no effect on use, and in those instances where there was an effect, changes were generally small. Clayton, Cattarello, and Johnstone (1996) conducted a five-year follow-up study of 23 schools randomly assigned DARE and 8 comparison schools. They found that there were short-term effects on attitudes towards drugs, resistance to peer pressure, and perceptions about peer substance use, but these effects disappeared within the five-year follow-up period. An even broader examination of evaluation studies of DARE conducted a decade later reaffirmed that it was ineffective at preventing drug use other than tobacco (West & O'Neal, 2004).

These small changes in use and attitudes in the short term, according to some critics, did not warrant the continued funding of DARE as a universal drug education program that, despite its demonstrated ineffectiveness, continued to grow in popularity, including having its own song. In response, the DARE programmers revised the curriculum in an attempt to improve program outcomes. Singh and colleagues (2011) compared six old DARE evaluations and one new evaluation and found that while the new DARE program had some effectiveness at influencing beliefs and attitudes, there was still no evidence of changes in actual substance-using behaviours. Both the old and new versions of DARE are based on a police model, focusing only on demand without any discussion of structural and environmental issues. DARE, like so much of the addiction field, remains focused on only the individual, without any consideration of the context of drug use; it is thus not much different from the "Just Say No" philosophy.

Why do school boards and educational decision-makers continue to select DARE as their drug education program when it has produced no demonstrable change? And why is there no government policy as to what educational programming is being delivered to students?

Gorman and Huber (2009) argue that supporters of programs like DARE selectively emphasize positive results while ignoring the negative or insignificant results of these programs. If people have no idea what is ineffective or potentially counterproductive then they cannot balance the costs with the small benefits. This helps to legitimate the continued use of ineffective programs, because some benefit is better than no benefit. While the programming of DARE is ineffective, its marketing is not, and is far superior to any other drug education program available. Moreover, with widespread law enforcement support, it is not surprising that DARE continues to be delivered despite its ineffectiveness.

Table 10.1 provides several alternative school-based prevention programs classified based on their level of prevention. While there are many other programs available, the programs here have been listed as effective or promising in two Canadian government-based reports. As the table indicates, there are more universal and selective programs than indicated programs. As well, some programs, such as Project TND (Toward No Drug Abuse) are cross-listed, in part because the objectives of the program can be adapted for different individual risk levels. However, this is also in part a reflection of a lack of consistency in how programs are classified and ways in which different researchers view these programs as having different applications. Of the programs listed, there are several initiatives developed in Canada. While this may appear promising for drug education in Canadian schools, the case study of Ontario schools at the end of the chapter suggests that effective or promising Canadian programs have historically been ignored in favour of more popular and sometimes locally developed programming that has yet to demonstrate effectiveness.

Table 10.1: School-Based Drug Education Categorized by Type of Prevention

Universal Programs	Selective Programs	Indicated Programs
All Stars	Creating Lasting Family Connections	Focus on Families
Alcohol Misuse Prevention Study	Lifestyles '94	Project SUCCESS (Schools Using Coordinated Community Efforts to Strengthen Students)
Illawara Program	Personal Growth Class	Project TND (Toward No Drug Abuse)
Project LST (Life Skills Training Program)	Project TND (Toward No Drug Abuse)	
Project ALERT	Seattle School Development Project Intervention (SOAR)	
STARS	Skills Training for College Students	
Making Decisions*	Social Competence Promotion Program for Young Adolescents	
Peer Support Program*	Aboriginal Shield*	
Student Alcohol and Drug Use Policy and School Curriculum Resources*	Opening Doors*	
Teens Against Drinking and Driving*	Families and Schools Together (FAST)*	
Tuning into Health*	Student Assistance for Everyone (SAFE)*	
Your Life: Your Choice!*		

*Canadian Program
Source: Adapted from Roberts et al. (2001) and National Crime Prevention Centre (2009).

Among the programs evaluated that are listed above, Project ALERT and Project LST were found to be promising and effective by Ghandi and colleagues (2007). Similarly, a more recent Canadian report by the National Crime Prevention Centre (2009) suggests that Project TND and Project SUCCESS are effective or promising indicated programs. The report further promotes the adoption of Project ALERT and Project LST as promising or effective universal school-based drug education programs. DARE and other similar universal programs that are widely adopted in Canada are not listed, as they have not proven to be effective, nor is their continued use in school-based programming supported by the research evidence. However, even programs that have proven to be effective are criticized for the manner in which effective programming is determined. Ghandi and colleagues (2007) found that programs considered as models of best practice—or at least promising in their outcomes—only needed to have two evaluations showing positive results. The outcomes need not be practical or important, just statistically significant. Moreover, most evaluations are conducted by the people who developed the program over relatively short follow-ups, leading many to be skeptical of the objectivity and longevity of the results.

In general, most evaluations of drug education programs do not show convincing evidence that drug education is worth the time and resources. Yet some researchers have argued that the focus on no use as the only possible positive outcome may not be the best approach to evaluating drug education programs, including DARE. As Midford (2000) argues, drug education evaluations have been focused on ideal outcomes rather than realistic ones, but drug education should be selected and evaluated based on the ability to have a positive impact on use and potential problems associated with use. More recently, Kyrrestad Strøm and colleagues (2014) conducted an evaluation that found that categorical outcomes of use versus no use, reflective of an abstinence-based approach, showed no effect; however, when use was seen as a continuous outcome—a harm reduction approach—there were small, positive changes. Thus, drug education program evaluations themselves may paradoxically be part of the problem, not the programs themselves.

Given the limited evaluations and the small changes to substance use outcomes for most drug education programs, it is questionable whether schools should be widely adopting these programs without some expectation that they will also conduct evaluations of the program upon completion and in the years that follow. However, given that drug education is not a formal requirement of school curriculum there is little impetus to do so. Mandating an evaluative component for all drug education programs would help to ensure that the best programs are being adopted, and that the ineffective programs are changed or eliminated; however, there is no provincial or national agency that has this authority.

10.3: MODELS OF DRUG EDUCATION

In addition to varying levels of prevention education based on risk, the content and modes of delivery of drug education programs vary considerably. Some programs provide knowledge about drugs, some on delaying or reducing use, while others are focused on reducing abuse and minimizing the harms associated with use (Cuijpers, 2003). There are four fundamental approaches to drug education: (1) information/knowledge models, (2) values/decision-making models, (3) social competency models, and (4) harm minimization/harm reduction models (Hawthorne, 2001).

Information/Knowledge Models

The oldest form of drug education is the information- or knowledge-based model, which became popular in the 1970s. There are two major forms of information/ knowledge delivery: basic factual information models and fear arousal information models. The former approach provides evidence-based information about drugs, their effects, and related harms; the main objective is to provide people with accurate information that will change their ideas about drugs and hopefully their drug decisions. The latter approach is premised on the idea that frightening people or making them anxious will help deter drug use. In isolation, information/knowledge approaches are ineffective at changing drug use outcomes, but they are effective at increasing awareness (Coggans, Evans, & O'Connor, 1999; Hawthorne, 2001). Thus, it is important that the information being provided to young people is accurate. Fear-arousing models are popular, even spawning television shows, but they do not produce long-term behaviour change and in fact produce more harm than no education at all (Petrosino, Turpin-Petrosino, & Buehler, 2013).

Values/Decision-Making Models

These approaches are also referred to as "life skills" or affective models. In the many variations of these educational models that have been developed, the focus is always on improving individual self-esteem, as the assumption is that youth who are lacking self-confidence are more likely to adapt to their situations with drug use. The focus of these approaches is on teaching young people to make healthy drug-wise decisions by teaching them alternative coping strategies and increasing their self-awareness (Coggans, Evans, O'Connor, 1999; Hawthorne, 2001; Lloyd, Joyce, Hurry, & Ashton, 2000). For some programs, a normative approach may also be incorporated. These strategies focus on providing facts about prevalence of use and challenging the perception that "everyone is doing drugs" (Roberts et al., 2009). The intention is to dispel the notion that all peers and adults are using substances; in turn, the individual will develop a different perception about drug use than is often the case from isolated experiences or rumours.

Social Competency Models

Social competency models, also referred to as social influence or resistance education, are founded on the assumption that individuals need to learn appropriate techniques in order to resist peer influence or pressure. These models use peers and/or community leaders, such as police officers, as the main facilitators, with the intention of exposing young people to "more realistic" socialization experiences (Hawthorne, 2001). Of all the models evaluated thus far, some researchers argue that these are the most promising, as they incorporate elements of both information and decision-making models while also being interactive (Tobler & Stratton, 1997). The paradox to this conclusion is that the classic example of a social influence model is also one that has been repeatedly demonstrated to be ineffective: DARE (Ennett, Tobler, Ringwalt, & Flewelling, 1994; Singh et al., 2011).

Harm Minimization/Harm Reduction Models

Harm minimization/harm reduction models are the most recent ones to be created. Their central idea is to deliver accurate information about the effects and harms of drugs while also providing opportunities for self-discovery, empowerment, and the general development of life-skills. Ultimately, this newest model combines elements of the previous three models, while also recognizing that abstinence may not be a realistic goal for drug education initiatives. The challenge with these models is the potential for educators to give the impression that they are condoning substance use and misuse (Hawthorne, 2001). However, if harm minimization/harm reduction is combined in a more comprehensive health education model, this issue of balancing tolerance with healthy decisions may become easier to manage and address (Hargreaves, 2011).

10.4: DRUG EDUCATORS: TEACHERS AND POLICE

While there are a variety of different people who may formally deliver drug education to young people, including parents, public health nurses, community leaders, counsellors, and members of AA (Cameron et al., 1999; Kulbok, Thatcher, Park, & Meszaros, 2012; Stanhope & Lancaster, 2013)—which in itself may be an issue—society's main drug educators remain police officers and teachers. Unfortunately, the evidence shows that there are limits to these professionals serving this function. Police officers must uphold and enforce the law, making open discussions around harm minimization and substance use, particularly illegal substance use, difficult if not impossible. Students are unlikely to participate in honest conversations about drugs out of fear that they may get into legal trouble. Not surprisingly, then, much of the information that young people actually internalize is from their peers and their own experiences rather than formal drug educators (Aldridge, Measham, & Williams, 2011; Hargreaves, 2011; Parker, Aldridge, & Measham, 1998).

There are several advantages to teachers delivering drug education, such as their rapport with students, their general understanding of classroom dynamics, and their background information on particular students in the class (Coggans, Evans, & O'Connor, 1999). However, teachers can also fail to deliver drug education in a manner that is deemed effective, accurate, and long lasting. Trained teachers combined with proven effective programs produce the best results, but this combination is rare. While the majority of teachers will teach the content, only a small proportion use effective delivery methods for this topic, and an even smaller proportion combine effective delivery with effective content (Ennett et al., 2003).

Admittedly, teachers are in a vulnerable position teaching their students about drugs, as there may be value conflicts that arise between the teacher and the curriculum resources, especially when the curriculum is geared towards abstinence only. While teachers may feel they need to teach their students about drugs in a manner that is more realistic than it is based in fear, they cannot do so when they are expected to follow an established syllabus. As long as drugs are illegal—as is every psychoactive drug for elementary and high school students except caffeine and inhalants—the public sentiment remains focused on abstinence as the only possible solution for preventing drug use and drug problems. Teachers often have little flexibility in this area, as they are in a trusted position of authority where they must uphold the law and maintain a relatively pro-social view of drugs, which has traditionally led to the demonization of all substances.

This is despite the fact that the primary reason for experimenting with drugs continues to be that it is a part of adolescence.

Another significant limitation with respect to teachers as primary drug educators is their lack of formal training in this area. Teacher's colleges and professional development days are not focused on how to best educate students about drugs, as typically drug knowledge and prevention is not a teachable credit offered during their own education. In fact, beyond personal experience and perhaps personal interest, we cannot assume that teachers have any education about drugs when they are charged with the task of educating their students.

Beyond personal experience, which is not the most valid or evidence-informed foundation for education, several researchers argue that there is a need for proper training of teachers if they are going to be involved in educating children and youth about substance use and misuse (Harris, 1998; Tupper, 2008b). As Tupper (2008b) contends, the limited education tools available to teachers in Canada are problematic in that they are not accurate and provide misleading suggestions on how to best educate young people about drugs and drug use. One viable suggestion has been to examine the ways in which sex education has evolved in Canada, and extrapolate the lessons learned from another highly contentious education debate (Tupper, 2008a).

For various practical and moral reasons, teachers will often adopt drug education programs that can be delivered by another authority who has historically wanted to fill this space: the police. This not only allows teachers to have a break from delivering lessons, but it also removes them from the uncomfortable position of not knowing the best way to deliver drug education without misleading young people, being hypocritical, or losing the respect of their students. For instance, many of the drug education programs being offered in schools, including DARE and Values, Influences, and Peers (VIP), are delivered by a community police officer. According to some researchers, police involvement in drug education helps build relationships with children and schools in general, which is a prominent reason why these authority figures continue to lead drug education programs, and why school boards continue to adopt these programs (Birkeland, Murphy-Graham, & Weiss, 2005).

However, using police as the sole drug educators in the school system may be counterproductive. As many students have anecdotally reported over the years, they do not feel comfortable asking police officers about drugs, as they are fearful of the response and the perceived consequences. They also do not feel that what they are being told by the police officers is entirely reflective of their experiences and beliefs concerning drugs. Many students actually feel as though they are less respectful of the police after their drug education, because they do not believe that they have been told the truth, while other students are utterly confused about which drugs are most harmful. When the main message being delivered is "Just Say No" or that all drugs are bad, it is difficult for individuals to make responsible and knowledge-based decisions. Instead, they rely on experiential and peer-based knowledge, which can pose significant risks (Beck, 1998; Parker, Aldridge, & Measham, 1998).

Understandably, the messages delivered by police are one-sided. It would be puzzling for a police officer to suggest that drug use is tolerable, given that most psychoactive substances are illegal, particularly for students in the school system. Moreover, it is understandable that police might highlight the negative consequences of substance use and misuse, as this is what they are most likely to experience as first responders in the community. Thus, their role as effective drug educators is inherently limited. Coggans, Evans, and O'Connor (1999) argue that police should not necessarily be the main deliverers of drug education; rather, they should adopt a supportive role. From this standpoint, the primary educators are well-trained teachers, who have had the opportunity to build a rapport with students and who have better background knowledge about them. Teachers are the most suitable educators, but again teachers face the dilemma of credibility versus pre-prepared curriculum. Drugs and drug use continue to be a morally charged issue with real legal consequences that should be understood by young people; thus, police can certainly play a part in educating them with respect to the law and safety, while supporting schools and teachers in whatever capacity is needed from a legal and safety standpoint. However, police involvement beyond these concerns should be limited. The remaining drug education, including information and knowledge awareness, building life skills and challenging norms, and social interaction and social competency, should be left for teachers to deliver to their students, despite the inherent limitations.

10.5: ONTARIO: THE CASE OF FAILED DRUG EDUCATION

In addition to the meagre evidence supporting current popularized drug education initiatives in schools across North America, there is a relative lack of consistency and standardization for deciding which drug education program is offered and who will deliver it in Ontario. Moreover, there are minimal curriculum expectations that students receive drug education in the same manner in which we provide other forms of health education, including sex education. In fact, beyond grade 9, when students are no longer required to take physical and health education, there is no expectation that students will receive any drug education unless a specific teacher decides to incorporate it in to their course.

During the months of May and June 2014, 133 randomly selected elementary schools across Ontario were contacted to identify what drug education, if any, was being offered at each selected school (Bruno & Csiernik, forthcoming). In Ontario there are 63 public and Catholic English-speaking school boards, with 3,566 elementary schools across the various boards. In addition to finding evidence that there is no consistent program being offered, the simple process of determining what program was being delivered proved to be quite difficult. Some of the schools insisted that the drug education being offered was similar across the entire school board, yet when individual schools within that board were contacted it was regularly discovered that one school was offering one program while another was offering a vastly different one. And other schools were not offering any drug education at all! Some school administrators (usually the secretaries) were unsure of what program was being offered and referred the inquiry to the school board; upon calling the school board, the researchers were advised to call individual schools and speak with individual principals. Interestingly, some schools did not want to disclose what drug education program they were offering unless it was authorized by the school board. In addition to this bureaucratic maze, and the obstruction or ignorance concerning a relatively simple question regarding a well-defined subject matter, several individuals simply did not have the time to answer "DARE" or "Project TND." In the end, there appeared to be a general sense from the school boards that individual schools propose using a specific program and the board provides approval. However, in a conversation with one principal, it was revealed that the individual teachers usually propose a particular program and the principal is responsible for approving or denying the request (Bruno & Csiernik, forthcoming).

Based on the information gathered from individual schools and school board administrators, two dominant drug education programs are primarily offered at schools across Ontario, with a handful of other programs offered in smaller numbers of schools (Table 10.2). Not surprisingly, despite the knowledge that exists, the most frequently adopted program was still DARE, at 30.1 percent (Table 10.3). The second most used program is Values, Influences, and Peers (VIP), with approximately 17 percent of schools using this program, despite the Ministry of Education in Ontario no longer endorsing this out-dated program. Interestingly, 16 percent were using a range of different programs, sometimes in addition to VIP or DARE, increasing the number of students who are being provided these popularized but unproven programs. Other programming initiatives in use included BRAVO, Kids in the Know, MADD, Racing Against Drugs, and Weeding Out Drugs. Interestingly, we could not find any evidence that either Kids in the Know or Weeding Out Drugs were specifically drug-related. Other schools reported limited drug education that was usually delivered by police officers, and only one school reported using a health nurse to deliver the education. Perhaps most surprising was the fact that the most common form of drug education in Ontario was to provide none at all. In fact, 38 percent of respondents reported they were not using any drug education programming (Bruno & Csiernik, forthcoming).

Several interesting conclusions can be drawn from this example. First and most prominently is the lack of cooperation among individual schools, administrators, and even school board officials, which indicates that there is still a reluctance to talk about drugs or drug education in any way, or acknowledge its presence in school environments. Second, there is no consistency across schools or within school boards as to which drug education program will be offered. This indicates a lack of provincial ministerial leadership on this topic. Third, there are still large proportions of schools that do not offer any form of drug education, despite the fact that many young people need this education in order to navigate their social experiences and that when drug use is delayed it is less likely to become a lifelong issue. Finally, there is limited consideration of the effectiveness of the drug education programs being delivered, as the most popular programs have been shown to be only minimally effective at best, and sometimes even counterproductive.

10.6: FUTURE OF DRUG EDUCATION: THE GOOD AND THE BAD

Over the past four decades, several different drug education programs have emerged, with varying degrees of effectiveness. The existing research suggests that the most effective programs are not widely offered, nor are they easily accessible in terms of cost and resources. Instead, DARE, an American program and one of the most criticized, continues to be offered across Canada and beyond. According to Dusenbury and Falco (1995), the success of DARE has been the result of the aggressive marketing and political support that the program has been able to establish and maintain. Despite the proven ineffectiveness of DARE, its wealth of resources means that it is easily identified by schools and school

Table 10.2: Drug and Alcohol Education Programs Currently Delivered in Ontario, 2014

Education Program	Description
DARE	Drug Abuse Resistance Education (DARE) was founded in 1983 in Los Angeles and is focused on teaching students about good decision-making skills so they can lead safe and healthy lives free from violence, substance abuse, and other dangerous behaviors. The program is led by police officers in classrooms and teaches children from kindergarten to grade 12, though it was originally designed for grades 5 and 6. The program consists of 17 one-hour sessions delivered each week. DARE's "Keeping it REAL" elementary curriculum is based on socio-emotional learning theory that highlights self-awareness/management, responsible decision-making, understanding others, relationships/communication skills, and handling responsibilities/challenges as core processes for healthy development. The program aims to teach youth impulse control, the risks and consequences of poor choices, and therefore encourages "more productive drug-free lives" (DARE America, 2016).
VIP	VIP stands for Values, Influences, and Peers. This program was introduced by the Ministry of Education and Training in Ontario in 1982 and has developed into a proactive partnership between the school community and the police. This is an awareness program targeting students in grades 6 to 8. The program highlights making good decisions, taking responsibility for actions, understanding that anyone can be influenced by peer pressure, self-respect/confidence, and respect for others. VIP covers a range of topics including drug awareness, bullying, Internet safety, social networking, and sexting (Guelph Police, 2015). Different police services offer varying numbers of sessions, though they usually range between seven and eight one-hour sessions delivered by police officers from the Community Services Unit. Classroom teachers deliver the remaining sessions.
BRAVO	Building Respect, Attitudes and Values with Others, or BRAVO, is a newer "Made in Halton" program that was developed out of the DARE program. It was created by the Halton District School Board, the Halton Catholic District School Board, and members of Halton independent schools. The program is delivered to grade 6 students by a team of Elementary School Liaison Officers (ESLOs). It consists of eight lessons, followed by a culminating activity and celebration. The program builds on topics presented in DARE, such as decision-making, peer relationships, and substance abuse (tobacco, marijuana, and alcohol), and features new areas of study, including bullying, cyber bullying, Internet safety, social media, and youth and the law (Halton Regional Police, 2015).

(continued)

Education Program	Description
Racing Against Drugs	Racing Against Drugs is a community-based drug and alcohol awareness program developed in partnership by the Royal Canadian Mounted Police, London Detachment, the staff and students of Saunders Secondary School in London, Ontario, The Whitlock/Abby Ford Quality Care racing team, and the Ford Motor Company of Canada. The objective is to utilize the sport of car racing to turn the attention of youth towards zero tolerance for drug use. It is considered a drug/alcohol awareness program geared toward grade 5 students. The program is held annually and is presented by substance abuse professionals, including police officers, educators, and addiction counsellors. It consists of four two-hour sessions held over the course of two days (RCMP, 2012).
MADD	This is a registered Canadian charitable organization aimed at reducing impaired drivers. MADD's youth program gives presentations to grades 7 to 12. There is a school assembly program, a DVD program for grades 4 to 6, a high school graduation event for grade 12 students, and several public awareness videos. The key theme of many MADD presentations is the dramatization of the consequences of impaired driving, ending with testimonials from real-life victims (MADD Canada, 2015).
Kids in the Know	This program, though identified as a drug education program by one school, is not a drug education program.
Weeding Out Drugs	Despite several searches, there was no public information available for this program.
Source: Bruno & Csiernik (forthcoming).	

Table 10.3: Percentage of Schools Offering Specific Drug and Alcohol Programming in Ontario, 2014

Program Offered	Frequency	Percentage
No education offered	50	37.6
DARE	40	30.1
VIP	22	16.5
Other	21	15.8
Total	**133**	**100**
Source: Bruno & Csiernik (forthcoming).		

boards as being the best choice for drug education. Many education decision-makers likely believe that if the program is so widely known and supported by politicians and the broader community, including law enforcement, then it must be effective. The problem, according to Dusenbury and Falco (1995), is that academics and researchers are often terrible marketers. Since the effective programs are not aggressively marketed by researchers, they are not well-known to education decision-makers. Furthermore, without marketing and political support, the effective programs often do not have the easily accessible resource support that comes with adopting DARE or VIP. If communities and policy-makers promoted and marketed more aggressively the programs that work, there is a better chance they could be more widely adopted.

Beyond marketing, it may appear puzzling that ineffective programs continue to be funded and offered in schools, though the case study of Ontario illustrates why this continues to occur. There needs to be a more consistent set of criteria for effective education, and school boards should be obliged to select programs that meet these general standards—standards set by provincial ministries of education based on empiricism, not marketing. Yet, as with most issues that are drug related, there is limited consistency in determining what criteria should be used to select effective programs. Some researchers suggest that interactive programs are superior to other forms of education (Coggans, Evans, & O'Connor, 1999; Cuijpers, 2003; United Nations Office on Drugs and Crime, 2009). In addition to interactive elements, others suggest smaller group size is important (Tobler & Stratton, 1997). Most recently, a Canadian report argued that interactive, evidence-based, and youth-focused programs are the best at reducing drug abuse, but that these programs must be taught by trained professionals, in smaller settings, with booster sessions offered for high-risk youth (National Crime Prevention Centre, 2009). Table 10.4 presents an American expert panel's recommendations for developing an effective drug education program, which could serve as a starting point for assessing appropriate curriculum.

Some of the most recent research on drug education has focused on developing what Dusenbury and Falco (1995) refer to as "additional components." In terms of media and technology, Twombly, Holtz, and Tessman (2008) found that the use of drug prevention–related multimedia tends to improve people's knowledge of drugs and drug abuse. The use of multimedia as a form of drug education, as long as it is realistic and evidence-based, may be an important way to relate to young people through a medium with which they are familiar and comfortable. Beyond increasing knowledge, Champion, Newton, Barrett, and Teesson (2013) reviewed seven different technology- or Internet-facilitated programs and concluded that

Table 10.4: Criteria for Effective Drug Education Programs

1. Research-based/theory-driven
2. Developmentally appropriate information about drugs
3. Social resistance skills training
4. Normative education
5. Broader-based skills training and comprehensive health education
6. Interactive teaching techniques
7. Teacher training and support
8. Adequate coverage and sufficient follow-up
9. Cultural sensitivity
10. Additional components (e.g., family, community, and media integration)
11. Evaluation

Source: Dusenbury & Falco (1995).

this may be a promising area for prevention of alcohol, tobacco, and cannabis use, but as with previous initiatives too little evaluation work has been completed. The findings indicated that six out of the seven programs led to a significant reduction in use. While technologically driven strategies may be helpful supplements, there is still significant importance to social relationships and ensuring that young people are obtaining a more comprehensive and engaging education about drugs than what a computer or digital device can offer. However, given the limitations of current face-to-face programs as discussed in this chapter, technological programs do not have to stretch far to achieve better outcomes.

Comprehensive drug education that incorporates media, family, schools, and the broader community appear to be the most promising approaches. According to Lloyd, Joyce, Hurry, and Ashton (2000), drug education programming should be continuous, thorough, and interactive, while also involving families and communities in the process. Other researchers have also found that the most promising areas of prevention include families and communities in their approaches (Cuijpers, 2003).

PARADOXES

1) What has been demonstrated to be effective in preventing drug use among adolescents is the least likely strategy to be employed in Ontario schools, whereas programs with no or negative outcomes are more likely to be implemented.

2) The least engaged educators in the lives of students are the most likely to provide drug education.

3) Drug education program evaluations may contribute to the problem of determining effectiveness more than the programs themselves.

4) A major paradox of drug education as a prevention strategy is the disconnect between political and public ideas about effective drug education and the actual evaluations of the programs being offered.

CRITICAL REFLECTIONS

1) What are the inherent strengths and limits of universal, selected, and integrated prevention efforts?

2) What forms of drug prevention education were you exposed to in high school? How effective was it in preventing drug use in your high school peer group?

3) Based upon the readings and your personal experience, design a drug prevention program that would have a meaningful impact upon high school students.

11 Legal Responses to Drugs and Drug Users

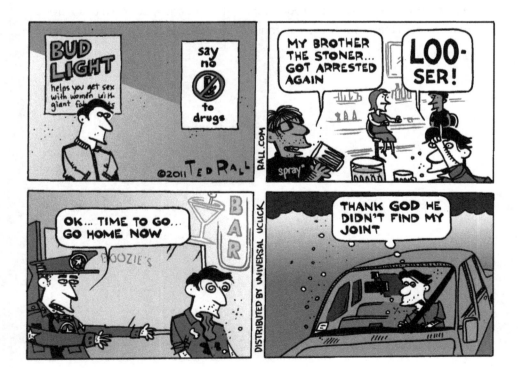

Figure 11.1: Why Does Society Tolerate and Encourage Booze Consumption While Obsessively Banning Marijuana?

Source: Copyright 2011 Ted Rall, all rights reserved, www.rall.com. Used by permission.

Despite the fact that drugs and drug use are more appropriately framed as biological, psychological, and sociological phenomena, the dominant approach to dealing with drugs and drug use remains the law and the criminal justice system. According to drug policy expert Patricia Erickson, this approach represents a central paradox in Canadian society, where "Canada has a strong public health tradition and has tended to reduce social conflicts through fairly equal access to health care, education, and social services," yet, when it comes to drugs and drug use, these more humane approaches are replaced with an unjustified commitment to criminalization (Erickson, 1999: 275).

Several hundred substances are prohibited under Canada's Controlled Drugs and Substances Act (CDSA), which carries criminal penalties for use, possession, distribution, trafficking, cultivation and manufacturing, and importing and exporting (Government of Canada, 1996, 2015a). Undoubtedly, our understanding of drugs and drug users is intimately connected with our notions of criminality, which of course itself is a social construct. When students are asked if alcohol or tobacco are drugs, the overwhelming response is "Yes, of course." However, when asked whether they and their friends do drugs on the weekend, the majority respond, "No, of course not." When challenged on these paradoxical responses, it becomes clear that they are academically aware that alcohol and tobacco are drugs, but socially drugs have come to mean substances that are prohibited under the law.

To understand the importance of law enforcement as a major priority for drugs and drug use, several researchers have examined the government's funding allocations to various areas related to substance use. In 2007, when the Conservative government launched its major policy initiative in this field, the National Anti-Drug Strategy, it was proclaimed that the focus would shift away from law enforcement and towards more harm reduction, treatment, and prevention. However, despite what was proffered, approximately two-thirds, or 63 percent, of all government funding relating to psychoactive drugs and drug use was allocated to law enforcement efforts, while just over a quarter of the total funding was divided amongst treatment, prevention, and harm reduction efforts (DeBeck, Wood, Montaner, & Kerr, 2009).

When compared, the amount of funding dedicated to law enforcement is 3 times the amount allocated to treatment, 18 times the amount given to prevention, and 28 times the amount devoted to harm reduction. Only 6 percent of all national funding is devoted to coordination and research, an area that should be given more attention if the government intends to create more effective laws and policies. Admittedly, this funding breakdown is not significantly different from previous government funding allocations. The difference, however, was the blatant and misleading commitment that the Conservatives were trying to convey to the public with the "new" National Anti-Drug Strategy.

Legal responses to psychoactive drugs and drug users exist on a continuum from complete prohibition to decriminalization to government-regulated legalization to complete legalization. Within each of these approaches there is variation in how the law is applied, if at all. Important considerations, according to some researchers, include to whom the laws will apply, under what conditions, for what substances, and why (Goldstein, 2001).

11.1: PROHIBITION

Prohibition, with respect to psychoactive drugs and drug use in Canada, is essentially criminalization. Drugs, the drug trade, and drug users are penalized under criminal law to varying degrees depending on the type of substance and type of infraction. In Canada, the Controlled Drugs and Substances Act (CDSA) is a criminal ststute, whereby any violation of the CDSA constitutes a criminal act necessitating some form of punishment, be it loss of income and assets or loss of personal freedom. As Chapters 2 and 5 illustrate, the history, politics, and legal classifications of certain substances under criminal law has little to do with the harms related to individual substances and more to do with the vested interests of particular groups in society, especially criminal justice organizations and officials. Not surprisingly, staunch advocates of prohibition have vested interests in maintaining a criminal justice approach to drugs; however, many are not willing to admit that this is the case, instead, continuing to fuel misrepresentations and punitive approaches to substance use (Griffin, Orbin, & Hayden, 2001).

Indeed, there are many legitimate health and social reasons for the continued prohibition of many psychoactive substances. One reasonable argument that is empirically supported is that there is a risk of increased substance use in the general population if prohibition were to be lifted (Caulkins, Kasunic, Kleiman, & Lee, 2014; Goldstein, 2001; Ledermann, 1956). However, it is impossible to accurately estimate if substance use would increase significantly and to what extent the health and social costs would increase in connection with these changes (MacCoun & Reuter, 2011). Moreover, many drug policy experts and economists argue that the costs associated with a potential increase in experimenters or even regular users still does not outweigh the costs associated with prohibition (Thornton, 2007).

However, there are some parallels that can be drawn from a licit drug when it is made more accessible. When Finland cut taxes on alcohol, on average deaths from alcohol use rose by eight per week, a 17 percent increase from 2003 (Koski, Sirén, Vuori, & Poikolainen, 2007), while in Norway a one-hour extension of bar closing hours led to an increase of violent nighttime weekend cases to an average of 20 per 100,000 people per year (Rossow & Norström, 2012). In Canada, when British Columbia allowed privatization of liquor stores in 2003, the total number of liquor stores per 1,000 residents quickly rose, which in turn was followed by an increase of alcohol-related deaths of 3.25 percent for each 20 percent increase in private store density (Stockwell et al., 2011). In contrast, alcohol-related disease mortality declined by 7 percent after a 1990 tax increase for spirits and beer in the state of New York (Delcher, Maldaono-Mollina, & Wagenaar, 2012).

Caulkins, Kasunic, Kleiman, and Lee (2014) distinguish two types of prohibition: de facto and de jure. *De facto* prohibition exists in practices, policies, and even market forces, but is not formally written in the laws. *De jure* prohibition, on the other hand, is written in the law with particular sanctions, but as we have learned from cannabis use rates, there is no guarantee that de jure prohibition will be widely practiced or upheld by citizens. Prohibitionist approaches can vary, from the traditional approach that uses criminal law to harshly sanction and stigmatize substance users to more pragmatic approaches that are focused on reducing harms associated with substance use, which does not need to involve the criminal justice system at all. Hall and West (2008) consider the example of tobacco regulation using a prohibitionist framework. They argue that de facto prohibition would be more likely to be implemented before du jure prohibition would ever be accepted. As was learned from alcohol prohibition, enshrining something in formal laws does not mean that people will stop doing it; in fact, there is likely to be significant backlash from individual users, civil libertarians, the tobacco industry, and even those who are concerned about the loss of tax revenue. However, regulations in conjunction with public health campaigns concerning where, when, and with whom it is legally permissible to smoke or purchase tobacco have been relatively easy to accomplish without significant resistance. Moreover, there is evidence to suggest that stricter regulations on tobacco availability, along with increasing its price through taxation, is effective at reducing the onset of tobacco use amongst youth (Gehrke, 2011; Spivak & Monnat, 2015). Conversely, formally enacting laws that attempt to completely eradicate smoking tobacco would be ineffective and subject to severe challenge from users, producers, and civil libertarians. As it stands, in Canada, tobacco is not a prohibited substance. However, it is becoming increasingly regulated through various policy changes, provincial regulations, and even municipal by-laws.

Much of the debate about the effectiveness or ineffectiveness of prohibition in the twenty-first century has focused on cannabis. From Caulkins, Kasunic, Kleiman, and Lee's (2014) classification, cannabis regulations are analogous to de jure prohibition, where there are formal laws restricting possession and use, cultivation, distribution, importation, and exportation; however, the rates of use and corresponding rates of imprisonment indicate that the laws do not deter people from using cannabis. Punitive laws restricting cannabis in Canada have long been questioned by researchers, yet strong political and moral forces continued to uphold these laws until 2017. If the empirical evidence suggests the laws are too punitive, how do such practices persist despite seemingly widespread resistance? A recent example from Sweden may help to explain.

Analyzing the discourses contained in two cannabis-related symposia in Sweden, a prohibitionist country, Månsson and Ekendahl (2015) found evidence of policy-makers, service providers, and other professionals presenting information in a way that continues to uphold problematic views of cannabis in order to legitimate continued prohibition. The researchers argued that the presenters of this information claimed to be the moral authorities, with superior scientific evidence that supported the continuation of prohibition. In order to rationalize this approach, youth become the main target of these claims, as it is believed that they are the most vulnerable and need to be protected. The researchers further concluded that using youth to legitimate a problematic view of substances such as cannabis may in fact be the mechanism by which prohibition will continue to be the dominant approach in many countries.

There are two recent examples of youth being the target of the prohibition debate in Canada. The first example is related to Conservative attack ads against the Liberals in the 2015 election campaign. This advertisement appears in Chapter 6 (Figure 6.2), and was accompanied by copious verbal claims made by the Conservatives throughout their campaign that sought to undermine the Liberal promise to legalize cannabis by claiming that Justin Trudeau wanted to make it easier for children and youth to access cannabis. However, as we discuss later in this chapter, this is not consistent with contemporary legalization policies. Nevertheless, the misunderstood aspects of legalization by the general public, in this case largely due to the misrepresentation of information, leads many to believe that this would occur if cannabis were to be legalized.

The second example involves the use of scientific research that targets the vulnerability of youth with respect to substance use. These examples, though not intentionally infused with moral messaging, includes research out of McGill University and more recently a study from Western University. The researchers at McGill found that cannabis use during adolescence induces behaviours that are similar to anxiety and depression in adulthood, and that these findings were isolated to adolescent use of cannabis, not adult use (Bambico, Nguyen, Katz, & Gobbi, 2009). Also related to the mental health of adolescents, researchers at Western University found that adolescent cannabis use mimics schizophrenic patterns in the brain that persist into adulthood; however, the same patterns do not develop from cannabis use in adulthood (Renard et al., 2017).

Undoubtedly, these studies are important for developing evidence-based policies and programs; however, there are several ways in which these studies may be used out of context to support the continued prohibition of cannabis. First, the emphasis on youth as the vulnerable group is in line with Månsson and Ekendahl's (2015) argument that prohibition will continue to exist as long as we can provide a compelling and compassionate reason for why policy-makers and society need to protect young people. From this standpoint, there is a false assumption that criminal law is somehow the only effective means of preventing young people from using substances. Secondly, the connection made between substance use and the risk of developing other mental health disorders, such as anxiety, depression, and schizophrenia—though important—is another way to induce fear in the general public about the unknown potential of developing these lifelong disorders as a result of decisions made as an adolescent. Again, prohibition offers an easy solution to avoid the potential risks, and fear of the unknown helps to legitimate responding with criminal sanctions.

Advantages and Disadvantages of Prohibition

In addition to the political and criminal justice interests that are served by prohibition, there are two important social advantages to prohibiting psychoactive substances. The first is that it reduces the number of users and overall consumption, because it is believed that illicit status is enough to deter many people from using in the first place (Goldstein & Kalant, 1990). Goldstein (2001) further argues that some drugs are inherently biologically dangerous and prohibiting them is in the best interests of society. However, determining which drugs are prohibited and which drugs are not needs to be founded on pharmacological evidence that carefully weighs the costs and the benefits of changing the legal status of the substance (such as lethal dose level).

A second benefit of prohibition is its ability to define moral boundaries and reinforce social values and norms (Duster, 1970; Goode & Ben-Yehuda, 2009; Lucas, 2009). Prohibiting psychoactive substances through the law indicates to citizens what will not be tolerated. By extension, those who violate the laws are criminalized and stigmatized, while those who abide by the law are by definition more virtuous and have a right to citizenship. Although the key to teaching people about responsible consumption may involve some element of moral boundary setting and establishing appropriate, moderate consumption patterns, the current prohibitionist practice of using the criminal law to define moral boundaries does not necessarily legitimate the use of punitive laws and practices (Husak, 2004). In fact, some would argue that we cannot legislate morality and expect positive changes and outcomes for the groups that are being criminalized (Duster, 1970), especially when drug laws are based more on race than on actual potential physical and psychological harm. A contemporary example of this is khat, which was legal in Canada until 1997 and then suddenly transformed into an illicit substance just as the Somali population of Canada, the primary users of this drug, began to increase. As in the past with opium and cocaine, prohibition was used as a way to discern who the "other" is in our society.

In contrast to the advantages of prohibition, there are several disadvantages to using the criminal justice system as a means of eradicating and controlling psychoactive substances and those who use them. Prohibition critics have highlighted several disadvantages, including the cost to taxpayers (Nadelmann, 1988; Weatherburn, 2014). As mentioned earlier, a large proportion of government tax revenues allocated to psychoactive drugs and drug users is dedicated to law enforcement, criminal justice administration, and the operation and maintenance of prisons. Unfortunately, these efforts are not alleviating drug problems in society, as the purpose is punishment and not rehabilitation, and some would even argue a criminal justice approach may make the problems worse (Erickson & Hyshka, 2010; Kellen, Powers, & Birnbaum, 2017). In addition to criminal justice costs, there are also significant social service and health care costs that could be alleviated if drugs and drug use were not as stigmatized.

A second related disadvantage of prohibition is the increase in total crime that results from various aspects of drug use and the drug trade (Nadelmann, 1988; Weatherburn, 2014). There are several ways in which crime increases when drugs are controlled through law enforcement. Under prohibition, production, sales, purchasing, and consuming drugs are all defined as crimes, which increases the total number of offences that occur each year. While the overall crime rate has decreased substantially in the past three decades, the total rate of drug offences has seen a corresponding increase of 52 percent (Cotter, Greenland, & Karam, 2015). Drug offences represent approximately 5 percent of all police reported crime, with 67 percent of drug offences being cannabis related and over half of all drug offences related to possession of cannabis. Additionally, other types of crimes committed in pursuit of earning money to purchase drugs increase when drugs are prohibited, including theft, human trafficking, and drug dealing. This is partially related to the increased likelihood of committing crimes while under the influence of drugs, and partly because of the inflated cost of drugs when they are illicit. Finally, there is a substantial amount of violence involved in the drug trade under prohibition, particularly because people involved have no legitimate recourse when wronged. Individuals must solve disputes on their own, usually through violent means (Werb et al., 2011).

Prohibition also encourages corruption, through police accepting bribes from drug dealers, stealing from drug dealers, and authorities dealing drugs themselves (Nadelmann, 1988; Weatherburn, 2014). This third disadvantage of prohibition is particularly challenging to estimate, as there are few people willing to admit that they have engaged in corrupt behaviours. As with the previous disadvantage, there are no civil options available to those involved in the drug trade being exploited by law enforcement.

Fourth, there are physical health risks and consequences that result from prohibition. Under prohibition, there is no quality control or any sort of regulatory standard for what is being sold to consumers. There is no assurance that a substance is uncontaminated, nor is there any guarantee that the potency will be the same as the previous purchase. These uncertainties pose a significant risk of tremendous physical harm for individual users and are a leading cause of drug-related overdoses and deaths.

The fifth major cost of prohibition is the undermining of morality (Nadelmann, 1988, 1989). Having a moral commitment to protecting members of society is an admirable goal; however, when the laws that are created to achieve these ends are disproportionately directed at particular groups of people and the means to achieve these goals undermine civil liberties, we need to question the measures we are willing to take to uphold a particular morality. Should family members, neighbours, and friends feel obliged to call the police if they know someone who is using or dealing drugs? What of counsellors and the harm reduction movement, working to aid those using drugs? Should people who use drugs be subject to undercover operations, surveillance, drug testing, and unlawful search and seizure practices? To engage in these questionable tactics runs counter to building a fair and equitable society.

Several additional limitations of prohibition, especially with respect to cannabis, were identified in the Le Dain Commission's final report in 1973:

- criminal records have a lasting impact on future opportunities and liberties;
- people are placed in a position where they must commit a crime or associate with criminals in order to use their drug of choice;
- criminalization facilitates the growth of deviant subcultures;
- prohibition undermines the credibility of drug education;
- criminalization creates disrespect for law and law enforcement;
- prohibition negatively influences law enforcement morale; and
- criminalization diverts police resources away from more important tasks.

Most recently, the Senate Special Committee on Illegal Drugs argued that "in addition to being ineffective and costly, criminalization leads to a series of harmful consequences" (Kenny & Nolin, 2002: 42). The report from the committee further recommended that cannabis in particular should be legalized and that proper practices for legal production and sale should be introduced, a recommendation that took a decade and a half, and a change in government, to consider.

An alternative approach to complete prohibition is to decriminalize personal use of psychoactive substances and continue to prohibit trafficking and manufacturing, a recommendation that was made by the majority of the Le Dain Commission (1973) members several decades ago and reiterated by the Senate Special Committee on Illegal Drugs (Kenny & Nolin, 2002). This approach would continue to criminally sanction those involved in the higher levels of the drug trade, while shifting away from defining users of psychoactive substances as criminals. When the majority of the members of the Le Dain Commission fully supported the decriminalization of cannabis, in particular, and further considered the decriminalization of other recreational psychoactive substances, it seemed that Canada was about to be the first nation to seriously reconsider the use of criminal law as a means of controlling personal drug use (Le Dain Commission, 1970, 1973). However, no legislative changes resulted from these recommendations until 2001, when the Marihuana Medical Access Program (MMAP) was introduced. Nearly three decades passed before any changes resulted and, truthfully, the outcome was not what the committee had originally advocated. Instead, what resulted from the MMAP was an alternative means of identifying people who consumed and produced their own cannabis, eventually criminalizing them on the basis of questionable bureaucratic inefficiencies and a presumption of illicit intentions amongst authorized MMAP patients (Lucas, 2009).

11.2: DECRIMINALIZATION

Many people tend to equate decriminalization with legalization (Bretteville-Jensen, 2006); however, they represent two different responses with distinct advantages and disadvantages. Decriminalization is a subcategory of a more general policy of depenalization, where penalties are changed or reduced. Decriminalization is essentially the removal of criminal penalties relating to the loss of personal freedom; those apprehended and charged are typically fined rather than incarcerated. Depenalization, on the other hand, can refer to any reduction or removal of penalties, both criminal and civil. Decriminalization is the term more often used with respect to illicit drug policies, though many countries and regions have different approaches that may or may not be considered decriminalization (Pacula et al., 2005).

Many view decriminalization and depenalization as a compromise between prohibition and legalization (Caulkins, Kasunic, Kleiman, & Lee, 2014). Like prohibition, there are many different ways in which countries or regions may implement it (Pacula et al., 2005). Some may reduce penalties associated with possession and use such that prison is not an option but the criminal status of the offence remains. Others may shift the focus from criminal to administrative or civil violations, whereby a system similar to traffic ticketing is used (Babor et al., 2010; Pacula et al., 2005). In some cases, individuals are given the option to enter a drug court initiative or community-based treatment program to deal with the underlying issue that led them to being caught with an illicit substance or engaging in a criminal act due to their drug use. Importantly, decriminalization only exists in its true form when all criminal penalties are removed, not just reduced, for drug use and possession offences.

In some places, decriminalization is considered de facto for some substances, usually cannabis, while other potentially "hard" drugs remain strictly prohibited (Fischer, Ala-Leppilampi, Single, & Robins, 2003). Another important distinction is the manner in which distribution and manufacturing are dealt with under the law, for in these circumstances de facto decriminalization does not apply. In fact, distribution and manufacturing are still considered criminal offences and carry fairly punitive penalties regardless of the substance. In the United Kingdom, in particular, cannabis use and possession are against the law but various discretionary measures have been put in place at various stages of the criminal justice system, from the police to the courts (Fischer Ala-Leppilampi, Single, & Robins, 2003). Since the laws state that cannabis is illegal, de facto decriminalization is only realized through discretionary criminal justice practices. There remains a risk of being held criminally responsible if an individual is continuously caught and warned.

In other countries, such as Portugal, de jure decriminalization has been formally recognized and upheld for purchase, use, and possession of all psychoactive substances, though distribution and production are still criminal offences. De jure decriminalization is when the law formally removes criminal penalties associated with drugs and drug use but still considers use an offence, usually as a civil or administrative violation (Fischer, Ala-Leppilampi, Single, & Robins, 2003). Under the Portuguese approach, substance use is viewed primarily as a health and social problem, not a criminal issue. However, the criminal justice system still plays a role in hearing cases and providing judgments on the appropriate course of action for individuals. People who do not abide by court orders risk facing formal criminal sanctions (Babor et al., 2010).

Advantages and Disadvantages of Decriminalization

Some have referred to decriminalization as a "middle path" or compromise between prohibition and legalization (Caulkins, Kasunic, Kleiman, & Lee, 2014). In this sense, there are a few important advantages to decriminalization over prohibition and legalization. The first advantage of decriminalization is that it has greater public support than legalization. For instance, an Angus Reid public opinion poll from 2012 indicated 57 percent of Canadians support legalizing cannabis (MacQueen, 2013). Not surprisingly, a more recent opinion poll of Canadians from Global News Ipsos showed that 65 percent of adults would like to see cannabis decriminalized (Armstrong, 2015). There is a possibility that there is confusion amongst citizens as to the differences between decriminalization and legalization as policy options; nevertheless, there is certainly evidence of a shift in attitudes, with decriminalization supported by more people than legalization. The extent to which decriminalization would be supported for other psychoactive substances beyond cannabis in Canada is unknown. However, if people were given more honest information about drugs and drug use, we could speculate that decriminalization might be preferred over prohibition.

Part of the reluctance to support legalization is founded on the assumption that making a substance legal suggests that it is now acceptable or at least tolerable. This creates a cognitive dissonance, and society questions the authority of leaders who have created policies and practices indicating these drugs were unsafe and were ruining communities. If they were wrong regarding this issue, what other policies and practices can now also be brought into question? A second advantage of decriminalization is that it does not support or condone drug use in the way that many people feel legalization does for alcohol and tobacco. This is also certainly supported by current licit drug interests, such as the brewing industry, who economically fear alternative competitive licit drug options. At the same time, decriminalization conveys the message that people who use drugs are not criminals in the same sense as people who commit murder, theft, or fraud. Of course, as not all substances are equally harmful, support for decriminalization is likely to vary by substance (Faupel, Horowitz, & Weaver, 2010).

Finally, under decriminalization, criminal sanctions still remain for trafficking and production without authorization. This directs law enforcement efforts to the supply rather than the demand for substances, which is better addressed with treatment and education. The current system of criminalizing drug use and possession, especially for cannabis, has led to a significant burden on the criminal justice system and few resources are being directly targeted at the sources; instead the focus is on drug users and street-level dealers, as they are the most visible, vulnerable, and easy targets.

Although decriminalization removes criminal penalties from possession and use, and depenalization reduces or removes penalties altogether, there are still many of the same limitations with decriminalization as there are with prohibition. Moreover, decriminalization does not necessarily remove legal sanctions, as there is still a possibility that civil law can regulate what is acceptable and what is prohibited. Like legalization, there are some who argue that removing or reducing criminal penalties will still increase the total number of people who experiment with certain drugs and will perhaps continue using (Bretteville-Jensen, 2006).

Debates also remain regarding the overall effectiveness of decriminalization in preventing individual and social harms. It is difficult to estimate what, if any, changes in use patterns are related to policy change or enforcement practices. In Australia and Portugal, where there were changes or reductions in penalties and the formal removal of criminal sanctions, the official records of drug use or possession charges actually increased after the policy changes (Fischer, Ala-Leppilampi, Single, & Robins, 2003; Weatherburn, 2014). These increases cannot be directly connected to the policy shift, as there is no way to control for the law enforcement practices that existed prior to the changes. However, there is some indication that the total number of drug users increased on the official record because the new enforcement practice of ticketing was easier to implement. The more important concern is whether or not the changes in policy resulted in greater individual and social harms, which is far more difficult to estimate.

Another related disadvantage is that the increased crime and physical harms of the illegal drug trade remain under decriminalization. While possession and use-related harms related to criminal justice responses would abate, the illicit market would still be unregulated, encouraging individual criminal involvement outside of drug use, corruption amongst law enforcement, and the systemic violence inherent in an illicit market (Faupel, Horowitz, & Weaver, 2010).

11.3: LEGALIZATION

Legalization, despite its seeming simplicity, is actually more complicated a concept than either prohibition or decriminalization, as there are three distinct approaches: free-market legalization, limited-distribution legalization, and medical legalization. Similar to decriminalization policies, legalization is de facto for some substances, usually cannabis, in some places, while other potentially "hard" drugs remain strictly prohibited, as is the case with heroin, cocaine, or crystal meth consumption. In some nations, the purchase and sale of cannabis is tolerated and available in predetermined authorized outlets, though still technically illegal (Fischer, Ala-Leppilampi, Single, & Robins, 2003). For instance, in the Netherlands, personal consumption of cannabis is tolerated and even sold in designated coffee shops. However, according to the law, it is still illegal to possess or sell cannabis. Owners of the well-known coffee shops are not immune to criminal penalties for their role in providing cannabis to customers, especially if there is an incident with a tourist. They must follow strict regulations concerning the amounts that they are selling to individuals and the amounts they have in their possession at any given time, or they may face severe sanctions (Babor et al., 2010). In this particular case, cannabis is considered de facto legalized because it is available in the market and there is rarely any enforcement against individual users.

De jure legalization can also come in many different forms. The most recent example of de jure legalization in the United States is cannabis in Colorado, Oregon, Alaska, and Washington state (Room, 2014). While cannabis is still federally illegal in the United States, individual states have the liberty of making their own regulations. Interestingly, federal statues supersede the state laws, still leaving the federal drug agencies with the authority to shut down and criminally charge individual users and distributors (Caulkins, Kasunic, Kleiman, & Lee, 2014). As well, presently the cannabis industry is a "cash only" enterprise, as by accepting a credit card a business would be breaking federal law. Moreover, these changes in state laws are in violation of international drug conventions, which hold greater power than the federal and state laws, suggesting international treaties will need to be addressed in the near future (Room, 2014).

Free-Market Legalization

Freedom and choice are central to a democratic capitalist society. Free-market legalization is founded on the notion of freedom with responsibility, which is akin to the founding principles of neo-liberalism, a sweeping global socio-political movement (Harvey, 2005). At the beginning of the twentieth century in Canada there were no restrictions on any substance, including alcohol, nicotine, opium, and cocaine, though there had been several attempts to ban alcohol. Of all the possibilities for legalization, free-market legalization is the most liberal of all the models. As Thomas Szasz (1992) argued, it is our human right to buy and sell drugs, regardless of the potential harms associated with such substances, for the notion of licit and illicit is at its foundation a social construct. Importantly, people who advocate for free-market legalization, even Szasz, are not advocating for children or other vulnerable groups who do not have the capacity to make rational decisions to have access to psychoactive substances. It is usually advocated by civil libertarians who believe that it is every adult citizen's right to choose what they consume and that psychoactive substances are like any other commodity that should be available for purchase in the market.

A current example of free-market legalization of a psychoactive substance in Canada is caffeine, which is available in a variety of different outlets and products across the country with no regulations. Despite the argument that even free-market legalization prevents access to children and others who may not have the capacity to understand the harms associated with certain substances, caffeine is widely available to children and adults alike. There are no regulations in place that limit access to children, even for highly caffeinated products such as energy drinks. One does not have to look far to find a Tim Hortons or Starbucks, where they can purchase caffeine in one of its most notable forms: coffee and tea. In addition to special coffee shops devoted to selling caffeine, convenience stores, grocery stores, and even vending machines provide ample opportunity for individuals to purchase caffeine in its many available forms.

Similarly, solvent and inhalants are among the most physically harmful psychoactive substances ever created, yet no one would ever consider placing broad societal restrictions on who can buy gasoline, whipping cream, rubber cement, or nail polish remover. In fact, these readily available substances are not even considered drugs, despite the fact that even short-term use causes brain damage and can lead to premature death regardless of a user's age.

Some argue that free-market legalization is not a viable solution for psychoactive substances that are currently controlled (Goldstein & Kalant, 1990; Jones, 2010). This is especially evident in our experiences with alcohol and tobacco, where economic business interests are not concerned about protecting the health of citizens, leading to substantial numbers of citizens consuming the substances and experiencing devastating effects. It is not the mere consumption that is necessarily problematic with these substances; rather, it is the negative health and social consequences that result from their use that is undesirable.

Limited-Distribution Legalization

According to some advocates of legalization, a limited distribution model with age restrictions and regulated outlets would be more effective and humane than the current criminal justice approach (Nadelmann, 1988). On a continuum of legalization practices ranging from completely unrestricted, as is the case with free-market legalization, to strictly regulated legalization, such as medical legalization, the limited-distribution model falls in the middle. Limited distribution refers not only to who can have access to substances but also where and when the substances can be sold.

In Canada, both alcohol and tobacco are legalized under a limited-distribution model, but the model differs by province and territory. While there are federal legislations guiding provincial decisions, each province and territory is responsible for setting regulations and controlling the distribution and access to alcohol. For instance, in Ontario, most alcohol is distributed through government-regulated outlets known as the Liquor Control Board of Ontario (LCBO). However, beer and wine are available through privately owned, but strictly controlled, retail outlets. The Beer Store in Ontario is the most common place to purchase beer, but a few retailers are authorized by the provincial government to sell smaller quantities of beer and wine, a model that is similar in other provinces, such as Quebec, where beer and wine are commonly available in grocery stores and convenience stores. The drinking age also varies by province, with a minimum legal drinking age of 18 in Quebec, Manitoba, and Alberta and 19 in the remaining provinces and territories (see Table 11.1).

The limited-distribution model is more relaxed for tobacco than for alcohol, though there are still restrictions. In all of the provinces and territories, tobacco sales are privatized, meaning the products are available in a variety of non-governmental outlets. Prior to the legislative crackdowns and tax increases in the late 1980s through to the early 1990s, tobacco was widely available and unmonitored (Studlar, 2002). Children could bring a note to the store and purchase cigarettes for their parents, and vending machines that dispensed cigarettes to anyone were located in various places with no monitoring. Since the legislative changes, tobacco control has become much more regulated, with severe penalties for retailers and individuals who violate the law. Under federal legislation enacted in 1997, the Tobacco Act, it is against the law to sell or provide individuals under the age of 18 with tobacco. Provincially, the minimum age to purchase tobacco varies from 18 to 19 years of age. In Alberta, Saskatchewan, Manitoba, Quebec, Yukon, and the Northwest Territories the minimum age to purchase tobacco is 18. The remaining provinces and territory set the limit at 19 (Pope, Chaiton, & Schwartz, 2015). Even more complicated is the ability of regions or municipalities to develop their own tobacco control regulations, concerning where smoking is or is not allowed (Studlar, 2002). Thus, in Canada, there are federal, provincial, and municipal laws that govern tobacco sales and use.

Though tobacco is currently more widely available than alcohol, the limited-distribution model of tobacco is becoming increasingly restrictive. This is opposed to alcohol distribution, which is becoming more relaxed in jurisdictions including British Columbia, Ontario, and Quebec. If public health is the foremost concern of policy-makers concerning tobacco, why is the same not true for alcohol? It seems there is a contradiction in the way different substances are treated under the law and both the market and the social acceptability of the substance have important roles to play.

Medical Legalization

Medical legalization is considered the most restrictive model of legalization. Along with pharmaceutical psychoactive drugs such as sedative-hypnotics and antidepressants, which are legal for medicinal purposes, there are only two other types of substances under the CDSA that fit a quasi-medicalized status in Canada: cannabis and opioids. While legalization has long been advocated for cannabis in Canada (Le Dain Commission, 1970), the only departure from criminalization has been the medical use of cannabis (Fischer, Kuganesan, & Room, 2015). The first formal attempt to medically legalize cannabis came in

Table 11.1: Tobacco and Alcohol Regulations by Province and Territories in Canada, 2016

Province/ Territory	Tobacco	Alcohol
Alberta	Banned smoking in public spaces and workplaces Tobacco display ban Illegal to sell to minors	Drinking Age: 18 Private retailer market Restaurants can apply for a liquor permit that will allow them to serve wine that customers bring themselves
British Columbia	Banned smoking in all public spaces and workplaces Displays of tobacco visible to people under the age of 19 banned in public areas Ventilated smoking rooms only permitted in nursing homes and care facilities Banned smoking in vehicles with children under 16 Smoking ban does not apply to hotel rooms	Drinking Age: 19 Beer, wine, and spirits are sold in provincially owned and private liquor stores. Craft beer can be purchased at the brewery.
Manitoba	Banned smoking in all public spaces and workplaces Banned retail displays of tobacco Restricted promotion and advertising of tobacco and tobacco-related products Banned smoking in vehicles with children under 16	Drinking Age: 18 Mix of government-run and private wine and beer stores Hotels are allowed to sell beer as licensed vendors
New Brunswick	Banned smoking in public spaces and workplaces Ventilated smoking rooms are not permitted Banned retail displays of tobacco Banned smoking in vehicles with children under 16	Drinking Age: 19 Restaurants can apply for a liquor permit that will allow them to serve wine that customers bring themselves

Province/ Territory	Tobacco	Alcohol
Newfoundland and Labrador	Banned smoking within public places Ventilated smoking rooms are permitted only in psychiatric facilities and long-term care facilities Sales of tobacco are prohibited in places such as retail stores that have a pharmacy, university and college campuses, and recreational facilities Banned smoking in vehicles with children under 16	Drinking Age: 19 Beer is available in various convenience stores Liquor and beer sold at provincially owned liquor store outlets Wine sold at provincially owned liquor store outlets
Nova Scotia	Banned smoking in public spaces and workplaces Ventilated smoking rooms are permitted in nursing homes and care facilities Banned retail displays of tobacco Banned smoking in vehicles with children under 19 Minors are prohibited from possessing tobacco products	Drinking Age: 19 Government-only markets
PEI	Banned smoking in public spaces and workplaces Ventilated smoking rooms are only allowed in long-term care facilities	Drinking Age: 19 Government-only markets
Ontario	Banned smoking in public spaces and workplaces Ban on retail displays of tobacco Banned smoking in vehicles with children under 16 Smoking prohibited province-wide on all bar and restaurant patios Tobacco sales prohibited on college and university campuses Many Ontario municipalities have passed smoke-free bylaws	Drinking Age: 19 Can purchase at the Beer Store, the Liquor Control Board of Ontario, Wine Racks, and select grocery retailers for beer Restaurants can apply for a liquor permit that will allow them to serve wine that customers bring themselves

(continued)

Province/ Territory	Tobacco	Alcohol
Quebec	Banned smoking in public spaces and workplaces The province eliminated designated smoking rooms The sale of electronic cigarettes is regulated like tobacco Prohibited to sell flavoured tobacco products, including menthol As of May 2016, smoking and e-cigarettes will be banned in certain vicinities	Drinking Age: 18 Can buy beer in corner stores and grocery stores Restaurants can apply for a liquor permit that will allow them to serve wine that customers bring themselves
Saskatchewan	Banned smoking in public places and workplaces Tobacco display ban Banned smoking in vehicles with children under 16	Drinking Age: 19 Beer, wine, and spirits are sold at provincially owned liquor stores, rural franchises licensed by the government, and in three privately owned stores.
Northwest Territories	Banned smoking in public places and workplaces	Drinking Age: 19
Nunavut	Banned smoking in public spaces and workplaces	Drinking Age: 19
Yukon	Banned smoking in public spaces and workplaces	Drinking Age: 19

2001 under the Marihuana Medical Access Program (MMAP). Over the course of a decade, the number of people accessing medical marijuana increased from 500 to over 30,000 (Health Canada, 2013b). In 2013, the MMAP was replaced with the Marihuana for Medical Purposes Regulations (MMPR) (Government of Canada, 2014). This newer legislation attempted to take away individual authorization to grow for personal consumption and place production under the control and regulation of authorized distributors. However, this was challenged and repealed by the Supreme Court of Canada (Health Canada, 2015). The current regulation, the Access to Cannabis for Medical Purposes Regulations, came into effect in 2016. This new regulation permits users with medical permission to grow cannabis for personal consumption, rather than requiring users to purchase from Health Canada–authorized distributors (Government of Canada, 2016).

These regulations, though important steps towards more sensible cannabis policy, are still not considered de jure legalization. While cannabis continues to be illegal for recreational purposes, it is de facto legalized for medically authorized uses (Fischer, Kuganesan, & Room, 2015). The formal introduction of regulations in 2002, 2013, and 2016 is still considered de facto legalization for medicinal purposes, as the substance being regulated, cannabis, is still criminally sanctioned for recreational users (Government of Canada, 2015a). Medical de facto legalization creates significant confusion amongst citizens as to the penalties and the increased availability of cannabis through various dispensaries that were authorized for medical purposes (Dauvergne, 2009; Leblanc, 2016).

With respect to opioids, Canadian researchers led a brief trial study from 2005 to 2008 called the North American Opiate Medication Initiative (NAOMI), which can be broadly classified as a medical legalization model (Oviedo-Joekes et al., 2008). NAOMI was conducted in Vancouver and Montreal to evaluate the feasibility and effectiveness of Heroin Assisted Treatment (HAT) in Canada. The results of the drug trial found that participants were less likely to use street drugs than those in a methadone maintenance program, and were also less likely to engage in criminal activity, increasing the likelihood of an eventual move towards abstinence (Nosyk et al., 2010). A follow-up, the Study to Assess Long-term Opioid Medication Effectiveness (SALOME), compared prescription heroin with hydromorphone. It too reported superior outcomes among those using the prescription heroin, which further reinforced the findings of earlier outcome studies from the United Kingdom, Germany, the Netherlands, and Switzerland (Ferri, Davoli, & Perucci, 2011).

The results of the two Canadian studies led to a recommendation by Health Canada to allow prescription heroin use among individuals not successfully using methadone. However, Conservative Health Minister Rona Ambrose objected to Health Canada's approval and introduced regulations intended to make prescribing the drug outside of clinical trials illegal. However, British Columbia Supreme Court Chief Justice Christopher Hinkson ruled against the minister of health, stating that risks would be reduced under this specialized medical program for the 202 SALOME participants authorized by Health Canada to receive the drug (Woo, 2014).

With the change in government it appears that properly screened individuals will be eligible for HAT programs, joining those participating in methadone maintenance and methadone treatment programs. There is a much greater emphasis on treatment, education, and respect for the individual user in harm reduction programs compared with law enforcement–informed approaches. Thus, public health medicalized approaches are indications of progress towards a non-criminalized model for psychoactive substances; however, we cannot be sure of the extent to which medicalizing substance use will be an effective alternative. Given that medicalization is synonymous with pathology, this fails to acknowledge the functional and even rewarding aspects of substance use for many people.

Advantages and Disadvantages of Legalization

In addition to some of the benefits and drawbacks of legalization mentioned above, there are several other advantages and disadvantages (Table 11.2). Advocates of legalization tend to draw on the counter evidence to prohibition and decriminalization to support their arguments. A key economic contention is that legalization would allow for the generation of tax revenue from the production and sale of psychoactive substances, creating new employment opportunities; similar to the current system with alcohol and tobacco, it would in turn provide greater amounts of public funding for health and social services. This action would also negate some of the economic resources and power of organized crime, though it would also inevitably shift this sector to search for other sources of revenue (Ducatti, 2012; Nadelmann, 1988). In addition, assuming that the appropriate public health strategies are used to ensure that there is not a corresponding increase in drug abuse, some argue that legalization will increase quality of life and general health amongst substance users, something that is clearly lacking when law enforcement is the primary focus. Quality control would also most likely be enhanced, as legal recourse would be possible if an impure substance was sold to consumers. Furthermore, shifting to a health and social welfare approach means there will be less government spending on law enforcement. Finally, in a legalized and regulated market, there will be less drug-related crime and corruption.

Two of the most significant disadvantages of legalization are the uncertainty and limited evidence supporting legalization of formerly illicit substances. Ledermann's (1956) work with alcohol indicates that the fewer the restrictions, the greater the increase in use. However, it is uncertain if legalization would result in increased drug abuse or dependence, as the existing evidence is conflicting and varies by time and place. Moreover, there are not enough cases of illicit drugs being totally legalized to know in advance, with any certainty, whether the negative aspects of drug use and abuse can be better controlled through something other than the criminal justice system (Goldstein & Kalant, 1990). Indeed, Taylor, Buchanan, and Ayres (2016) warn that following through with more pragmatic approaches that have not demonstrated effectiveness is not much different than continuing with punitive prohibitive approaches that are ineffective. Evidence should be the driving force of drug policy, not ideology, even if it is seemingly pragmatic. We have to ensure that the responses, regardless of whether or not they appear to makes sense, do not create more harm.

Medical legalization, such as HAT and NAOMI, are the closest examples of current illicit substances for which we have long-term evidence on their effectiveness from controlled trials. However, there are limitations in using this as a standard for other illicit substances. The number of people who access these services is relatively small and there is no evidence to suggest that this method would be effective for other substances (MacCoun & Reuter, 2011). Goldstein (2001) further argues that not all substances should be treated equally, as some pose greater physical harms than others and should be strictly prohibited, while the prohibition of some other substances clearly undermines the integrity of our laws. Conducting a comprehensive cost-benefit analysis of the pharmacological, toxicological, sociological, and historical evidence, Goldstein and Kallant (1990) argue that changing the legal status of currently illegal drugs would make drug problems worse, not better, in most cases.

Recent examples of cannabis legalization from Washington and Colorado will likely offer significant insight into legalization of cannabis in particular, though again, we should not assume that these experiences will apply to all places at all times. As Canadians intently watch to see what unfolds, it is likely that the potential positive and negative consequences of legalization will be delayed, and will only become fully evident in years to come, as occurred with other substances such as barbiturates and benzodiazepines. However, preliminary evidence suggests that the key to effective legalization for individuals is public health, not free-market capitalism (Room, 2014).

11.4: CONCLUSION

There are several different legal responses to psychoactive substances that are presently being applied. In some cases, drugs are deemed socially acceptable and even promoted in society, as is the case with alcohol and caffeine. In other cases, despite being legal, some substances are becoming less tolerated and more stigmatized, as is the case with tobacco, while some are simply ignored, like solvents. Beyond these legally available substances, there are several other psychoactive substances that are used both medicinally and recreationally, though many of

Table 11.2: Advantages and Disadvantages of Different Types of Legal Responses

Legal Response	Advantages	Disadvantages
Prohibition	• Reduces the number of users and overall consumption • Defines moral boundaries and reinforces social values and norms	• Cost • Increase in total crime • Encourages corruption • Physical health risks and consequences • Undermines morality • Criminal records have a lasting impact on future opportunities and liberties • People are placed in a position where they must commit a crime or associate with criminals in order to use their drug of choice • Growth of deviant subcultures • Undermines credibility of drug education • Creates disrespect for law and law enforcement • Negatively influences law enforcement morale • Diverts police resources
Decriminalization	• Greater public support than for legalization • Does not support or condone drug use • Criminal sanctions still remain for trafficking and production without authorization	• Some indication that the total number of drug users increases • Increased crime and physical harms of the illegal drug trade remain in place
Legalization	• Generation of tax revenue from the production and sale of psychoactive substances • Quality of life and general health amongst substance users	• Uncertainty • Limited evidence to support legalization of formerly illicit substances

them are strictly prohibited under Canadian law. As this chapter illustrates, there is a broad continuum of practices when it comes to regulating substances, from prohibition to decriminalization to legalization. Most of the debate centres on prohibition versus legalization, yet decriminalization also has great support (Thornton, 2007; Armstrong, 2015). Evidence of the effectiveness of each of these approaches is relatively limited, with the exception of prohibition. We have clearly seen that prohibition does not work in its current form, yet remains a dominant response not only in Canada but also globally. However, the evidence on decriminalization is also mixed, even in countries that have adopted this approach for all psychoactive substances (Hughes & Stevens, 2012). In general, there is limited evidence on which to base future decisions about psychoactive substances and the role of law enforcement. As drug policy experts have aptly argued: "Changing the legal status of a drug is no silver bullet; it's more 'trading the devil you know for the devil you don't know'" (Caulkins, Kasunic, Kleiman, & Lee, 2014: 285). Based on the lessons we have learned from over a century of prohibition, is this a risk we should be willing to take? Probably. For, just like the recommendation from solution-focused therapy, if something, works do more of it—but if it doesn't work, do something different.

PARADOXES

1) Despite the extensive biological, psychological, and sociological research that frames drug use in Canada, the dominant approach remains a criminal justice model.

2) Despite the extensive biological, psychological, and sociological research that frames drug use in Canada, the criminal justice system receives the majority of drug-related funding.

3) Canada has a strong public health tradition and has tended to reduce social conflicts through fairly equal access to health care, education, and social services, yet when it comes to drugs and drug use, these more humane approaches are replaced with an unjustified commitment to criminalization.

CRITICAL REFLECTIONS

1) Why, in the twenty-first century, are psychoactive drugs still viewed primarily thorough a criminal justice lens?

2) Differentiate between decriminalization and legalization. Which approach has the best arguments for implementation in Canada?

3) Disregard the current socially constructed status of the following psychoactive agents and, using only the facts, discuss what legal status you would recommend for the following substances and why:

   i)   Heroin and methadone

   ii) Barbiturates and alcohol

   iii) Coca, Ritalin, and nicotine

   iv) LSD and cannabis

   v)   Lithium and anabolic steroids

12 International Drug Policies

As the previous chapter illustrated, there is significant variation under the law in how drug policies and practices are upheld in Canada and internationally. In terms of legal responses to drugs and drug users, the vast majority of countries use variations of prohibition or decriminalization rather than legalization. This is not coincidental. Beyond country-specific laws and policies, there are three international drug conventions that govern the worldwide response to drugs and drug users, all of which are intended to restrict the types of approaches to drugs and drug users that are considered appropriate (Dion, 1999; Room, 2012). However, dealing with substance use and the drug trade requires flexibility and a recognition that various places and time periods require different responses (Reinarman, 2004). Thus, not all regulations are followed in all countries, making these nations vulnerable to consequences from the international community if they are too lenient with their drug regulations. The purpose of this chapter is to provide an international overview of policies used to control drugs and drug users. A brief overview of international drug conventions and the limitations that these agreements place on countries is provided, followed by examples of three countries with punitive drug policies and three countries with more pragmatic approaches.

12.1: INTERNATIONAL DRUG CONVENTIONS

There are three international drug conventions that currently govern the worldwide response to policies governing drugs and drug users. Each convention covers a range of substances and activities related to both the supply and demand of most, but not all, psychoactive drugs. One unintended outcome has been the rise in development of new synthetic drugs that fall outside any of the existing conventions.

The Single Convention on Narcotic Drugs was not the first international agreement concerning psychoactive substances; however, it is the oldest of all the international treaties on drugs that is still enforced. Originally ratified in 1961, the Single Convention was later amended by the Geneva Protocol in 1972 (United Nations, 1972). The Single Convention governs the legitimate use, treatment, production, and trade of opium, coca, cannabis, and any of the related derivatives of these three substances. The only permitted use, production, and trade of these three types of substances is for medical and scientific purposes, which are also strictly regulated. Recreational use, production, and distribution is prohibited and nations are dictated to punish these actions under their respective criminal laws (Room & Reuter, 2012).

The Single Convention was created with the intended objective of protecting public health while still ensuring adequate supplies of medically useful substances were available to countries in need (United Nations, 1972). The convention contains four drug schedules that have been continuously updated, though none of these schedules directly correspond with the schedules contained in Canada's Controlled Drugs and Substances Act (Government of Canada, 2015a). Interestingly, under the Single Convention countries must abide by a minimum set of regulations concerning the production and use of opium, coca, and cannabis; however, there are no restrictions on individual countries imposing stricter measures or more severe sanctions (Dupras, 1998).

Though Canada is a party to the Single Convention and its amendments, our government was not one of the original signatories. Canada waited until 1976 to agree to the Single Convention and even then expressed reservations regarding restrictions on importing and exporting some of the listed substances. There were also concerns about extraditing individuals charged with drug trafficking within Canadian borders to other signatory nations, due to the harsher penalties placed upon those convicted in other countries, including capital punishment (United Nations, 1972).

In the interim, the Vienna Convention on Psychotropic Substances was enacted in 1971, which extended the international regulations beyond opium, coca, and cannabis to include additional psychoactive substances, including commonly prescribed pharmaceutical medications (United Nations, 1971). Similar to the Single Convention, the Vienna Convention contains four drug schedules. However, the substances contained in the Vienna Convention refer more to psychoactive substances that are prescribed by doctors, with only a few exceptions. The Vienna Convention sets out regulations relating to hallucinogens, tetrahydrocannabinol (THC), amphetamines, barbiturates, hypnotics, tranquilizers, and some additional analgesics. Each of the restricted substances is classified based on the drug's apparent therapeutic value. Drugs classified as Schedule I are deemed to have no therapeutic value, which includes hallucinogens and THC. Drugs classified as Schedule IV are deemed useful for therapeutic purposes, including analgesics, hypnotics, and tranquilizers. The classification schemes are puzzling, as there appears to be limited consistency in how the drugs are classified. The Single Convention has four schedules for which there is no clear rationale, while the Vienna Convention does attempt to make clear distinctions within its four schedules—but without indicating what evaluative criteria were used in the decision-making process. The most obvious example is THC, the psychoactive component of cannabis, which is listed in the Vienna Convention but not included in the Single Convention under cannabis restrictions. Furthermore, the current classification of psychoactive substances under Canada's CDSA does not directly correspond to the 1971 Vienna Convention.

The third and most recent international drug treaty is the Convention against Illicit Traffic in Narcotic Drugs and Psychotropic Substances, ratified in 1988 at the height of the War on Drugs rhetoric (United Nations, 1988). This international law extends drug control to precursor substances and places greater emphasis on the collaborative efforts of countries attempting to eliminate the illicit trafficking of the substances contained in all three conventions.

The actual authority of the conventions is not much different than other international treaties, with vast differences between intentions and actual implementation. Rohypnol, which became known as the date rape drug, was a legal prescription drug in Mexico and illegal in the rest of North America, but if you had a Mexican prescription you could travel with the drug without its confiscation into Canada or the United States. The president of Bolivia, Evo Morales, was a coca farmer before moving into politics, and the nation depends on coca production for its economy. Likewise, khat is an economic staple of Kenya, yet illegal in North America, while ketamine (Special K), which has severe restrictions in the West, is vital in developing nations as it is among the least expensive and easiest to produce anesthetics. Similarly, Canada's CDSA conflicts with several of the stated conventions, which has led some drug experts to argue that instead of the conventions changing, the more likely course of events will involve individual countries denouncing or withdrawing from the agreements and then seeking to rejoin them with reservations (Room, 2012).

The lack of actual authority of the conventions also results in minimal protections against extremely punitive actions that some countries take against their own citizens (Bewley-Taylor, 2013; Dupras, 1998). In contrast to what could be considered barbaric treatment of drug users, other nations are moving away from the "War on Drugs" mentality and are becoming more pragmatic, tolerating recreational use of psychoactive substances through legalization or decriminalization and focusing on education and treatment rather than criminalization and punishment. Though there needs to be flexibility in international agreements to allow for individual countries to respond to drug issues independently, there also needs to be a basic expectation that countries cannot purposefully harm citizens for drug offences, either by being too punitive with users or too lenient with traffickers. In addition, there needs to be some form of quality control over the creation of new synthetic drugs developed purely for recreational use.

12.2: PUNITIVE POLICIES

There is significant variation in the policies and practices related to drugs and drug use, even among countries that are known for severe responses to drugs. While there are many reasons why different countries have distinct approaches, two common themes amongst the more punitive countries are economic trade and the role of the state in individual lives. Russia, China, and Iran are three notable examples of nations that have punitive policies. In Russia, drug policies are reflective of the challenges of free-market trade and the transition to a democratic state that has occurred since the fall of the Iron Curtain in 1989 (Paoli, 2002). For China and Iran, researchers and the government alike argue that free-market trade and geographic location are the major issues contributing to drug availability and the significant rise of drug use problems (Nissaramanesh, Trace, & Roberts, 2005; Wen, 2014).

Russia

Since the collapse of the Soviet Union in 1991, Russia has seen an enormous growth in drug trade and use; prior to this time, drug use and abuse was not reported as a significant societal problem. Cannabis and heroin are the two most commonly used illicit substances in Russia, though alcohol remains the most prominent public health issue (Koposov, Ruchkin, Eisemann, & Sidorov, 2002; Leon et al., 2007). Some researchers have argued that the transition to a market-based economy and a democratic state have led to a surge in heroin use in particular (Paoli, 2002), yet methadone and other substitution treatments for opioid dependence are banned (Lancet, 2011). Moreover, there are strict regulations, even for terminally ill patients requiring pain medications (Clark, 2015), which has also contributed to a rise of the black market for opium-based substances.

Particularly concerning are the reported lifetime use rates for heroin among adolescents, which is estimated to be around 6 percent, a rate that is significantly higher than most other countries, such as Canada, which hovers around 1 percent (Paoli, 2002; Young et al., 2011). Russia's response to drugs and drug use continues to resemble the Soviet Union approach, rather than a human rights or health-based approach (Kramer, 2011). Similar to other countries that employ punitive responses to drugs, the goal for Russia is to completely remove drugs from society, and the government believes that the only conceivable means of achieving this objective is through coercive and repressive measures, such as forced treatment, extended police powers, and imprisonment (Sarang, Rhodes, Sheon, & Page, 2010; Lancet, 2011). Police and government corruption, along with fear among citizens, further perpetuate the drug problems in Russia (Kramer, 2011).

While Russia's punitive policies towards drugs and drug users are problematic for their use of law enforcement, imprisonment, and forced abstinence-based treatments, there are far worse conditions in other countries, where the death penalty is routinely used for questionable drug-offending behaviour.

China

China is considered the world leader for the number of people executed and sentenced to death each year, many of whom are believed to have committed drug offences, mostly trafficking (Gallahue et al., 2012). However, it is unknown how many executions take place, and the offences for which an individual is convicted is not always clear, as the judicial and political realms continually intermingle. There are no estimates for capital punishment as the figures remain a state secret; thus, it is impossible to know the extent to which death penalties are imposed and enforced. What is known is that drug trafficking still remains on the list of 55 offences in the country where an offender can be sentenced to death. More troubling is the fact that once an offender is accused of an offence in China, she or he is certain to be convicted (Gallahue et al., 2012).

Drug problems and punitive responses in China are not a new phenomenon. China's drug policies and practices in the early twentieth century were mostly concerned with widespread opium production and use, a remnant of the Opium Wars with England. In an attempt to control and completely eradicate opium and other illicit substances, production and consumption were controlled through punitive state control, which included the use of the death penalty, a practice that continues today. These strict state controls were practiced for several decades, and from the 1950s through to the late-1970s China officially became a "drug free" society (Lu, Miethe, & Liang, 2009). However, in the early 1980s, China's once restricted economy became more open to global trade, and the drug problems of the early twentieth century returned, this time with heroin and methamphetamines (Wen, 2014). The increased integration into the global economy negated China's ability to respond to the drug trade and drug use in the same manner it had in the past, closing all of its borders and strictly controlling the actions of the people. A return to the previous approach of complete eradication was no longer possible, yet punitive punishment-based responses to drugs and drug use continued. Penalties for drug users ranged from fines or detainment for first-time offences to detainment in a re-education through labour (REL) centre for one to three years (Xiao, Yang, Zhou, & Hao, 2015), and capital punishment for drug trafficking offences.

In 2008, under China's Anti-Drug Law, there was a formal shift to a seemingly more humane, health-based approach, which included abolishing REL and instituting compulsory isolated rehabilitation for drug users. However, in practice the response remains punitive and focused on law enforcement efforts to control drug use (Xiao, Yang, Zhou, & Hao, 2015). Moreover, the new rehabilitation model still resembles REL in the way programming is administered, not to mention that treatment approaches are vastly underfunded and often delivered by unqualified personnel (Yang, Zhou, Hao, & Xiao, 2014; Wen, 2014). The irony here is that cigarette consumption in China accounts for more than 2 trillion cigarettes smoked per year, out of a worldwide total of approximately 6 trillion, and that use of tobacco is actively encouraged because it is a major source of government revenue (Jha, & Peto, 2014).

Iran

Sharing a border with Afghanistan, the world's largest producer of opium, Iran has become a major transit country for the distribution of opium to other drug markets in Russia, Europe, and the Persian Gulf (Nissaramanesh, Trace, & Roberts, 2005). Combined with strict regulation and enforcement, the geographic location of Iran has resulted in large numbers of Iranians using and abusing opioid drugs, especially heroin. Opium and its derivatives are not the only substances that are strictly controlled in Iran; unlike many other countries, alcohol is also prohibited, with similar punitive punishments used to control the people (Ghiabi, 2015). Laws against alcohol were enacted following the 1979 revolution under the Islamic legal term of *hudud*, or "crimes against God," though in one cross-sectional study of 8,175 Iranians living in Tehran aged 15 to 35, the rate of alcohol abuse was reported at 25.7 percent (Hamdieh, Motalebi, Asheri, & Boroujerdi, 2009), which is far greater than in Western nations.

While Iran has made numerous attempts to control drug problems over the past four decades, the response has not always been so punitive. Some researchers argue that, since the shift to a religious state, anti-drug campaigns are responsible for the severe treatment of not only those who are involved in the drug trade but also those who use drugs (Ghiabi, 2015). Historically, strict enforcement had been justified through international drug agreements, but the revolution replaced this with a more fervent message that described drug use as "moral deviancy, anti-revolutionary behaviour and westoxification" (Ghiabi, 2015: 141).

Some of the most severe penalties used in Iran include life imprisonment and capital punishment. In fact, Iran ranks second in the world after China for the use of the death penalty, and drug offences are a large proportion of the total number of executions. However, unlike China, there are estimates available for the number of Iranians sentenced to death each year, though it is unknown how accurate these estimates truly are. Iran Human Rights (2015) reported that 648 Iranians were executed in the first half of 2015, with 463 cases a direct result of drug offences. This amounts to almost 100 more executions for drug offences than in the entire preceding year.

Beyond capital punishment and lengthy prison sentences, punitive drug enforcement in Iran also involves routine mandatory drug screening that takes place before being allowed to marry, obtain a driver's licence, or apply for a government position (Nissaramanesh, Trace, & Roberts, 2005). Testing positive for drugs, including alcohol, results in being officially registered as a drug user and subject to further discrimination and suspicion by the state. If one is found in possession of a drug, then judges have the discretion to determine if the individual is involved in trafficking, which can lead to the death penalty. Multiple convictions for alcohol offences can also lead to the death penalty.

12.3: PRAGMATIC POLICIES

While punitive approaches to drugs and drug users rest on the notion that societies can be "drug free" if the consequences are harsh enough, countries with more practical policies tend to recognize that no amount of law enforcement or public shaming is going to completely eradicate drugs from society. This view is pragmatic given that human use of psychoactive drugs predates written texts, and none of the hundreds of attempts at prohibition have succeeded in eliminating drug use (Csiernik, 2016). Pragmatic approaches are evident to varying degrees in the practices and policies of Portugal, the Netherlands, and Uruguay. Each of these countries illustrates a different form of pragmatism, ranging from policies that apply to all drugs, that distinguish between the harmfulness of certain drugs, and that apply to a specific drug, namely cannabis.

Portugal

On July 1, 2001, Portugal became the first country in the modern world to decriminalize the use and possession of small amounts of all illicit psychoactive drugs. Portugal's national drug strategy sought to address the negative effects of substance use, abuse, and dependence using a public health model of harm minimization. The decriminalization of drug use and the possession of small amounts was only one aspect of a much broader strategy focused on dealing with drugs and the related health and social issues (van Beusekom, van het Loo, & Kahan, 2002).

The history behind this bold step to decriminalize all psychoactive substances has been traced back to Portugal's 1974 revolution, when the former Fascist dictatorship was replaced with a democracy. This shift resulted in increased individual freedom and uncertainty, as initially occurred in Russia, along with significant economic growth. However, it also resulted in more visible increases in drug use and drug trade under a less authoritarian regime. By the 1990s, there was widespread agreement that Portugal was facing a significant drug problem that needed to be addressed, though there were no official sources of data to support the claim that drugs and drug use had become increasingly problematic leading up to the formal policy changes (van het Loo, van Beusekom, & Kahan, 2002).

Even with limited empirical support, Portugal launched a national commitment to reducing the harms associated with drugs, and has maintained this approach ever since its enactment in 2001. This was in part due to deteriorating economic conditions and the realization that this small nation did not have sufficient finances to police individual users as well as all of its land and sea borders against drug traffickers, and thus a new initiative was needed to protect its citizens. The new approach entailed decriminalization, whereby drug possession and use became administrative rather than criminal offences (van het Loo, van Beusekom, & Kahan, 2002). Rather than the traditional enforcement approach where police, lawyers, and judges are left to deal with and negotiate penalties concerning drug offences, in Portugal, Commissions for the Dissuasion of Drug Addiction (CDTs) hear the cases and make treatment recommendations specific to the individual and the offence. Each commission consists of three members: two are health professionals appointed by the minister of health, and may be physicians, psychologists, psychiatrists, or social workers; the third member is a legal professional appointed by the minister of justice (Laqueur, 2015). While the administrative nature of a drug offence applies to all substances, the commissions who hear individual cases are expected to take into consideration the severity and type of drug, the place and pattern of use, and the general circumstances of the individual (van Beusekom, van het Loo, & Kahan, 2002).

Those who celebrate the success of decriminalization in Portugal claim there have been significant reductions in HIV infections, less heroin use, a decline in the total number of young people aged 15 to 19 using drugs, an increase in people entering treatment, and an increase in large-scale drug seizures (Hawkes, 2011). The most dramatic and undeniable change, though not necessarily directly related to use, has been the shift in attitude towards drugs and drug use, from that of a criminalized and stigmatized issue to a public health issue with an emphasis on treatment rather than punishment (Hawkes, 2011; Laqueur, 2015).

Others have been more skeptical of the true changes that decriminalization has brought to Portugal. Laqueur (2015) highlights several limitations of decriminalization, including the increase in the number of non-addicted or non-problematic young users of cannabis being overly represented in the commission hearings, as well as a significant reduction in drug trafficking convictions under the criminal law, suggesting the liberalization of the laws has extended beyond use and possession to allow greater latitude to those involved in the drug trade. Moreover, while there have been notable reductions in heroin use, there have been corresponding and concerning increases in cannabis and cocaine use in Portugal, especially amongst older people (Hawkes, 2011).

The true effectiveness of decriminalization in Portugal is difficult to assess because, as Laqueur (2015: 746) states, "the de jure legal change largely codified de facto practices." Essentially, this means that Portugal's practices had already shifted from a punitive, criminalizing approach to a more pragmatic treatment-based approach before decriminalization came into formal effect. In addition, Portugal did not collect population data on drugs or drug use prior to 2001. Thus, it is difficult to ascertain exactly what changes are directly related to this policy shift and what changes are the result of other factors. Regardless of the criticisms and the lack of a priori evidence to support such a dramatic policy shift, the change in how drugs and drug users are perceived and treated is an important step towards resolving both individual and societal oppression associated with drugs and drug use.

Over the past decade, researchers and policy-makers all over the world have been monitoring the outcomes of Portugal's approach to drugs and drug users to determine its effectiveness (Hawkes, 2011; McCaffrey, 2010; Russoniello, 2012). However, as some more cautious scholars have noted, what works in one country does not necessarily work in another. They further argue that cross-cultural research is important to develop a better understanding of the approaches that work and under what conditions (MacCoun & Reuter, 2002).

Netherlands

Another approach, long considered effective and admired from afar, is the Dutch policy surrounding cannabis and other supposedly "soft" drugs. The Netherlands is the best known example of liberalized drug policy, especially with respect to cannabis. Both academics and the general public often refer to the Netherlands as an example of an alternative, pragmatic approach to drugs and drug users. However, the practices and policies today are not as liberal as many believe, partially because of the international criticism that has targeted the Dutch, and partially because what is written in policy does not always translate into practice (Rigter, 2006).

Prior to the 1960s, cannabis and other recreational substance use was not considered a widespread problem in the Netherlands. However, as drug use became more popular or perhaps more visible, the Dutch government launched a commission to investigate the potential outcomes of widespread cannabis and other recreational substance use. The primary concern of the committee was the use of the criminal justice system in dealing with mostly young cannabis and experimental drug users, who were likely to slow down or quit using illicit substances altogether as they entered adulthood (Cohen, 2001), a pattern noted in other Western nations (Waxman & Csiernik, 2010). Similar to the conclusions made by the Le Dain Commission (1973) in Canada around the same time, the Baan Commission in the Netherlands recommended that the possession and use of recreational psychoactive substances be decriminalized. While Canada never made the recommended changes, the new Dutch policies were among the first attempts to focus on reducing the harms associated with recreational drug use.

The most well-known practice of the Dutch drug policy is the practice of de facto legalization of cannabis products, which has been in effect since the 1970s. Since this initial change in policies and practices, the Netherlands has often been criticized and simultaneously celebrated for focusing on decriminalizing individual possession and use with various non-criminal interventions. The distinction between hard and soft drugs under the Dutch policies was premised on the idea that tolerating and making available less harmful substances, such as marijuana and hashish, will prevent people from seeking out alternatives in the illicit market that may be more harmful, such as heroin and cocaine (Spapens, Müller, & van de Bunt, 2015). In the event that people began using harder drugs, the focus was on reducing the harms associated with use through treatment and maintenance programs.

Criticisms of the Dutch drug policies have focused on the widespread availability of cannabis and the younger age limit for gaining access to cannabis than what many people find acceptable. For instance, as a result of widespread international criticism, the age limit to purchase cannabis products increased in 1995 from 16 to 18 years old, and general policing and regulating of coffee shops licenced to sell cannabis also increased (Cohen, 2001; Spapens, Müller, & van de Bunt, 2015). Of course, this change led to unintended consequences, which is the norm when only the supply side is considered in implementing any drug policy: the changes to the age regulations resulted in younger users resorting to the illicit market to obtain cannabis, which further put them in contact with other hard drugs through association with drug dealers, an outcome that is considered undesirable to many authorities (Spapens, Müller, & van de Bunt, 2015). Changes to the policing and regulating of coffee shops have resulted in many being shut down in recent years, and as is the case with youth, more are seeking out alternative, higher risk sources to obtain cannabis as its supply becomes more limited; in other words, these new policies do nothing to address demand (van Ooyen-Houben & Kleemans, 2015).

The increased availability that came with the new drug policy did not result in increased use, nor did it lead to a confirmation of the gateway hypothesis, which has since fallen into disrepute. Instead, what many have found is that some people might be more inclined to experiment with cocaine or other "hard" drugs, but beyond that there is no clear indication of a progression to harder drugs simply because cannabis is de facto legalized (Cohen, 2001). The Netherlands has similar rates of youth cannabis use as Canada, while the adult prevalence of life-time cannabis use is substantially lower in the Netherlands compared to Canada (Boak, Hamilton, Adlaf, & Mann, 2013; EMCDDA, 2015; Health Canada, 2013a; UNODC, 2012).

However, the most recent changes in policy in the Netherlands indicate that international criticisms are beginning to have a regressive effect on the long-standing tradition of pragmatic, humanistic approaches to drugs and drug use. Where the Dutch practice has been to normalize and de-stigmatize drugs and drug users, the newest policy directions from 2009 indicate a shift towards mor-alizing substance use, an approach that is all too familiar in North America (Euchner, Heichel, Nebel, & Raschzok, 2013) and reflects the growing neo-liberal trend across Western nations. Given the decades of normalized policies and practices, however, the Netherlands should serve as evidence that liberal-izing policies towards certain substances and not others does not inevitably lead to widespread use (Cohen, 2001), nor does it mean that society will disintegrate. Moreover, countries with longstanding punitive, prohibitionist policies and prac-tices that moralize drugs and drug use should serve as important warnings to the Netherlands that greater punishment and enforcement does not resolve drug issues entirely, and can result in significant negative consequences for both indi-viduals and societies (van Ooyen-Houben & Kleemans, 2015).

Uruguay

In May of 2011, the first official draft of Uruguay's Bill 534 was introduced, pro-posing the legalization of the possession and cultivation of cannabis for personal use, including for recreational purposes. Over the course of five years, the coun-try developed a comprehensive cannabis policy that legalizes and regulates not only possession and cultivation but also sales and distribution (Faubion, 2013). Uruguay is not the first jurisdiction to practice legalization of a previously illicit substance; however, it is the first country to make a formal attempt at a nation-wide drug policy legalizing cannabis since the introduction of global prohibition in the 1960s.

Unlike the Netherlands, where de facto legalization for personal use and possession has been in practice for several decades but distribution and traffick-ing remains illegal, Uruguay's approach legalizes and regulates both the market and personal possession. Individuals are allowed to grow their own cannabis if they register with the government, and they can purchase cannabis if they go through a fingerprinting process to ensure that they do not purchase more than 480 grams each year. The Uruguayan approach to cannabis is focused on public health and government control. As a result, there are bans on cannabis-impaired driving, similar to alcohol-impaired driving, with a legal THC limit of 10 ng/mL when operating a motor vehicle. Tax revenues generated from sales are directly funnelled back into public health initiatives, and there is a ban on promoting and advertising cannabis (Spithoff, Emerson, & Spithoff, 2015).

At this time, the long-term effectiveness of Uruguay's legalization of cannabis is yet to be determined. However, it seems that drug policy officials in Uruguay are wise in taking a cautious and evidence-based approach, a lesson many countries have learned from the histories of tobacco and alcohol regulation. However, it is unclear where these changes place Uruguay in light of the international conventions prohibiting the recreational use of substances such as cannabis (Room, 2012). How do these fundamental shifts in drug policy begin to undermine the authority and effectiveness of the international conventions, which are undeniably out of date with the current climate surrounding drugs and drug use?

12.4: CONCLUSION

This chapter has reviewed drug policies and practices in six different countries, ranging from extremely punitive approaches that include capital punishment to fairly pragmatic and lenient approaches that recognize the normalcy of drug use for some people under certain conditions. Central to variations in global responses are social, political, economic, and geographic considerations, demonstrating the importance of the sociological perspective in understanding drugs and drug use in society. The concluding chapter considers Canada's position on the punitive-pragmatic continuum in both policy and practice.

PARADOXES

1) Implementation of the international drug conventions by different signatory nations has led to the creation of both punitive and pragmatic national drug policies.

2) Even in the Netherlands, where pragmatic approaches have shown to be effective for decades, there is no guarantee that these approaches will remain in effect. Evidence does not necessarily guide decisions on whether to use pragmatic or punitive responses to drugs and drug users.

3) The international drug conventions, in their current form, do not take into account decades of international research proving that punitive prohibition does not work; yet these conventions are still the standard by which signatory nations must abide. This limits the capacity of nations to enact regulations that are potentially more effective without compromising their status and image from an international standpoint.

4) International drug conventions limit the ability of countries to use pragmatic responses outside of the law, yet there is no limit to the punitive responses they can use. This is despite the fact that we know the punitive responses are not effective.

CRITICAL REFLECTIONS

1) What have been the driving factors behind the creation of international drug conventions?

2) What is the primary intent of international drug conventions? How do they lead to both punitive and pragmatic national policies being created?

3) Which of the international drug conventions do you think is the most harmful? Which is the least harmful? Explain what aspects of the conventions are useful.

4) If you were in charge of how the international drug conventions should be revised, what would you change to ensure that the international interests of the United Nations would be preserved? How would you balance the pragmatism envisioned by some countries with the punitive force used in others?

13 Canada's Drug Policies

The purpose of this concluding chapter is to provide an overview of policies used to control drugs and drug users in Canada by highlighting the central argument of this book: that Canada's current approach to drugs and drug users is conflicting and paradoxical. Determining how Canada is best characterized within a punitive versus pragmatic framework, relative to other countries, is not a simple task. According to policy experts, and to common sense, Canada is not located at the far end of the spectrum with the most punitive countries, such as China, Iran, or Russia (Mosher & Akins, 2014). While some international researchers and policy-makers view Canada's drug laws and treatment of drug users as being pragmatic (Goodwin, 2003/2004; Mosher, 2011), the perspective from within Canada suggests that our laws have been closer to the punitive end of the scale, particularly during the years that Stephen Harper's Conservatives were in power (Cavalieri & Riley, 2012; Erickson & Hyshka, 2010; Fischer, 1999; Hathaway & Ericskon, 2003; Hyshka, 2009; Hyshka et al., 2012; Khenti, 2014; Williams, 2010). Hence, there is considerable disagreement in the characterizations of Canada's approach to drugs and drug use. We are certainly not as pragmatic as most Canadian drug experts would like to see (Cavalieri & Riley, 2012), though this does appear to be changing with the 2017 announcement that the federal government will introduce legislation to legalize cannabis in Canada. The proposed legislation, referred to as the Cannabis Act, will finally realize what many drug policy experts have been advocating for since the 1960s.

Herein lies one of the central paradoxes of drugs and drug use in Canada: we are a nation that has simultaneously been pragmatic and punitive. We have also been a leader and a follower when it comes to our position on international drug policies discussed in previous chapters. The reality is that there are a significant number of individuals and organizations committed to reducing the harms associated with psychoactive substances, but there is also a lack of political commitment and sometimes significant political resistance to changing our decades-long crime control approach (Erickson, 1998; Valleriani & MacPherson, 2015). According to Guy Dion (1999: 15):

> Since the 1960s we have witnessed a dual movement: on the one hand, there is an intensification of controls as well as a tightening of the application of these controls on both the national and the international levels and, at the same time, an increasingly organized opposition is emerging to the prohibitionist system from various groups of individuals, academics and non-government treatment organizations.

This "dual movement" supports the paradoxical aspects of drugs and drug use that have framed this book. Even after half a century of diligent research and advocacy for the health and well-being of those most directly and indirectly affected by drugs and drug use, the tension between political and socio-legal control and individual rights and freedoms continues. The political will to fundamentally change our approach has remained elusive.

Goode's (1989) classic examination of the 1980s drug panic in the United States offers a potentially useful explanation for why there are conflicting approaches to drugs and drug use in Canada, and how these competing approaches continue to persist. Drugs in contemporary society are both objectively threatening and socially constructed. While Goode does not address Canada's approach to drugs and drug users as conflicting or puzzling, central to his argument is that drugs and drug use are more than just social constructions. There is a real biological change that occurs to the human mind and body when psychoactive drugs are consumed, be it for medical or recreational purposes, which can be observed and measured. There is an empirical, objective reality that exists independent from what laws are created, what education and treatment is offered, and how people are affected. Drugs exist. Undoubtedly, some drugs can have devastating consequences for some individuals who use them both chronically and acutely, the people with whom all users are associated, and the broader communities and societies in which they are embedded. This empirical reality is evident regardless of how drugs are framed. Population-based evidence confirms that psychoactive drugs can be dangerous, including alcohol, tobacco, and even caffeine (Kerrigan & Lindsey, 2005; Rehm et al., 2006). However, the way in which we have come to view certain drugs negatively or punitively is a social construction (Goode, 2008), especially as the vast majority of psychoactive drug use does not lead to long-term harm for the individual user or society. There is nothing inherently criminal about drugs or drug use; nor is there any reasonable justification for why we have spent over a century criminalizing and stigmatizing drugs and drug users, instead of dealing with the issues through a holistic public health and social lens.

13.1: ADVOCATES FOR PUNITIVE APPROACHES

Who or what is responsible for the continuation of harsh, moralized treatment of substance users and the perception of the substances themselves? Goode and Ben-Yehuda (1994) suggest three possible explanations: the grassroots theory, the elite-engineered theory, and the interest group theory. The grassroots approach is driven by public sentiment towards drugs and drug use. However, in Canada, there is no official way in which public attitudes towards drugs and drug use is consistently or representatively measured. Thus, it is impossible to determine the true extent to which public attitudes are responsible for the punitive approaches adopted. However, it could be argued that a lack of public resistance to a harsh criminal-justice approach indicates a passive public acceptance of the current laws and policies. The election of a string of politically conservative governments in Canada, though never by a majority of Canadians, through the beginning of the twenty-first century also indirectly supports this view.

The second explanation for continued punitive treatment of drugs and drug users is the elite-engineered theory. Central to this perspective are political interests and the need to divert public attention away from other potentially problematic issues facing society. This approach has been particularly prominent during the early part of the twenty-first century as Canada experienced a significant economic recession, yet the Harper government still managed to justify the passing of the Safe Streets and Communities Act and the amendment of the CDSA to include lengthier prison sentences for relatively minor drug infractions.

Undoubtedly, these changes and the consequences for the justice system are costly, and were compounded by issues related to the recession, such as unemployment, family breakdown, and criminal charges and convictions. Nevertheless, the elite-engineered explanation cannot exist without additional support from other groups. As Jensen and Gerber (1993) were able to show, Conservative leader Brian Mulroney's attempt to wage a War on Drugs in Canada in the late 1980s failed because there was inadequate public support.

The third and final explanation for punitive approaches to drugs is called the interest group theory (Goode & Ben-Yehuda, 1994). Interest groups have diverse concerns and objectives concerning drugs and drug use, which sometimes makes their impact less obvious than political leaders or grassroots advocates who explicitly attack a specific drug or group of users. Interest groups include the media, police, religious groups, and educational organizations. Each of these groups have a vested interest in demonizing drugs (Hammersley & Reid, 2002). For the media, sensationalism and a perceived threat posed by drugs or drug users themselves sells stories and makes money. For the police, drugs and drug use help justify increased funding and the development of more specialized task forces devoted to combatting drugs. Religious groups and educational organizations use drugs to define social boundaries, "properly" socialize members of society, and maintain group cohesion in a multicultural nation.

13.2: ADVOCATES FOR PRAGMATIC APPROACHES

Who or what challenges this moralized, punitive status quo? There are many individuals and organizations committed to a more realistic and compassionate treatment of substance use and abuse. Advocates of pragmatic approaches to drugs and drug use can include individuals with personal drug experiences, concerned citizens, medical professionals, drug researchers, some government officials, legal professionals including lawyers, and police officers. Some examples of notable advocates and organizations supporting more pragmatic approaches in Canada include the following:

- Marc Emery, also known as the "Prince of Pot," longstanding advocate of legalization
- Jack Layton, former New Democrat Party leader
- Justin Trudeau, prime minister of Canada, who formally included legalization of cannabis as a major campaign platform

- Canadian Students for Sensible Drug Policy, a grassroots network of young people concerned about the current drug policy approaches and the impact they have on both individuals and communities (www.cssdp.org)
- Canadian Foundation for Drug Policy, a non-profit organization founded by leading experts in drug policy across Canada and offers "a forum for the exchange of views among those interested in reform of drug policies" (www.cfdp.ca)
- Canadian Drug Policy Coalition, who, in partnership with the Centre for Applied Research in Mental Health and Addiction at Simon Fraser University, is considered "an independent civil society network of organizations and individuals working to improve Canada's drug policies" (www.drugpolicy.ca)
- Law Enforcement Action Partnership (formerly Law Enforcement Against Prohibition), an organization composed of individuals concerned about the harms associated with drug policy and criminal justice, is more developed in the United States and the United Kingdom than in Canada; anyone can be a member, though only those with a previous background in law enforcement can represent the group through meetings and presentations (www.lawenforcementactionpartnership.org)
- Canadian Harm Reduction Network (CHRN), a virtual community of individuals and organizations focused on reducing the social, health, and economic harms associated with drugs and drug policies (www.canadianharmreduction.com)

13.3: WHAT IS THE OFFICIAL APPROACH TO DRUGS AND DRUG USE IN CANADA?

Canada's first drug laws were primarily constructed based upon issues of morality and race, and unfortunately current approaches have nearly as ignoble a foundation. While American President Richard Nixon launched his own War on Drugs in 1971, in part to have another weapon against his political opponents and in part to distract from losing the war in Vietnam, it was Ronald Reagan who would bring this term to global attention a decade later. When Brian Mulroney was elected prime minister in 1984, he quickly aligned himself ideologically, politically, and personally with President Reagan, and among the initiatives he brought to Canada was our own War on Drugs.

The first nationwide strategy to address drugs and drug use in Canada was introduced in 1987, with the announcement of a $210 million five-year plan devoted to tackling the supply and demand for drugs across the country. One year later the first national non-governmental agency focused on substance use, the Canadian Centre on Substance Abuse (CCSA), was established. Prior to 1988, addiction issues had been solely a provincial concern and left to the hands of provincial ministries and affiliated agencies such as the Addictions Foundation of Manitoba, Alberta Alcohol and Drug Abuse Commission, and Addiction Research Foundation of Ontario (now the Centre for Addiction and Mental Health). Upon its creation, the mission of the CCSA was to increase awareness of and participation in reducing the harms associated with substance abuse by promoting evidence-based information on effective programming related to substance abuse. The goals of CCSA are to:

- promote and support consultation and co-operation among governments, the business community and labour, professional, and voluntary organizations in matters relating to alcohol and drug abuse;
- contribute to the effective exchange of information on alcohol and drug abuse;
- facilitate and contribute to the development and application of knowledge and expertise in the alcohol and drug abuse field;
- promote and assist in the development of realistic and effective policies and programs aimed at reducing the harm associated with alcohol and drug abuse; and
- promote increased awareness among Canadians of the nature and extent of international efforts to reduce alcohol and drug abuse and supporting Canada's participation in those efforts (Government of Canada, 1985/2016).

Over the next two decades, Canada's National Drug Strategy evolved into what is known as the four-pillar approach, including prevention, treatment, harm reduction, and enforcement (Collin, 2006; Cavalieri & Riley, 2012). In parallel, CCSA was working with researchers, medical professionals, policy experts, front-line workers, law enforcement authorities, legal professionals, and government representatives to create a National Framework for Action to Reduce the Harms Associated with Alcohol and Other Drugs and Substances in Canada (Figure 13.1) (Canadian Centre on Substance Abuse, 2005). The goal of this collaborative effort was to produce a national plan to reduce the harms associated with drugs and drugs use in society, which was a promising shift from the traditional criminal justice approach.

However, as this movement towards a holistic view of substance use was taking shape through this collaborative process, the Harper government launched its own National Anti-Drug Strategy (NADS) in 2007, in essence rejecting the initiatives previous governments had supported. NADS was a joint initiative of 12 federal departments and agencies, led by the Department of Justice and not Health Canada (Government of Canada, 2014). Using the Department of Justice as the principal agency speaks directly to the perspective of drug policy in Canada and stands in contrast to the National Framework. The other ten contributing groups to the NADS were:

1. Public Safety Canada
2. Public Prosecution Service of Canada
3. Royal Canadian Mounted Police
4. Canada Border Services Agency
5. Correctional Service of Canada
6. Foreign Affairs and International Trade Canada (Foreign Affairs, Trade and Development)
7. Public Health Agency of Canada
8. Public Works and Government Services Canada
9. Canada Revenue Agency
10. Financial Transactions and Reports Analysis Centre of Canada

While the stated objectives of the NADS are to prevent use, treat dependency, reduce production and distribution of illicit drugs, and address prescription drug abuse, in examining the list of members, an emphasis on criminality and prosecution rather than prevention and treatment is clearly evident. This is further evidenced by the fact that the National Anti-Drug Strategy replaced the former drug strategy and removed harm reduction as a central aim of the government's efforts to address drugs in society (Government of Canada, 2007). What further underscores this paradox in Canada is that while the National Framework developed in 2005 remains central to the CCSA, it does not formally promote the National Drug Strategy, even though the government continues to fund the CCSA and support its mandate. As well, while the CCSA was promoting harm reduction programs, the Harper government was attempting to shutter Canada's only safe injection sites and heroin-assisted treatment program through formal court proceedings. In addition to trying to prevent harm reductionist measures from being implemented

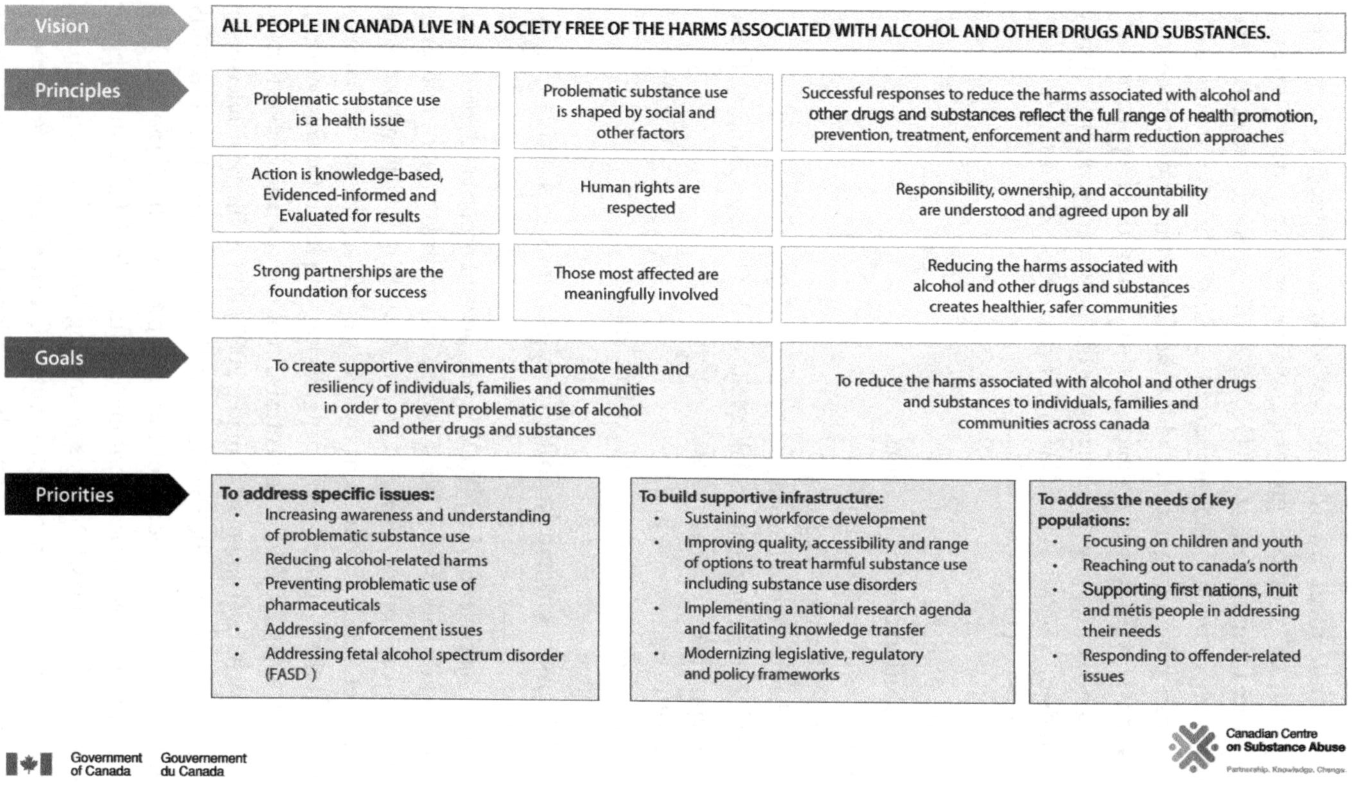

Vision

ALL PEOPLE IN CANADA LIVE IN A SOCIETY FREE OF THE HARMS ASSOCIATED WITH ALCOHOL AND OTHER DRUGS AND SUBSTANCES.

Principles

- Problematic substance use is a health issue
- Action is knowledge-based, Evidenced-informed and Evaluated for results
- Strong partnerships are the foundation for success
- Problematic substance use is shaped by social and other factors
- Human rights are respected
- Those most affected are meaningfully involved
- Successful responses to reduce the harms associated with alcohol and other drugs and substances reflect the full range of health promotion, prevention, treatment, enforcement and harm reduction approaches
- Responsibility, ownership, and accountability are understood and agreed upon by all
- Reducing the harms associated with alcohol and other drugs and substances creates healthier, safer communities

Goals

- To create supportive environments that promote health and resiliency of individuals, families and communities in order to prevent problematic use of alcohol and other drugs and substances
- To reduce the harms associated with alcohol and other drugs and substances to individuals, families and communities across canada

Priorities

To address specific issues:
- Increasing awareness and understanding of problematic substance use
- Reducing alcohol-related harms
- Preventing problematic use of pharmaceuticals
- Addressing enforcement issues
- Addressing fetal alcohol spectrum disorder (FASD)

To build supportive infrastructure:
- Sustaining workforce development
- Improving quality, accessibility and range of options to treat harmful substance use including substance use disorders
- Implementing a national research agenda and facilitating knowledge transfer
- Modernizing legislative, regulatory and policy frameworks

To address the needs of key populations:
- Focusing on children and youth
- Reaching out to canada's north
- Supporting first nations, inuit and métis people in addressing their needs
- Responding to offender-related issues

Government of Canada / Gouvernement du Canada

Canadian Centre on Substance Abuse
Partnership. Knowledge. Change.

Figure 13.1: National Framework for Action to Reduce the Harms Associated with Alcohol and Other Drugs and Substances in Canada

Source: Canadian Centre on Substance Abuse (2005). Used by permission.

within Canada, there was an active resistance to mentioning harm reduction policies at international proceedings (Webster, 2014). Thus, while the CCSA continues to actively and officially promote the National Framework (Figure 13.1), the Government of Canada continues to actively and officially promote the National Anti-Drug Strategy through three defined action plans on prevention, treatment, and enforcement—but not harm reduction (Table 13.1).

13.4: THE MISSING COMPONENT IN CANADA'S CURRENT NATIONAL ANTI-DRUG STRATEGY: HARM REDUCTION

Even though the National Anti-Drug Strategy of 2007 eliminated harm reduction as one of the four main areas of focus (Government of Canada, 2007; Valleriani & MacPherson, 2015), this approach still remains central to the objectives of the CCSA, other professionals and programs operating across the country, and the National Framework developed in 2005. Thus, while the Harper Government no longer officially supported this more pragmatic approach to drugs, there were many ongoing efforts focused on reducing harms associated with drugs, from front-line workers to organizational practices to policy developments from within provinces and territories (Cavalieri & Riley, 2012).

Harm reduction is among the most misunderstood approaches to drug treatment, as many believe that it condones and even promotes drugs use (Cheung, 2000; Single, 1995; Watkin, Rowe, & Csiernik, 2010). This, however, is not the case. Harm reduction combines public health and human rights, while recognizing that the complete elimination of drugs and drug use is an unrealistic goal (Des Jarlais, 1995; Erickson, Riley, Cheung, & O'Hare, 1997; Erickson, 1995; Erickson & Hathaway, 2010; Reinarman, 2004). While some argue that harm reduction must be driven by the user (Hathaway & Tousaw, 2008), others have suggested that harm reduction is a diverse movement ranging from individuals to communities to broader public policy (Marlatt, Larimer, & Witkiewitz, 2012) (Figure 13.2).

Conceptually, harm reduction is a philosophy, a policy approach, and a series of actual programming options; this also contributes to the confusion about what the term actually means. Moreover, given that harm reduction originally emerged as a grassroots movement, its institutionalization has resulted in the misappropriation of some of the originally intended goals, for example by abstinence-based programs who claim they are the most effective harm reduction initiatives (Cavalieri & Riley, 2012). Broadly defined, *harm reduction* is "a set of compassionate and pragmatic approaches for reducing harm associated

Table 13.1: Canada's National Anti-Drug Strategy Action Plans

Prevention Action Plan	• Aims to prevent illicit drug use and prescription drug abuse
	• Funds the development and implementation of community-based interventions and initiatives
	• Provides information directly to youth as well as to their parents and other concerned adults through the Internet
	• Supports development of awareness materials and provision of awareness sessions
Treatment Action Plan	• Aims to treat those with drug dependencies
	• Supports efforts to improve treatment systems, programs, and services
	• Enhances treatment and support for First Nations and Inuit peoples
	• Supports treatment programs for youth in the justice system with drug-related problems
	• Provides support for the use of drug treatment courts, which offer an alternative to the traditional justice system for offenders who have committed non-violent crimes motivated by their addictions
	• Supports research on new treatment models and on the consequences of illicit drug use
Enforcement Action Plan	• Aims to combat the production and distribution of illicit drugs
	• Provides funding to the RCMP to expand its efforts to help locate, investigate, and shut down organizations involved in the production and distribution of illicit drugs
	• Gives additional resources to the Public Prosecution Service of Canada to provide legal advice to law enforcement at the investigative stage and to effectively prosecute those involved with the production and distribution of illicit drugs
	• Increases the number of Health Canada inspectors and investigators to ensure accurate and timely analysis of suspected illicit drugs seized by law enforcement
	• Increases the capacity of Canada Border Services Agency to inhibit the cross-border movement of precursor chemicals and illicit drugs
	• Helps law enforcement stop the flow of money that organized crime makes from the illicit drug trade
	• Improves the ability of Canadian law enforcement officials to conduct joint investigations with the US
	• Ensures that serious penalties are in place for serious drug crimes
Source: Government of Canada (2007).	

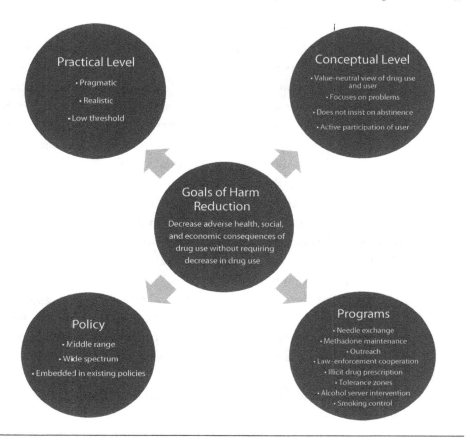

Figure 13.2: Harm Reduction Model

Source: Adapted from Cheung (2000).

with high-risk behaviours and improving quality of life" (Marlatt, Larimer, & Witkiewitz, 2012: 5). According to a special ad hoc committee of the Centre for Addiction and Mental Health (Erickson, Butters, & Walko, 2002), harm reduction can be understood as having six guiding principles or themes:

1. Pragmatism: substance use is inevitable and to a certain extent it is normal, so we need to tolerate substance use as a social reality that does not necessitate stigma.
2. Focus on harms: rather than attempting to eliminate substance use from society, harm reduction aims to reduce the harmful consequences of use without the requirement that users must reduce their use or completely abstain.

3. Prioritization of goals: substance use goals are set out according to what is feasible and what can be achieved immediately, instead of focusing on long-term possibilities and objectives.

4. Flexibility and maximization of intervention options: contrary to traditional approaches that use a one-size-fits-all model, such as the 12 steps of Alcoholics Anonymous, the harm reduction approach recognizes that individual and environmental contexts require flexible approaches and options, as well as recognizing the potential need for multiple approaches to be used collaboratively.

5. Autonomy: substance use is seen as a personal choice for which individuals need to be empowered to take responsibility. This should not be misunderstood as blaming the victim; instead, harm reduction sees the individual as an active agent, capable of making decisions with the support of a broader community.

6. Evaluation: central to harm reduction is innovative and creative approaches that can be evaluated and proven effective through specific identification of what harms are being addressed and the extent to which harms are being reduced for both the individual and the broader community.

For harm reduction to be successful, there needs to be a balance between public health and human rights (Reinarman, 2004), including a balance between compassion and control (Erickson, Butters, & Walko, 2002). Unfortunately, under Canada's more dominant punitive prohibition approach, public health, human rights, compassion, and control have all been compromised. Our formal national initiative, the National Anti-Drug Strategy, misleads the public into believing that our government is committed to a balanced, holistic approach to drugs and drug use; however, a closer examination of the amount of support each area receives indicates the government has one major priority and a couple of other priorities that are deemed less significant. The funding allotments for what was intended to be an inclusive approach to drugs and drug users disproportionately supports law enforcement efforts, at the expense of limited research funding, prevention, treatment, and harm reduction (DeBeck, Wood, Montaner, & Kerr, 2009). The following is the breakdown of the Canadian dollar amounts and percentage of funding that was allocated to each category from 2007 to 2008:

- Law Enforcement: $282.1 million, 70 percent of annual funding
- Treatment: $67.6 million, 17 percent of annual funding

- Other (Research and Coordination): $26.1 million, 7 percent of annual funding
- Prevention: $14.7 million, 4 percent of annual funding
- Harm Reduction: $9.7 million, 2 percent of annual funding

Approximately two-thirds of all the funding directed to drugs and drug use is being used for law enforcement efforts, while the remaining one third is divided amongst prevention, treatment, harm reduction initiatives, and research, which directly reflects the coalition of government agencies that compose the NADS. This funding formula clearly calls attention to our priorities as a nation: Canada in the twenty-first century has continued to follow a punitive policy path promoting and funding criminalization over harm reduction, prevention, and treatment. From a national and provincial government standpoint, law enforcement and social control have prevailed over pragmatism and compassion. Despite increases in knowledge, the funding allocation under Canada's National Anti-Drug Strategy has not significantly differed from previous funding formulas. However, there is clear evidence in policy arenas that this strategy is not going to work: it hasn't worked in the past and it is not congruent with national and international research on how to respond to drug use issues (Valleriani & MacPherson, 2015). Moreover, the explicit removal of harm reduction from the official national response to drugs has sent a clear message regarding the lack of concern for drug users and their lives.

13.5: THE FUTURE

Since the departure of the Conservative leadership in Canada on October 19, 2015, no changes to the National Anti-Drug Strategy have been made. The newly elected Liberals have committed to legalizing cannabis as a part of their platform promises (Liberal Party of Canada, 2016), and new safe injection facilities have been proposed for communities across the country including Victoria, Saskatoon, Thunder Bay, Toronto, Ottawa, and Montreal (Biber, 2016; CBC News, 2016a, 2016b; Cleverly, 2014; Duffy, 2016; Fiddleman, 2015). However, beyond these initiatives, there has been no formal discussion of actually changing the national strategy and delivering a more effective approach to drugs and drug use beyond the proposed Cannabis Act. Unfortunately, the lack of coordinated efforts from national, provincial, and regional governments continues to highlight the challenges that Canada faces moving forward with sensible drug policies, including harm reduction (Valleriani & MacPherson, 2015).

It is evident both nationally and internationally that psychoactive drug use is a multi-faceted phenomenon that cannot be dealt with in a one-size-fits-all model. Using the law and international treaties to govern country-specific issues is only part of the solution. There needs to be a more holistic approach to drugs and drug use that recognizes the complexities of this biopsychosocial phenomenon, and both demand and supply side issues need to be addressed by comprehensive policies. Nations in both Europe and South America have taken the policy lead, shifting away from a punitive approach toward pragmatic and humanistic endeavours. In moving forward in the Canadian context, we need to acknowledge the paradox that has been created between knowledge and practice. Beyond the biological and psychological elements of drug demand there are social, political, and economic differences both within and between countries that must be carefully examined if Canada is to adopt an approach that actually addresses its needs and does not respond to fear. However, we must still be cautious when considering policy initiatives that have been adopted elsewhere, as the outcomes produced by these different approaches are not easily measurable; in many instances, we need to accept that there is no single policy approach guaranteed to be successful with issues pertaining to psychoactive drugs and psychoactive drug users. However, there is certainty that the current paradoxical situation is not addressing local, provincial, or national needs, and that a revised policy initiative is needed in order to enhance the future health and well-being of Canadians.

PARADOXES

1) Canada's drug policies have been simultaneously pragmatic and punitive. The reality is that there are a significant number of individuals and organizations committed to reducing the harms associated with substances, but there is also a lack of political commitment and sometimes significant political resistance to changing our decades-long crime control approach.

2) In Canada's experience, there has been an intensification of controls as well as a tightening of the application of these controls on both the national and international levels, while at the same time an increasingly organized opposition to the prohibitionist system from various groups of individuals, academics, and non-government treatment organizations.

3) There is a significant disconnect between the laws governing drugs and drug users in Canada and how drugs and drug use are viewed in treatment.

4)   The most significant paradox remains between knowledge and policies and practices. What we empirically know, and what the evidence indicates, is neither what consistently drives policy nor what becomes practice.

CRITICAL REFLECTIONS

1)   What factors have led Canadian drug policy to be historically more aligned with punitive rather than pragmatic nations?

2)   What factors prevent knowledge from being transferred to policy and best practices?

3)   What policy recommendations would you make, not from your beliefs but rather from the empirically based information in this book, to move Canada towards being a more pragmatic nation with respect to psychoactive drugs?

APPENDIX A

CANADIAN CANNABIS LEGALIZATION HIGHLIGHTS (BY PROVINCE / TERRITORY)
(as of March 16th, 2018)
Note: All jurisdictions will maintain the federal 30g possession limit (non-medical)

	British Columbia*	Alberta	Saskatchewan	Manitoba	Ontario	Quebec
Name of Provincial Bill/Act (or link to released framework)	https://news.gov.bc.ca/releases/2018PSSG0006-000151	An Act to Control & Reg. Cannabis – Royal Assent Dec.15/17 (no proclamation date yet)	Bill 121 – The Cannabis Control (Saskatchewan) Act – 1st Reading Mar.14/18	Bill 11 (Safe & Responsible Retailing of Cannabis Act) (2nd reading) and Cannabis Harm Prevention Act	Cannabis Act, 2017 and Ontario Cannabis Retail Corporation Act, 2017 (no proclamation dates yet)	Bill 157 (Cannabis Regulation Act) - Hearings before Committee on Health & Social Services
Min. Age	19	18	19	19	19	18
Transport Restrictions	Must be in a sealed package, or inaccessible to vehicle occupants	Closed package out of reach of driver & occupants	Possession in vehicle solely for transport to place of lawful use or storage	In trunk or behind last seat	Must be packed in closed baggage or as per regs.	
Recreational Consumption Restrictions	Permitted where tobacco smoking is permitted but not where children are present (beaches, parks,playgrounds) or in vehicles	Not at hospital, school, daycare, etc. or wherever smoking is prohibited	No public consumption – consumption of lighted cannabis in private places may be limited by regulation	No consumption in vehicle or enclosed public spaces	No consumption in public, at workplace or in vehicle or boat	Prohibition at enumerated enclosed and public spaces
Provincial Distributor	BC Liquor Distribution Branch	Alberta Gaming and Liquor Commission	Private, regulated by Sask Liquor & Gaming Auth.	Liquor, Gaming and Cannabis Authority (with private distr's)	Ontario Cannabis Retail Corporation	Société des alcohols du Québec
Permitted Retailer(s)	Public and Private	Private. Applications open March 6	Private, regulated by Sask Liquor & Gaming Auth.	Delta9/Canopy NAC Hiku/BOBHQ 10552763 Can.Corp.	Ontario Cannabis Retail Corporation	Société Québécoise du Cannabis
Number of Retail Locations	No cap on licences, but municipalities must approve locations	250 retail licences anticipated in Yr. 1	Up to 51 permits in 32 communities		40 stores by July 2018; 80 by July 2019; 150 by 2020	15 physical stores at outset
Retail Location Restrictions	No co-location with alcohol or tobacco. Cannabis & accessories only in urban areas	No co-location with anything other than cannabis accessories	Co-location w access./ ancill. items only – communities can opt out -no minors	Municipalities can prohibit retail sales – no co-location with alcohol	Unclear whether municipalities can delay or prohibit retail	Restrictions may be imposed by regulation
Online Sales	Yes, by govt	Yes, by govt	Yes, by private retailers	Yes, by private retailers	Yes, by govt	Yes, by govt
Announced LP Supply Deals	RFI published March 13th – closes March 27th	Expression of interest process closed Feb.12		Tilray to supply NAC		MedReleaf Hydropothecary Canopy, Aurora Aphria, Tilray
Home Grow Restrictions	No visible plants from public space. No growing in daycare homes. Landlords and strata councils may restrict	Expected to be permitted in regulations	Permitted as per Cannabis Act. Proposed that landlords may set & enforce cannabis rules	No home growing permitted	Permitted as per Cannabis Act	No home growing permitted. Private possession of >150g prohibited

* Based on announced framework only – no bill introduced yet
FOR INFORMATIONAL PURPOSES ONLY. THIS DOES NOT CONSTITUTE LEGAL ADVICE.
© Brazeau Seller Law, 2018. Prepared by Trina Fraser, Partner and CannaLaw® group leader.

Newfoundland & Labrador	New Brunswick	Nova Scotia*	Prince Edward Island*	Yukon	Northwest Territories	Nunavut*
Bill 23 (Act to Amend the Liquor Corporation Act) – Royal Assent on Dec.7/17	Bill 16 (*Cannabis Control Act*) & Bill 17 (*Cannabis Mgmt Corp Act*) 3rd readings on Feb.2/18	https://novascotia.ca/cannabis/	https://www.princeedwardisland.ca/en/service/cannabis-legislation	Bill 15, *Cannabis Control and Regulation Act*, 1st reading on March 8/18	Bill 6, *Cannabis Legalization and Regulation Implementation Act*–2nd reading Mar.1/18 –now before standing committee	https://www.gov.nu.ca/sites/default/files/final_modified_text_r_pt_-_regulating_cannabis_in_nunavut-eng.pdf
19	19	19	19	19	19	19
	Restriction only on consumption within a vehicle		Packages must be secured & inaccessible to anyone in vehicle	Must be in closed container & inaccessible to occupants	Must be unopened or resealed & inaccessible to occupants	Must be in closed packaging and inaccessible to occupants
Private residences only	Private dwelling w consent of occupant or vacant land w consent of owner or occupant only		Private residences only (with potential for designated spaces)	For now, restricted to privately owned residences and adjoining property, where owner consents	Permitted on private property (with LL permission) and in restricted public areas	Same as tobacco -also restricted in vehicles, school grounds, hospitals, playgrounds
Newfoundland and Labrador Liquor Commission	Cannabis Management Corporation	Nova Scotia Liquor Corp (NSLC)	PEI Liquor Control Commission (PEILCC)	Government of Yukon	NWT Liquor Commission	Nunavut Liquor Commission (NULC)
Private (public only where no private retailer) Tweed to have 4 locations	New subsidiary of NB Liquor under name "CannabisNB"	NSLC	PEILCC	Private (but govt to start)	NWT Liquor Commission	Public and Private
RFP for retailers closes March 29/18 41 stores expected	11 locations by July/18; 20 locations by September/18	9 locations	Four in 2018 (Charlottetown, Summerside, Montague, West Prince)	One government-owned location to start	Initially, within existing liquor stores	No physical locations in 2018
No co-location/ shared access with pharmacy - no adjacent lounge where alcohol served	>300m from schools	Co-location with existing liquor stores, but in separate area	Stand-alone government-owned locations – No advertising	No co-location with alcohol sales	Municipalities can prohibit retail sales / est. restrictions via plebiscite	Proposed that 'dry' communities will not be permitted
By govt for now www.ShopCannabisNL.com	Yes, by govt	Yes, by govt	Yes, by govt	Yes, by govt	Yes by govt but only where no liquor store	Yes, by govt asap after legalization
Canopy Growth	Organigram, Canopy, Zenabis, Nuuvera	RFI closed February 23rd	Organigram, Canopy, Canada's Island Garden			
	Indoors in separate locked space. Outdoors in locked encl. at least 1.52m high	Permitted as per *Cannabis Act*		Permitted as per *Cannabis Act*	Permitted as per *Cannabis Act*	Ability for landlords and condo corps to restrict home growing are being considered

REFERENCES

Abbott, A. (2000). *Alcohol, tobacco and other drugs: Challenging myths, assessing theories, individualizing interventions* (1st ed.). Washington, DC: National Association of Social Workers Press.

ABC News. (2006, 22 March). Drug high from "dusting" is fatal for one teen. Retrieved from http://abcnews.go.com/GMA/AmericanFamily/story?id=1752729

ABC News. (2012, 1 June). Face-eating cannibal attack may be latest in string of 'bath salts' incidents. Retrieved from http://abcnews.go.com/Blotter/face-eating-cannibal-attack-latest-bath-salts-incident/story?id=16470389

Adlaf, E. M., Begin, P. & Sawka, E. (2005). *Canadian addiction survey (CAS): A national survey of Canadians' use of alcohol and other drugs. Prevalence of use and related harms detailed report.* Ottawa, ON: Canadian Centre on Substance Abuse.

Adlaf, E. M., Demers, A. & Gliksman, L. (2005). *Canadian campus survey 2004.* Toronto, ON: Centre for Addiction and Mental Health.

Adrian, M. (2003). How can sociological theory help our understanding of addictions? *Substance Use & Misuse, 38*(10), 1385–1423.

Agger, B. (1991). Critical theory, poststructuralism, postmodernism: Their sociological relevance. *Annual Review of Sociology, 17,* 105–131.

Agic, B. & McKenzie, K. (2013). *The health equity office: 2011–2013 report.* Toronto, ON: Centre for Addiction and Mental Health.

Agnew, R. (1992). Foundation for a general strain theory of crime and delinquency. *Criminology, 30*(1), 47–88. doi:10.1111/j.1745-9125.1992.tb01093.x

Agrawal, A. & Lynskey, M. T. (2008). Are there genetic influences on addiction: Evidence from family, adoption and twin studies. *Addiction, 103*(7), 1069–1081. doi:10.1111/j.1360-0443.2008.02213.x

Akers, R. L., Krohn, M. D., Lanza-Kaduce, L. & Radosevich, M. (1979). Social learning and deviant behavior: A specific test of a general theory. *American Sociological Review, 44*(4), 636–655.

Akers, R. L. (1996). Is differential association/social learning cultural deviance theory? *Criminology,* 34(2), 229–247.

Alaggia, R. & Csiernik, R. (2017). Coming home: Rediscovering the family in addiction treatment in Canada. In R. Csiernik & W. S. Rowe (Eds.), *Responding to the oppression of addiction: Canadian social work perspectives* (3rd ed., pp. 76–94). Toronto, ON: Canadian Scholars.

Albonetti, C. A. (1997). Sentencing under the federal sentencing guidelines: Effects of defendant characteristics, guilty pleas, and departures on sentence outcomes for drug offenses, 1992–1992. *Law and Society Review, 31*(4), 789–822.

Alcoholics Anonymous. (2012). *2011 membership survey.* New York, NY: Alcoholics Anonymous World Service.

Alcoholics Anonymous. (2015). *Estimated worldwide AA individual and group membership.* Retrieved from http://www.aa.org/assets/en_US/smf-132_en.pdf

Aldridge, J., Measham, F. & Williams, L. (2011*). Illegal leisure revisited: Changing patterns of alcohol and drug use in adolescents and young adults.* London, UK: Routledge.

Aldridge, J., Parker, H. & Measham, F. (1998). Rethinking young people's drug use. *Health Education, 98*(5), 164–172. doi:10.1108/09654289810229636

Alexander, B. (1987). The disease and adaptive models of addiction: A framework evaluation. *Journal of Drug Issues, 17*(1), 47–66.

Alexander, P. (2005, 27 July). "Dusting" is the new killer high for teens. *NBC News.* Retrieved from http://www.today.com/id/8714725/ns/today/t/dusting-new-killer-high-teens/#.U-rLC6jbbeY

Allen, J. P., Chango, J., Szwedo, D., Schad, M. & Marston, E. (2012). Predictors of susceptibility to peer influence regarding substance use in adolescence. *Child Development, 83*(1), 337–350. doi:10.1111/j.1467-8624.2011.01682.x

American Psychiatric Association. (2000). *Diagnostic and statistical manual of mental disorders* (IV-TR ed.). Arlington, VA: American Psychiatric Publishing.

American Psychiatric Association. (2013). *Diagnostic and statistical manual of mental disorders* (5th ed.). Arlington, VA: American Psychiatric Publishing.

Anderson, E. (1999). *Code of the street: Decency, violence and the moral life of the inner city.* New York, NY: W. W. Norton & Company Inc.

Antone, J. & Csiernik, R. (2017). The role of culture in prevention. In W. S. Rowe & C. Rick (Eds.), *Responding to the oppression of addiction: Canadian social work perspectives* (3rd ed., pp. 60–73). Toronto, ON: Canadian Scholars' Press.

Arbour-Nicitopoulos, K. P., Kwan, M. Y. W., Lowe, D., Taman, S. & Faulkner, G. E. J. (2010). Social norms of alcohol, smoking, and marijuana use within a Canadian university setting. *Journal of American College Health, 59*(3), 191–196. doi:10.1080/07448481.2010.502194

Arendt, M., Mortensen, P., Rosenberg, R., Pedersen, C. & Waltoft, B. (2008). Familial predisposition for psychiatric disorder: Comparison of subjects treated for cannabis-induced psychosis and schizophrenia. *Achieves of General Psychiatry, 65*(11), 1269–1274.

Armstrong, J. (2015). Majority of Canadians support decriminalizing marijuana: Poll. *Global News.* Retrieved from http://globalnews.ca/news/2173919/majority-of-canadians-support-decriminalizing-marijuana-poll

Asbridge, M., Hayden, J. A. & Cartwright, J. L. (2012). Acute cannabis consumption and motor vehicle collision risk: Systematic review of observational studies and meta-analysis. *British Medical Journal, 344,* e536.

Aseltine, R. H., Jr. (1995). A reconsideration of parental and peer influences on adolescent deviance. *Journal of Health and Social Behavior, 36*(2), 103–121.

Atkinson, A. M., Bellis, M. & Sumnall, H. (2013). Young peoples' perspective on the portrayal of alcohol and drinking on television: Findings of a focus group study. *Addiction Research & Theory, 21*(2), 91–99. doi:10.3109/16066359.2012.687795

Avants, Brian B., Hurt, H., Giannetta, J. M., Epstein, C. L., Shera, D. M., Rao, H., Wang, J. & Gee, J. C. (2007). Effects of heavy in utero cocaine exposure on adolescent caudate morphology. *Pediatric Neurology, 37*(4), 275–279.

Babbie, E. (2016). *The practice of social research* (14th ed.). Boston, MA: Cengage Learning.

Babor, T., Caulkins, J., Edwards, G., Fischer, B., Foxcroft, D., Humphreys, K., Obot, I., Rehm, J., Reuter, P., Room, R., Rossow, I. & Strang, J. (2010). *Drug policy and the public good.* New York, NY: Oxford University Press.

Bachman, J. G., Johnston, L. D. & O'Malley, P. M. (1998). Explaining recent increases in students' marijuana use: impacts of perceived risks and disapproval, 1976 through 1996. *American Journal of Public Health 88*(6), 887–892.

Bahr, S. J., Hawks, R. D. & Wang, G. (1993). Family and religious influences on adolescent substance abuse. *Youth and Society, 24*(4), 443–465.

Bahr, S. J., Hoffmann, J. P. & Yang, X. (2005). Parental and peer influences on the risk of adolescent drug use. *The Journal of Primary Prevention, 26*(6), 529–551. doi:10.1007/s10935-005-0014-8

Bailey, L. (2005). Control and desire: The issue of identity in popular discourses of addiction. *Addiction Research and Theory 13*(6): 535–543. doi:10.1080/16066350500338195

Baker, T. E. (2011). Barbiturates. In M. A. Kleiman. & J. E. Hawdon (Eds.), *Encyclopedia of drug policy* (pp. 85–89). Thousand Oak, CA: Sage Publications.

Ball, D. (2007). Addiction science and its genetics. *Addiction,103*(3), 360-367. doi:10.1111/j.1360-0443.2007.02061.x

Ball, S. A., Carroll, K. M., Canning-Ball, M. & Rounsaville, B. J. (2006). Reasons for dropout from drug abuse treatment: Symptoms, personality, and motivation. *Addictive Behaviors, 31*(2), 320–330. doi:10.1016/j.addbeh.2005.05.013

Bambico, F. R., Nguyen, N. T., Katz, N. & Gobbi, G. (2009). Chronic exposure to cannabinoids during adolescence but not during adulthood impairs emotional behaviour and monoaminergic neurotransmission. *Neurobiology of Disease, 37*(3), 641–655. doi:10.1016/j.nbd.2009.11.020

Bandura, A. (1977). *Social learning theory.* Englewood Cliffs, NJ: Prentice-Hall.

Barfield-Cottledge, T. (2015). The triangulation effects of family structure and attachment on adolescent substance use. *Crime & Delinquency, 61*(2), 297–320. doi:10.1177/0011128711420110

Barnes, G. M., Hoffman, J. H., Welte, J. W., Farrell, M. P. & Dintcheff, B. A. (2007). Adolescents' time use: Effects on substance use, delinquency and sexual activity. *Journal of Youth and Adolescence, 36*(5), 697–710. doi:10.1007/s10964-006-9075-0

Barnes, G. M., Reifman, A. S., Farrell, M. P. & Dintcheff, B. A. (2000). The effects of parenting on the development of adolescent alcohol misuse: A six-wave latent growth model. *Journal of Marriage and Family, 62*(1), 175–186. doi:10.1111/j.1741-3737.2000.00175.x

Bears Augustyn, M. & McGloin, J. M. (2013). The risk of informal socializing with peers: Considering gender differences across predatory delinquency and substance use. *Justice Quarterly, 30*(1), 117–143. doi: 10.1080/07418825.2011.597417

Beccaria, C. (1764). *On crimes and punishments.* Indianapolis, IN: Hackett Publishing Co.

Beck, J. (1998). 100 years of "just say no" Versus "Just Say Know": Reevaluating drug education goals for the coming century. *Evaluation Review, 22*(1), 15–45. doi:10.1177/0193841X9802200102

Becker, H. S. (1953). Becoming a marihuana user. *American Journal of Sociology, 59*(3), 235–242.

Becker, H. S. (1963). *Outsiders: Studies in the sociology of deviance.* New York, NY: Free Press.

Bègue, L. & Roché, S. (2009). Multidimensional social control variables as predictors of drunkenness among French adolescents. *Journal of Adolescence, 32*(2), 171–191. doi:10.1016/j.adolescence.2008.04.001

Bell, K. & Salmon, A. (2012). Good intentions and dangerous assumptions: Research ethics committees and illicit drug research. *Research Ethics*, 8(4), 191–199.

Benowitz, N. L. & Fredericks, A. B. (2009). Nicotine. In P. Korsmeyer & H. R. Kranzler (Eds.), *Encyclopedia of drugs, alcohol & addictive behavior* (3rd ed., Vol. 3, pp. 134–139). Detroit, MI: Macmillan Reference USA.

Bentham, J. (1789). *An introduction to the principles of morals and legislation.* London, UK: The Athlone Press.

Berberian, R. M., Gross, C., Lovejoy, J. & Paparella, S. (1976). The effectiveness of drug education programs: A critical review. *Health Education & Behavior, 4*(4), 377–398.

Bernburg, J. G. & Thorlindsson, T. (2001). Routine activities in social context: A closer look at the role of opportunity in deviant behavior. *Justice Quarterly, 18*(3), 543–567. doi:10.1080/07418820100095011

Best, D. W. & Wilson. (2014). Patterns of family conflict and their impact on substance use and psychosocial outcomes in a sample of young people in treatment. *Vulnerable Children and Youth Studies, 9*(2), 114–122. doi:10.1080/17450128.2013.855858

Bewley-Taylor, D. R. (2013). Towards revision of the UN drug control conventions: Harnessing like-mindedness. *International Journal of Drug Policy, 24*(1), 60–68. doi:10.1016/j.drugpo.2012.09.001

Biber, F. (2016, 13 April). Saskatoon tribal council calls for study into safe injection sites. *CBC News Saskatoon.* Retrieved from http://www.cbc.ca/news/canada/saskatoon/health-injection-site-1.3534914

Birkeland, S., Murphy-Graham, E. & Weiss, C. (2005). Good reasons for ignoring good evaluation: The case of the drug abuse resistance education (D.A.R.E.) program. *Evaluation and Program Planning, 28*(3), 247–256. doi:10.1016/j.evalprogplan.2005.04.001

Blackwell, J. C. (1988). Sin, sickness, or social problem? The concept of drug dependence. In J. C. Blackwell & P. G. Erickson (Eds.), *Illicit drugs in Canada* (pp. 158–174). Toronto, ON: Nelson.

Boak, A., Hamilton, H. A., Adlaf, E. M. & Mann, R. E. (2013). *Drug use among Ontario students, 1977–2013: Detailed OSDUHS findings.* CAMH Research Document Series No. 36. Toronto, ON: Centre for Addiction and Mental Health.

Bouchard, M., Morselli, C., Gallupe, O., Easton, S., Descormiers, K., Turcotte, M. & Boivin, R. (2012). *Estimating the size of the Canadian illicit meth and MDMA markets: A multi-method approach.* No. 024. Ottawa, ON: Public Safety Canada.

Bourgois, P. (2000). Disciplining addictions: The bio-politics of methadone and heroin in the United States. *Culture, Medicine and Psychiatry, 24*(2), 165–195.

Bourgois, P. & Bruneau, J. (2000). Needle exchange, HIV infection, and the politics of science: Confronting Canada's cocaine injection epidemic with participant observation. *Medical Anthropology, 18*(4), 325–350.

Boyd, N. (1983). The dilemma of Canadian narcotics legislation: The social control of altered states of consciousness. *Contemporary Crises, 7*(3), 257–269. doi:10.1007/BF00729160

Boyd, N. (1984). The origins of Canadian narcotics legislation: the process of criminalization in historical context. *Dalhousie Law Journal, 8*(1), 102–137.

Boyd, N. (1998). Rethinking Our Policy on Cannabis. *Policy Options, 19,* 31–33.

Boyd, S. & Carter, C. I. (2014). *Killer weed: Marijuana grow ops, media and justice.* Toronto, ON: University of Toronto Press.

Boyle, M. H., Sanford, M., Szatmari, P., Merikangas, K. & Offord, D. R. (2001). Familial influences on substance use by adolescents and young adults. *Canadian Journal of Public Health, 92*(3), 206–209.

Brady, K. (2012). Comorbid anxiety and substance use disorders. In J. C. Verster, K. Brady, M. Galanter & P. Conrod (Eds.), *Drug abuse and addiction in medical illness: Causes, consequences and treatment* (pp. 267–274). New York, NY: Springer.

Brain, K., Parker, H. & Carnwath, T. (2000). Drinking with design: Young drinkers as psychoactive consumers. *Drugs: Education, Prevention & Policy, 7*(1), 5–20. doi:10.1080/713660094

Branstetter, S. A., Furman, W. & Cottrell, L. (2009). The influence of representations of attachment, maternal-adolescent relationship quality, and maternal monitoring on adolescent substance use: A 2-year longitudinal examination. *Child Development, 80*(5), 1448–1462. doi:10.1111/j.1467-8624.2009.01344.x.

Bretteville-Jensen, A. L. (2006). To legalize or not to legalize? Economic approaches to the decriminalization of drugs. *Substance Use & Misuse, 41*(4), 555–565. doi:10.1080/10826080500521565

Briar, S. & Piliavin, I. (1965). Delinquency, situational inducements, and commitment to conformity. *Social Problems, 13*(1), 35–45. doi:10.2307/799304

Briones, A., Cumsille, F., Henao, A. & Pardo, B. (2013). *The drug problem in the Americas.* Washington, DC: Organization of American States.

British Columbia Ministry of Children and Families Services. (1998). *Community action guide: Working together for the prevention of Fetal Alcohol Syndrome.* Retrieved from http://www.motherisk.org/fas1/resources/articles/community.pdf

Bruno, T. & Csiernik, R. (forthcoming). Politics, marketing and the lack of evidence in drug education in schools: A case study of school-based drug education programs in Ontario, Canada.

Bruser, D. & Bailey, A. (2012, 26 September). ADHD drugs suspected of hurting Canadian kids. *Toronto Star.* Retrieved from http://www.thestar.com/news/canada/2012/09/26/adhd_drugs_suspected_of_hurting_canadian_kids.html

Bryden, J. (2014, 18 June). "Conservatives attack Trudeau's marijuana stand in by-election." *The Globe and Mail.* Retrieved from https://www.theglobeandmail.com/news/politics/conservatives-attack-trudeaus-marijuana-stand-in-by-election/article19216247/

Bucossi, M. M. & Stuart, G. L. (2009). Amphetamines. In G. L. Fisher & N. A. Roget (Eds.), *Encyclopedia of substance abuse prevention, treatment, & recovery* (pp. 70–71). Thousand Oaks, CA: Sage Publications.

Burgess, R. L. & Akers, R. L. (1966). A differential association-reinforcement theory of criminal behavior. *Social Problems 14*(2), 128–147.

Burgmann, T. (2012, 16 January). B.C. ecstasy deaths: Teen overdose may be latest in string of deaths. *Canadian Press.* Retrieved from http://www.huffingtonpost.ca/2012/01/16/bc-ecstasy-deaths_n_1209266.html

Butters, J. E. (2002). Family stressors and adolescent cannabis use: A pathway to problem use. *Journal of Adolescence, 25*(6), 645–654. doi:10.1006/jado.2002.0514

Butters, J. E. (2005). Promoting healthy choices: the importance of differentiating between ordinary and high risk cannabis use among high-school students. *Substance Use & Misuse, 40*(6), 845–855.

Calcagnetti, D. J. (2009). Cocaine and crack. In G. L. Fisher & N. A. Roget (Eds.), *Encyclopedia of substance abuse prevention, treatment, & recovery* (pp. 194–196). Thousand Oaks, CA: Sage Publications.

Cameron, R., Brown, K. S., Best, J. A., Pelkman, C. L., Madill, C. L., Manske, S. R. & Payne, M. E. (1999). Effectiveness of a social influences smoking prevention program as a function of provider type, training method, and school risk. *American Journal of Public Health, 89*(12), 1827–1831.

Canadian Broadcasting Corporation (Producer). (1993, 28 January). *Davis Inlet: Innu community in crisis.* [Video/DVD]. CBC Digital Archives.

Canadian Centre on Substance Abuse. (2005). *National framework for action to reduce the harms associated with alcohol and other drugs and substances in Canada.* Retrieved from http://www.ccsa.ca/Resource Library/NatFra_1stEdition_chart_eng.pdf

Canadian Centre on Substance Abuse. (2007). *Substance abuse in Canada: Youth in focus.* Ottawa, ON: Canadian Centre on Substance Abuse. Retrieved from http://www.ccsa.ca/Resource%20Library/ccsa-011521-2007-e.pdf

Canadian Centre on Substance Abuse. (2009). *Substance abuse in Canada: Concurrent disorders.* Ottawa, ON: Canadian Centre on Substance Abuse.

Canadian Press. (2012, 20 September). Gas-sniffing on the rise in Natuashish. *Canadian Press.* Retrieved from http://o.canada.com/news/gas-sniffing-on-the-rise-in-natuashish

Canadian Press. (2016, 18 November). Opioid addiction, overdose and death: A Canadian crisis by the numbers. Retrieved from http://thechronicleherald.ca/canada/1416840-opioid-addiction-overdose-and-death-a-canadian-crisis-by-the-numbers

Carlson, S. R., Johnson, S. C. & Jacobs, P. C. (2010). Disinhibited characteristics and binge drinking among university student drinkers. *Addictive Behaviors, 35*(3), 242–251. doi:10.1016/j.addbeh.2009.10.020

Carpentier, P. J. (2012). ADHD. In J. C. Verster, K. Brady, M. Galanter, & P. Conrod (Eds.), *Drug abuse and addiction in medical illness* (pp. 285–296). New York, NY: Springer.

Carstairs, C. (2006). *Jailed for possession: Illegal drug use, regulation, and power in Canada, 1920–1961.* Toronto, ON: University of Toronto Press.

Catalano, R. F., Fleming, C. B., Haggerty, K. R., Oesterle, S. & White, H. R. (2010). Romantic relationship status changes and substance use among 18- to 20-year-olds. *Journal of Studies on Alcohol and Drugs, 71*(6), 847–856.

Caulkins, J. P., Kasunic, A., Kleiman, M. & Lee, M. A. C. (2014). Understanding drug legalization. *International Public Health Journal, 6*(3), 283.

Cavalieri, W. & Riley, D. (2012). Harm reduction in Canada: The many faces of regression. In R. Pates & D. Riley (Eds.), *Harm reduction in substance use and high-risk behaviour: International policy and practice.* London, UK: Wiley-Blackwell.

CBC News. (2005, 16 June). Parents warned of "dusting" solvent abuse. *CBC News.* Retrieved from http://www.cbc.ca/news/technology/parents-warned-of-dusting-solvent-abuse-1.568836

CBC News. (2006, 10 April). Cold remedies removed over crystal meth concerns. *CBC News.* Retrieved from http://www.cbc.ca/news/technology/cold-remedies-removed-over-crystal-meth-concerns-1.598787

CBC News. (2012, 31 January). Alberta deaths linked to ecstasy-like drug: Victims think they are taking ecstasy, but actually ingesting "Dr. Death." *CBC News Calgary.* Retrieved from http://www.cbc.ca/news/canada/calgary/8-alberta-deaths-linked-to-ecstasy-like-drug-1.1166437

CBC News. (2012, 24 June). Calgary "bath salts" drug incident sends 2 to hospital: User overpowered police in city's 1st reported incident of drug's use. *CBC News Calgary.* Retrieved from http://www.cbc.ca/news/canada/calgary/calgary-bath-salts-drug-incident-sends-2-to-hospital-1.1176067

CBC News. (2016a, 12 May). Safe-injection sites should open in Toronto, top health official to recommend. *CBC News Toronto.* Retrieved from http://www.cbc.ca/news/canada/toronto/toronto-safe-injection-1.3488700

CBC News. (2016b, 4 February). Thunder Bay to study whether safe injection site is needed. *CBC News Thunder Bay.* Retrieved from http://www.cbc.ca/news/canada/thunder-bay/thunder-bay-drug-strategy-1.3433545

CBS Miami. (2012, 27 June). Medical examiner: Causeway cannibal not high on bath salts. *CBS Miami.* Retrieved from http://miami.cbslocal.com/2012/06/27/medical-examiner-causeway-cannibal-not-high-on-bath-salts

Chambliss, W. J. (1994). Why the US government is not contributing to the resolution of the nation's drug problem. *International Journal of Health Services, 24*(4), 675–690.

Champagne, D. (2015). Centering Indigenous nations within Indigenous methodologies. *Wicazo Sa Review, 30*(1), 57–81. doi:10.5749/wicazosareview.30.1.0057

Champion, K. E., Newton, N. C., Barrett, E. L. & Teesson, M. (2013). A systematic review of school-based alcohol and other drug prevention programs facilitated by computers or the Internet. *Drug and Alcohol Review,* 32(2), 115–123.

Cheung, Y. W. (2000). Substance abuse and developments in harm reduction. *Canadian Medical Association Journal 162*(12), 1697–1700.

Clark, A. E. & Lohéac, Y. (2007). "It wasn't me, it was them!" social influence in risky behavior by adolescents. *Journal of Health Economics, 26*(4), 763–784.

Clark, F. (2015). Russia's war on drugs leaves patients without pain relief. *The Lancet, 386*(9990), 231–232.

Clark, H., Shamblen, S., Ringwalt, C. & Hanley, S. (2012). Predicting high risk adolescents' substance use over time: The role of parental monitoring. *The Journal of Primary Prevention, 33*(2–3), 67–77.

Clayton, R. R., Cattarello, A. M. & Johnstone, B. M. (1996). The effectiveness of Drug Abuse Resistance Education (Project DARE): 5-year follow-up results. *Preventive Medicine, 25*(3), 307–318. doi:10.1006/pmed.1996.0061

Cleverly, B. (2014, 26 June). *Safe injection site for Victoria gaining acceptance, mayor says.* Retrieved from http://www.timescolonist.com/news/local/safe-injection-site-for-victoria-gaining-acceptance-mayor-says-1.1160307

Cloward, R. A. & Ohlin, L. E. (1960). Delinquency and opportunity: A theory of delinquent gangs. *The Sociological Quarterly, 2*(3), 222–224.

Coggans, N., Evans, R. & O'Connor, L. (1999). Drug education and effectiveness: The contribution of the police service to work in schools. *Early Child Development and Care, 157*(1), 109–145.

Cohen, L. E. & Felson, M. (1979). Social change and crime rate trends: A routine activity approach. *American Sociological Review, 44*(4), 588–608.

Cohen, P. (2001). Liberal pot policies have mixed results in Netherlands. *Canadian Speeches, 15*(3), 23.

Collin, C. (2006). *Substance abuse issues and public policy in Canada: Canada's federal drug strategy.* Ottawa, ON: Parliamentary Information and Research Service.

Corrigan, P. W., Watson, A. C. & Miller, F. E. (2006). Blame, shame, and contamination: The impact of mental illness and drug dependence stigma on family members. *Journal of Family Psychology, 20*(2), 239–246.

Cosgrove, L. & Krimsky, S. (2012). A comparison of *DSM*-IV and *DSM*-5 panel members' financial associations with industry: A pernicious problem persists. *PLOS Medicine, 9*(3), e1001190. doi:10.1371/journal.pmed.1001190

Cosgrove, L., Krimsky, S., Vijayaraghavan M. & Schneider L. (2006). Financial ties between DSM-IV panel members and the pharmaceutical industry. *Psychotherapy and Psychosomatics, 75*(2), 154–160.

Cotter, A., Greenland, J. & Karam, M. (2015). Drug-related offences in Canada, 2013. *Juristat.* Catalogue no. 85-002-X. Ottawa, ON: Minister of Industry.

Courtwright, D. T. (2011). Language-use disorder: Comment on DSM-V's proposed "addiction and related disorders" and Charles O'brien's "addiction and dependence in DSM-V." *Addiction, 106*(5), 878–879. doi:10.1111/j.1360-0443.2010.03285.x

Cruz, S. (2011). The latest evidence in the neuroscience of solvent misuse. *Substance Use and Misuse, 46*(1), 62–67.

Csiernik, R. (2010). Is Alcoholics Anonymous of value for social work practitioners? In R. Csiernik & W. S. Rowe (Eds.) *Responding to the oppression of addiction: Canadian social work perspectives* (2nd ed., pp. 55–65). Toronto, ON: Canadian Scholars' Press.

Csiernik, R. (2014a). *Just say know: A counsellor's guide to psychoactive drugs.* Toronto, ON: Canadian Scholars' Press.

Csiernik, R. (2014b). *Workplace wellness: Issues and responses.* Toronto, ON: Canadian Scholars' Press.

Csiernik, R. (2016). *Substance use and abuse: Everything matters* (2nd ed.). Toronto, ON: Canadian Scholars' Press.

Csiernik, R. & Birnbaum, R. (2017). *Practising social work research: Case studies for learning* (2nd ed.). Toronto, ON: University of Toronto Press.

Csiernik, R. & Rowe, W. S. (2017). *Responding to the oppression of addiction: Canadian social work perspectives* (3rd ed.). Toronto, ON: Canadian Scholars.

Csiernik, R. Bhakari, M. & Koop-Watson, R. (2017). Many paths to prohibition: Drug policy in Canada. In R. Csiernik and W.S. Rowe (Eds.), *Responding to the oppression of addiction: Canadian social work perspectives* (3rd ed., pp. 396–414). Toronto, ON: Canadian Scholars.

Csiernik, R., Rowe, W. & Watkin, J. (2017). Prevention as controversy: Harm reduction. In R. Csiernik & W. S. Rowe (Eds.), *Responding to the oppression of addiction: Canadian social work perspectives* (3rd ed., pp. 28–47). Toronto, ON: Canadian Scholars.

CTV News. (2014, 3 July). "Killer heroin" prompts warning for Montreal drug users. *CTV News Montreal*. Retrieved from http://montreal.ctvnews.ca/killer-heroin-prompts-warning-for-montreal-drug-users-1.1898387

Cuijpers, P. (2003). Three decades of drug prevention research. *Drugs: Education, Prevention, and Policy, 10*(1), 7–20. doi:10.1080/0968763021000018900

Dallas, R., Field, M., Jones, A., Christiansen, P., Rose, A. & Robinson, E. (2014). Influenced but unaware: Social influence on alcohol drinking among social acquaintances. *Alcoholism: Clinical and Experimental Research, 38*(5), 1448–1453. doi:10.1111/acer.12375

DARE America. (2016). *DARE: Teaching students decision making for safe and healthy living*. Retrieved from http://www.dare.org/about-d-a-r-e

Dauvergne, M. (2009). Trends in police-reported drug offences in Canada. *Juristat, 29*(2), 1C.

DeBeck, K., Wood, E., Montaner, J. & Kerr, T. (2009). Canada's new federal "National Anti-Drug Strategy": An informal audit of reported funding allocation. *International Journal of Drug Policy, 20*(2), 188–191. doi:10.1016/j.drugpo.2008.04.004

Delcher, C., Maladaono-Mollina, M. & Wagenaar, A. (2012). Effects of alcohol taxes on alcohol-related disease mortality in New York State from 1969 to 2006. *Addictive Behaviors, 37*(7), 783–789. doi:10.1016/j.addbeh.2012.02.019

Des Jarlais, D. C. (1995). Editorial: Harm reduction: A framework for incorporating science into drug policy. *American Journal of Public Health, 85*(1), 10–12. doi:10.2105/AJPH.85.1.10

Deutsch, A. R., Chernyavskiy, P., Steinley, D. & Slutske, W. S. (2015). Measuring peer socialization for adolescent substance use: A comparison of perceived and actual friends' substance use effects. *Journal of Studies on Alcohol and Drugs, 76*(2), 267–277. doi:http://dx.doi.org/10.15288/jsad.2015.76.267

Dion, G. A. (1999). *The structure of drug prohibition in International law and in Canadian law*. Retrieved from http://www.parl.gc.ca/content/sen/committee/371/ille/presentation/dion-e.htm

Ducatti Flister, L. (2012). The economic case for marijuana legalization in Canada. *Journal of Alternative Perspectives in the Social Sciences, 5*(1), 96–100.

Duffy, A. (2016, 6 April). Battle lines drawn on proposed safe injection site for Ottawa. *Ottawa Citizen*. Retrieved from http://ottawacitizen.com/news/local-news/battle-lines-drawn-on-proposed-safe-injection-site-for-ottawa

Duncan, S. C., Duncan, T. E. & Strycker, L. A. (2006). Alcohol use from ages 9 to 16: A cohort-sequential latent growth model. *Drug and Alcohol Dependency, 81*(1), 71–81. doi:10.1016/j.drugalcdep.2005.06.001

Dupras, D. (1998). *Canada's international obligations under the leading international conventions on the control of narcotic drugs.* Ottawa, ON: Library of Parliament. Retrieved from https://sencanada.ca/content/sen/committee/371/ille/library/dupras-e.htm

Dusenbury, L. & Falco, M. (1995). Eleven components of effective drug abuse prevention curricula. *The Journal of School Health, 65*(10), 420–425. doi:10.1111/j.1746-1561.1995.tb08205.x

Duster, T. (1970). *The legislation of morality: Law, drugs and moral judgment.* New York, NY: Free Press.

Dyck, E. (2010). *Psychedelic psychiatry: LSD from clinic to campus.* Baltimore, MD: John Hopkins University Press.

Dyck, E. & Bradford, T. (2012). Peyote on the prairies: Religions, scientists, and Native-newcomer relations in Western Canada. *Journal of Canadian Studies, 46*(1), 28–52. doi:10.1353/jcs.2012.0003

Ehlers, C. L. (2007). Variations in ADH and ALDH in Southwest California Indians. *Alcohol Research & Health, 30*(1), 14–17.

Elikkottil, J., Gupta, P. & Gupta, K. (2009). The analgesic potential of cannabinoids. *Journal of Opioid Management, 5*(6), 341–357.

Elkins, I. J., King, S. M., McGue, M. & Iacono, W. G. (2006). Personality traits and the development of nicotine, alcohol, and illicit drug disorders: Prospective links from adolescence to young adulthood. *Journal of Abnormal Psychology, 115*(1), 26–39. doi:10.1037/0021-843X.115.1.26

Elliott, D. S., Huizinga, D. H. & Ageton, S. S. (1985). *Explaining delinquency and drug use.* Beverly Hills, CA: Sage Publications.

EMCDDA (European Monitoring Centre for Drugs and Drug Addiction). (2015). *European drug report: Trends and developments.* Retrieved from http://www.emcdda.europa.eu/system/files/publications/974/TDAT15001ENN.pdf

Eng, M. Y., Luczak, S. E. & Wall, T. L. (2007). ALDH2, ADH1B, and ADH1C genotypes in Asians: A literature review. *Alcohol Research & Health, 30*(1), 22–27.

Engels, R. C. M. E., Overbeek, G. J., Larsen, H. & Granic, I. (2010). Imitation of alcohol consumption in same-sex and other-sex dyads. *Alcohol and Alcoholism, 45*(6), 557–562. doi:10.1093/alcalc/agq053

Ennett, S. T., Ringwalt, C. L., Thorne, J., Rohrbach, L. A., Vincus, A., Simons-Rudolph, A. & Jones, S. (2003). A comparison of current practice in school-based substance use prevention programs with meta-analysis findings. *Prevention Science, 4*(1), 1–14. doi:10.1023/A:1021777109369

Ennett, S. T., Tobler, N. S., Ringwalt, C. L. & Flewelling, R. L. (1994). How effective is drug-abuse resistance education? A metaanalysis of project dare outcome evaluations. *American Journal of Public Health, 84*(9), 1394–1401.

Enoch, M. (2011). The role of early life stress as a predictor for alcohol and drug dependence. *Psychopharmacology, 214*(1), 17–31.

Ensminger, M. E. & Everett, J. (2001). Vulnerability as cause of substance abuse. In R. Carson-DeWitt (Ed.), *Encyclopedia of drugs, alcohol & addictive behavior* (2nd ed., Vol. 3, pp. 1319–1322). New York, NY: Macmillan Reference USA.

Erickson, K. G., Crosnoe, R. & Dornbusch, S. M. (2000). A social process model of adolescent deviance: Combining social control and differential association perspectives. *Journal of Youth and Adolescence, 29*(4), 395–425. doi:10.1023/A:1005163724952

Erickson, P. (1992). Recent trends in Canadian drug policy: The decline and resurgence of prohibitionism. *Daedalus, 121*(31), 239–239.

Erickson, P. G. (1995). Harm reduction: What it is and is not. *Drug and Alcohol Review 14*(3), 283–285.

Erickson, P. G. (1998). Neglected and rejected: A case study of the impact of social research on Canadian drug policy. *The Canadian Journal of Sociology, 23*(2/3), 263–280. doi:10.2307/3341968

Erickson, P. G. (1999). A persistent paradox: Drug law and policy in Canada. *Canadian Journal of Criminology, 41*(2), 275.

Erickson, P. G., Butters, J., & Walko, K. (2002). *CAMH and harm reduction: A Background paper on its meaning and application for substance use issues.* Retrieved from http://www.camh.ca/en/hospital/about_camh/influencing_public_policy/public_policy_submissions/harm_reduction/Pages/harmreductionbackground.aspx

Erickson, P. G. & Hathaway, A. D. (2010). Normalization and harm reduction: Research avenues and policy agendas. *International Journal of Drug Policy, 21*(2), 137–139. doi:10.1016/j.drugpo.2009.11.005

Erickson, P. G. & Hyshka, E. (2010). Four decades of cannabis criminals in Canada: 1970–2010. *Amsterdam Law Forum, 2*(4).

Erickson, P., Riley, D., Cheung, Y. W. & O'Hare, P. (1997). *Harm reduction: A new direction for drug policies and programs.* Toronto, ON: University of Toronto Press.

Etienne, M. & Brownbill, K. (2010). Understanding the ultimate oppression: Alcohol and drug addiction in Native Land. In R. Csiernik & W.S. Rowe (Eds.) *Responding to the oppression of addiction: Canadian social work perspectives* (2nd ed., pp. 256–273). Toronto, ON: Canadian Scholars' Press.

Euchner, E.-M., Heichel, S., Nebel, K. & Raschzok, A. (2013). From "morality" policy to "normal" policy: Framing of drug consumption and gambling in Germany and the Netherlands and their regulatory consequences. *Journal of European Public Policy, 20*(3), 372–389. doi:10.1080/13501763.2013.761506

Evans, R. (1999). Parents involvement in drug prevention and education: A comparative study of programme effectiveness in the UK and USA. *Early Child Development and Care, 150*(1), 69–95. doi:10.1080/0300443991500107

Farah, M., Betancourt, L., Shera, D., Savage, J., Giannetta, J., Brodsky, N., Malmud, E. & Hurt, H. (2008). Environmental stimulation, parental nurturance and cognitive development in human. *Developmental Science, 11*(5), 793–801.

Faubion, J. (2013). Reevaluating drug policy: Uruguay's efforts to reform marijuana laws. *Law and Business Review of the Americas, 19*(3), 383–408.

Faupel, C. E. (1991). *Shooting dope: Career patterns of hard-core heroin users.* Gainsville, FL: University of Florida Press.

Faupel, C. E., Horowitz, A. M. & Weaver, G. S. (2010). *The sociology of American drug use* (2nd ed.). New York, NY: Oxford University Press.

Fell, J. C. & Voas, R. B. (2006). Mothers against drunk driving (MADD): The first 25 years. *Traffic Injury Prevention, 7*(3), 195–212.

Ferri, M., Davoli, M. & Petrucci, C. (2011). Heroin maintenance for chronic heroin-dependent individuals. *Cochrane Database of Systemic Reviews, 12*, CD003410. doi:10.1002/14651858.CD003410.pub4

Fiddleman, C. (2015, 4 June). Coderre wants safe injection sites by this fall in Montreal. *Montreal Gazette*. Retrieved from http://montrealgazette.com/news/local-news/coderre-wants-safe-injection-sites-by-this-fall

Filiault, S. & Drummond, M. (2010). "Muscular, but not 'roided out'": Gay male athletes and performance-enhancing substances. *International Journal of Men's Health, 9*(1), 62–81.

Filley, C. (2013). Toluene abuse and white matter: A model of toxic leukoencephalopathy. *Psychiatric Clinics of North America, 36*(2), 293–302.

Finegood, B. (2011). Freebase. In M. A. Kleiman. & J. E. Hawdon (Eds.), *Encyclopedia of drug policy* (pp. 309–310). Thousand Oak, CA: Sage Publications.

Fischer, B. (1999). Prohibition, public health and a window of opportunity: An analysis of Canadian drug policy, 1985–1997. *Policy Studies, 20*(3), 197–210. doi:10.1080/01442879908423778

Fischer, B., Ala-Leppilampi, K., Single, E. & Robins, A. (2003). Cannabis law reform in Canada: Is the "saga of promise, hesitation and retreat" coming to an end?! *Canadian Journal of Criminology & Criminal Justice, 45*(3), 265–297.

Fischer, B., Chin, A. T., Kuo, I., Kirst, M. & Vlahov, D. (2002). Canadian illicit opiate users' views on methadone and other opiate prescription treatment: An exploratory qualitative study. *Substance Use & Misuse, 37*(4), 495–522. doi:10.1081/JA-120002807

Fischer, B., Erickson, P. G. & Smart, R. G. (1996). The new Canadian drug law: One step forward, two steps backward. *International Journal of Drug Policy, 7*(3), 172–179.

Fischer, B., Kuganesan, S. & Room, R. (2015). Medical marijuana programs: Implications for cannabis control policy—observations from Canada. *International Journal of Drug Policy, 26*(1), 15–19. doi:10.1016/j.drugpo.2014.09.007

Fischman, M. W. (2009). Cocaine. In P. Korsmeyer & H. R. Kranzler (Eds.), *Encyclopedia of drugs, alcohol & addictive behavior* (3rd ed., Vol. 1, pp. 326–331). Detroit, MI: Macmillan Reference USA.

Flanagan, C. A., Stout, M. & Gallay, L. S. (2008). It's my body and none of your business: Developmental changes in adolescents' perceptions of rights concerning health. *Journal of Social Issues, 64*(4), 815–834. doi:10.1111/j.1540-4560.2008.00590.x

Fleming, C. B., White, H. R. & Catalano, R. F. (2010). Romantic relationships and substance use in early adulthood: An examination of the influences of relationship type, partner substance use, and relationship quality. *Journal of Health and Social Behavior, 51*(2), 153–167.

Fong, G. W. (2001). *Relating the five-factor model of personality and severity of alcoholism*. Dissertation, ProQuest, UMI Dissertations Publishing.

Forchuk, C., Jensen, E., Csiernik, R., Ward-Griffin, C., Ray, S., Montgomery, P. & Wan, L. (2011). Exploring differences between community-based women and men with a history of mental illness. In

C. Forchuk, R. Csiernik & E. Jensen (Eds.), *Homelessness, housing and mental health: Finding truths–creating change* (pp. 243–256). Toronto, ON: Canadian Scholars' Press.

Foucault, M. (1967). *Madness and civilization: A history of insanity in the age of reason.* London, UK: Tavistock.

Foucault, M. (1973) *The birth of the clinic: An archaeology of medical perception.* London, UK: Routledge.

Foucault, M. (1999). *Religion and culture.* London, UK: Routledge.

Foucault, M., Rabinow, P. & Hurley, R. (1997). *Power: The essential works of Michel Foucault, 1954–1984.* New York, NY: New Press.

Fox, N. (1999). Postmodern reflections on "risk," "hazards" and life choices. In D. Lupton (Ed.), *Risk and sociocultural theory: New directions and perspectives* (pp. 12–33). Cambridge, UK: Cambridge University Press.

Francis, A., Alaggia, R. & Csiernik, R. (2010). Multiple barriers: The intersection of substance abuse in the lives of women seeking help for intimate partner violence. In R. Csiernik & W. S. Rowe (Eds.), *Responding to the oppression of addiction: Canadian social work perspectives* (2nd ed., pp. 197–214). Toronto, ON: Canadian Scholars' Press.

Fraser, T. (2018). Canadian cannabis legalization highlights (by province/territory). Brazeau Seller Law, Ottawa, ON. Retrieved from https://pbs.twimg.com/media/DVXjjVzUQAAi7W4.jpg:large

Fulkerson, J., Pasch, K., Perry, C. & Komro, K. (2008). Relationships between alcohol-related informal social control, parental monitoring and adolescent problem behaviors among racially diverse urban youth. *Journal of Community Health, 33*(6), 425–433. doi:10.1007/s10900-008-9117-5

Fuller-Thomson, E., Katz, R. B., Phan, V. T., Liddycoat, J. P. M. & Brennenstuhl, S. (2013). The long arm of parental addictions: The association with adult children's depression in a population-based study. *Psychiatry Research, 210*(1), 95–101. doi:10.1016/j.psychres.2013.02.024

Gallahue, P., Gunawan, R., Rahman, F., El Mufti, K., Din, N. U. & Felten, R. (2012). *The death penalty for drug offences: Global overview 2012: Tipping the scales for abolition.* Retrieved from http://www.countthecosts.org/sites/default/2012-Death-Penalty-Report.pdf

Gallupe, O. & Bouchard, M. (2013). Adolescent parties and substance use: A situational approach to peer influence. *Journal of Criminal Justice, 41,* 162–171. doi:http://dx.doi.org/10.1016/j.jcrimjus.2013.01.002

Garriguet, D. (2008). Beverage consumption of Canadian adults. *Health Reports, 19*(4), 23–29.

Gatehouse, J. (2013, 3 May). When science goes silent: With the muzzling of scientists, Harper's obsession with controlling the message verges on the Orwellian. *Macleans.* Retrieved from http://www.macleans.ca/news/canada/when-science-goes-silent

Gehrke, R. (2011, 1 August). Utah tobacco sales drop nearly 10 million packs. *Salt Lake Tribune.* Retrieved from http://www.sltrib.com/sltrib/politics/52273720-90/tax-sales-million-tobacco.html.csp

Ghandi, A. G., Murphy-Graham, E., Petrosino, A., Chrismer, S. S. & Weiss, C. H. (2007). The devil is in the details: Examining the evidence for "proven" school-based drug abuse prevention programs. *Evaluation Review, 31*(1), 43–74. doi:10.1177/0193841X06287188

Ghiabi, M. (2015). Drugs and revolution in Iran: Islamic devotion, revolutionary zeal and republican means. *Iranian Studies, 48*(2), 139–163. doi:10.1080/00210862.2013.830877

Giffen, P. J., Endicott, S. J. & Lambert, S. (1991). *Panic and indifference: The politics of Canada's drug laws: A study in the sociology of law.* Ottawa, ON: Canadian Centre on Substance Abuse.

Glaser, F. B. (1999). The unsinkable project MATCH. *Addiction, 94*(1), 34–36.

Goffman, E. (1963). *Stigma: Notes on the management of spoiled identity.* New York, NY: Simon & Schuster.

Goldstein, A. (2001). *Addiction: From biology to drug policy* (2nd ed.). New York, NY: Oxford University Press.

Goldstein, A. & Kalant, H. (1990). Drug policy: Striking the right balance. *Science, 249*(4976), 1513–1521. doi:10.1126/science.2218493

Goode, E. (1989). The American drug panic of the 1980's: Social construction or objective threat? *Violence, Aggression, and Terrorism 3*(4), 327–348.

Goode, E. (1999). *Drugs in American society* (5th ed.). New York, NY: McGraw-Hill.

Goode, E. (2008). *Drugs in American society* (7th ed.). New York, NY: McGraw-Hill.

Goode, E. & Ben-Yehuda, N. (1994). Moral panics: Culture, politics, and social construction. *Annual Review of Sociology, 20*, 149–171.

Goode, E. & Ben-Yehuda, N. (2009). *Moral panics: The social construction of deviance* (2nd ed.). Oxford, UK: Wiley-Blackwell.

Goodwin, D. W., Schulsinger, F., Knop, J., Mednick, S. & Guze, S. B. (1977). Psychopathology in adopted and non-adopted daughters of alcoholics. *Archives of General Psychiatry, 34*(9), 1005–1009. doi:10.1001/archpsyc.1977.01770210019001

Goodwin, D. W. Schulsinger, F., Møller, N., Hermansen, L., Winokur, G. & Guze, S. B. (1974). Drinking problems in adopted and non-adopted sons of alcoholics. *Archives of General Psychiatry, 31*(2), 164–169. doi:10.1001/archpsyc.1974.01760140022003.

Goodwin, K. G. (2003/2004). Is the end of the war in sight: An analysis of Canada's decriminalization of marijuana and the implications for the United States "war on drugs." *Buffalo Public Interest Law Journal, 22*, 199–236.

Gorman, D. M. & Huber, J. C. (2009). The social construction of "evidence-based" drug prevention programs: A reanalysis of data from the Drug Abuse Resistance Education (DARE) program. *Evaluation Review, 33*(4), 396–414. doi:10.1177/0193841X09334711

Gottfredson, M. & Hirschi, T. (1990). *A general theory of crime.* Stanford, CA: Stanford University Press.

Government of Canada. (1908a). *The opium act. Statutes of Canada, c. 50.*

Government of Canada. (1908b). *The proprietary or patent medicine act. Statutes of Canada, c. 56.*

Government of Canada. (1911). *The opium and drug act. Statutes of Canada, c. 17.*

Government of Canada. (1920). *An act to amend the opium and narcotic drug act. Statutes of Canada, c. 31.*

Government of Canada. (1921). *An act to amend the opium and narcotic drug act. Statutes of Canada, c. 42.*

Government of Canada (1922). *An Act to amend The Opium and Narcotic Drug Act. Statutes of Canada, c. 36.*

Government of Canada. (1923). *An act to prohibit the improper use of opium and other drugs. Statutes of Canada, c. 22.*

Government of Canada. (1929). *The opium and narcotic drug act. Statutes of Canada, c. 49.*

Government of Canada. (1961). *Narcotic control act. Statutes of Canada, c. 35*.

Government of Canada. (1985/2016). *Consolidation: Canadian centre on substance abuse act, Statutes of Canada, c. 49* (4th Supp.). Retrieved from http://laws-lois.justice.gc.ca/PDF/C-13.4.pdf

Government of Canada. (1996). *Controlled drugs and substances act. Statutes of Canada, c. 19*. Retrieved from http://laws-lois.justice.gc.ca/eng/acts/c-38.8

Government of Canada. (2007). *National anti-drug strategy*. Retrieved from http://www.healthycanadians. gc.ca/anti-drug-antidrogue/index-eng.php

Government of Canada. (2012). *Safe streets and communities act: Targeting serious drug crime*. Retrieved from https:// www.canada.ca/en/news/archive/2012/11/safe-streets-communities-act-targeting-serious-drug-crime.html

Government of Canada. (2014). *Marihuana for medical purposes regulations*. Retrieved from http://www.laws- lois.justice.gc.ca/eng/regulations/SOR-2013-119

Government of Canada. (2015a). *Consolidation: Controlled drugs and substances act. Statutes of Canada, 1996, c. 19*. Retrieved from http://laws-lois.justice.gc.ca/eng/acts/C-38.8

Government of Canada. (2015b). *Harper government highlights royal assent of the drug-free prisons act*. Retrieved from http://news.gc.ca/web/article-en.do?nid=988999

Government of Canada. (2016). *Access to cannabis for medical purposes regulations*. Retrieved from http://laws. justice.gc.ca/eng/regulations/SOR-2016-230/

Government of Canada. (2017). *Consolidation: Controlled drugs and substances act. Statutes of Canada, 1996, c. 19*. Retrieved from http://laws-lois.justice.gc.ca/eng/acts/C-38.8

Government of Prince Edward Island. (2002). Prince Edward Island Liquor Control Commission: LCC history. Retrieved from http://liquorpei.com/about-peilcc/history

Grant, B. F. (2000). Estimates of US children exposed to alcohol abuse and dependence in the family. *American Journal of Public Health, 90*(1), 112–115.

Grant, J. (2009). A profile of substance abuse, gender, crime, and drug policy in the United States and Canada. *Journal of Offender Rehabilitation, 48*(8), 654–668. doi:10.1080/10509670903287667

Grant, K. (2014, 7 July). Opioid use increases after oxycodone crackdown. *Globe and Mail*. Retrieved from http://www.theglobeandmail.com/life/health-and-fitness/healthopioid-use-increases-after-oxycodone- crackdown/article19501813

Green, M. (1979). A history of Canadian narcotics legislation. *University of Toronto Faculty of Law Review, 49*, 42–79.

Griffin, D., Orbin, D. & Hayden, G. (2001). Why drug prohibition must NOT be lifted. *Canadian Speeches, 15*(3), 7.

Grof, S., Goodman, L. E., Richards, W. A. & Kurland, A. A. (1972). LSD-assisted psychotherapy in pa- tients with terminal cancer. *International pharmacopsychiatry, 8*(3), 129–144.

Grunwell, J. (1998). Ayahuasca tourism in South America. *Newsletter of the Multidisciplinary Association for Psychedelic Studies, 8*(3), 59–62.

Gudonis-Miller, L. C., Lewis, L., Tong, Y., Tu, W. & Aalsma, M. C. (2012). Adolescent romantic cou- ples influence on substance use in young adulthood. *Journal of Adolescence, 35*(3), 638–647. doi:10.1016/j. adolescence.2011.08.011

Guelph Police. (2015). *Values, influences, peers (VIP).* Retrieved from http://www.guelphpolice.ca/en/crime-prevention-and-safety/vip-values-influences-peers.asp

Gulmatico-Mullin, M. L. & Cross, C. L. (2009). Opioids. In G. L. Fisher & N. A. Roget (Eds.), *Encyclopedia of substance abuse prevention, treatment, & recovery* (pp. 660–664). Thousand Oaks, CA: Sage Publications.

Hagele, C., Friedel, E., Kienast, T. & Kiefer, F. (2014). How do we "learn" addiction? Risk factors and mechanism getting addicted to alcohol. *Neuropsychobiology, 70*(1), 67–70.

Hall, W. & West, R. (2008). Thinking about the unthinkable: A de facto prohibition on smoked tobacco products. *Addiction, 103*(6), 873–874. doi:10.1111/j.1360-0443.2007.02129.x

Hallowell, G. (2013). Prohibition. *The Canadian Encyclopedia.* Toronto, ON: Historica Foundation.

Halton Regional Police. (2008). *Building respect, attitudes and values with others (BRAVO).* Retrieved from http://www.haltonpolice.ca/COMMUNITYPOLICING/BRAVO/Pages/default.aspx

Hamdieh, M., Motalebi, N., Asheri, H. & Boroujerdi, A. (2009). Prevalence of alcohol and drug abuse in young people, 15–35 years old, living in Tehran, Iran. *Pejouhesh dar Pezeshki, 32*(4), 315–319.

Hammersley, R. & Reid, M. (2002). Why the pervasive addiction myth is still believed. *Addiction Research & Theory, 10*(1), 7–30. doi:10.1080/16066350290001687

Hanson, G. R. (2009). Central Nervous System Stimulants. In G. L. Fisher & N. A. Roget (Eds.), *Encyclopedia of substance abuse prevention, treatment, & recovery* (pp. 166–170). Thousand Oaks, CA: Sage Publications.

Hargreaves, P. (2011). Making the case for drug education. *Criminal Justice Matters, 84*(1), 16–18. doi:10.1080/09627251.2011.576021

Harris, S. (1998). Drug education for whom? *Journal of Education for Teaching, 24*(3), 273–284. doi:10.1080/02607479819791

Harrison, L. (1997). The validity of self-reported drug use in survey research: An overview and critique of research methods. *NIDA Research Monograph, 167,* 17–36.

Hart, C. L. & Ksir, C. (2015). *Drugs, society & human behavior* (16th ed.). New York, NY: McGraw-Hill Education.

Harter, S. L. (2000). Psychosocial adjustment of adult children of alcoholics: A review of the recent empirical literature. *Clinical Psychology Review, 20*(3), 311–337. doi:10.1016/S0272-7358(98)00084-1

Harvey, D. (2005). *A brief history of neoliberalism.* New York, NY: Oxford University Press.

Hathaway, A. D. (2015). *Drugs and Society.* Toronto: Oxford University Press.

Hathaway, A. D. & Erickson, P.G. (2003). Drug reform principles and policy debates: Harm reduction prospects for cannabis in Canada. *Journal of Drug Issues, 33*(2), 465–495. doi:10.1177/002204260303300209

Hathaway, A. D. & Tousaw, K. I. (2008). Harm reduction headway and continuing resistance: Insights from safe injection in the city of Vancouver. *International Journal of Drug Policy, 19*(1), 11–16. doi:10.1016/j.drugpo.2007.11.006

Hawdon, J. E. (1996). Deviant lifestyles: The social control of daily routines. *Youth and Society, 28*(2), 162–188. doi:10.1177/0044118X96028002002

Hawkes, N. C. (2011). Highs and lows of drug decriminalisation. *British Medical Journal, 343*(7829), 874–875. doi:http://dx.doi.org/10.1136/bmj.d6881

Hawthorne, G. (2001). Drug education: myth and reality. *Drug & Alcohol Review, 20*, 111–119. doi:10.1080/09595230125182

Health Canada. (2008). *Methadone maintenance treatment.* Retrieved from http://www.hc-sc.gc.ca/hc-ps/ pubs/adp-apd/methadone-treatment-traitement/index-eng.php#fnb20

Health Canada (2011). *Canadian alcohol and drug use monitoring survey: Summary results for 2011.* Retrieved from http://www.hc-sc.gc.ca/hc-ps/drugs-drogues/stat/_2011/summary-sommaire-eng.php

Health Canada. (2012). *Canadian alcohol and drug use monitoring survey: Summary results for 2012.* Ottawa, ON: Health Canada. Retrieved from http://www.hc-sc.gc.ca/hc-ps/drugs-drogues/stat/_2012/summary -sommaire-eng.php

Health Canada. (2013a). *Canadian tobacco, alcohol and drugs survey (CTADS): Summary of results for 2013.* Retrieved from http://healthycanadians.gc.ca/science-research-sciences-recherches/data-donnees/ctads- ectad/index-eng.php

Health Canada. (2013b). *Harper government announces new medical marihuana regulations.* Retrieved from http://www.hc-sc.gc.ca/ahc-asc/media/nr-cp/_2013/2013-79-eng.php

Health Canada. (2015, 31 March). *Medical marijuana.* Retrieved from http://www.hc-sc.gc.ca/dhp-mps/ marihuana/index-eng.php

Health Canada. (2016). *A framework for the legalization and regulation of cannabis in Canada: Final report of the task force on cannabis legalization and regulation.* Retrieved from http://healthycanadians.gc.ca/task-force- marijuana-groupe-etude/framework-cadre/alt/framework-cadre-eng.pdf

Heath, A. C. (1995). Genetic influences on alcoholism risk: A review of adoption and twin studies. *Alcohol Health & Research World, 19*(3), 166.

Hirschi, T. (1969). *Causes of Delinquency.* Berkeley, CA: University of California Press.

Hobbes, T. (1651). *Leviathan.* London, UK: Continuum.

Hoffman, S. J. & Habibi, R. (2016). Commentary: International legal barriers to Canada's marijuana plans. *Canadian Medical Association Journal, 188*, E215–E216. doi:10.1503/cmaj.160369

Holman, C. (2011). Surfing for a shaman: Analyzing an ayahuasca website. *Annals of Tourism Research, 38*(1), 90–109.

Homma, Y., Chen, W., Poon, C. & Saewyc, E. (2012). Substance use and sexual orientation among East and Southeast Asian adolescents in Canada. *Journal of Child & Adolescent Substance Abuse, 21*(1), 32–50. doi:1 0.1080/1067828X.2012.636687

Hong, R. Y. & Paunonen, S. V. (2009). Personality traits and health-risk behaviours in university students. *European Journal of Personality, 23*(8), 675–696. doi:10.1002/per.736

House, Y. C. (2003). *"The grandmother of marijuana prohibition": The myth of Emily Murphy and the criminaliza- tion of marijuana in Canada.* Unpublished PhD Dissertation, Queen's University (Canada), Kingston, ON.

Howatt, W. A. (2003). Choice theory: A core addiction recovery tool. *International Journal of Reality Therapy, 22*(2), 12–15.

Hughes, C. E. & Stevens, A. (2012). A resounding success or a disastrous failure: Re-examining the inter- pretation of evidence on the Portuguese decriminalisation of illicit drugs. *Drug and Alcohol Review, 31*(1), 101–113. doi:10.1111/j.1465-3362.2011.00383.x

Humphreys, K. & Moos, R. (1996). Reduced substance-abuse-related health care costs among voluntary participants in Alcoholics Anonymous. *Psychiatric Services, 47*(7), 709–713. doi:10.1176/ps.47.7.709

Hundleby, J. D. (1987). Adolescent drug use in a behavioral matrix: A confirmation and comparison of the sexes. *Addictive Behaviors, 12*(2), 103–112. doi:10.1016/0306-4603(87)90017-7

Hunt, S. & Kilmer, J. (2009). Alcohol. In G. L. Fisher & N. A. Roget (Eds.), *Encyclopedia of substance abuse prevention, treatment, & recovery* (pp. 31–35). Thousand Oaks, CA: Sage Publications.

Hunter, R. G. (2009). Rohypnol. In P. Korsmeyer & H. R. Kranzler (Eds.), *Encyclopedia of drugs, alcohol & addictive behavior* (3rd ed., Vol. 3, pp. 435–436). Detroit, MI: Macmillan Reference USA.

Hurt, H., Brodsky, N., Roth, H., Malmud, E. & Giannetta, J. (2005). School performance of children with gestational cocaine exposure. *Neurotoxiology and Teratology, 27*(2), 203–211.

Hurt, H., Giannetta, J., Korczkowski, M., Hoang, A., Tang, K., Beancourt, L., Brodsky, N., Shera, D., Farah, M. & Detre, J. (2008). Functional magnetic resonance imaging and working memory in adolescents with gestational cocaine exposure. *Journal of Pediatrics, 152*(3), 371–377.

Hurt, H., Malmud, E., Betancourt, L., Braitman, L., Brodsky, N. & Giannetta, J. (1997). Children with in utero cocaine exposure do not differ from control subjects on intelligence testing. *Achieves of Pediatric Adolescent Medicine, 151*(12), 1237–1241.

Hurt, H., Malmud, E., Betancourt, L., Brodsky, N. & Giannetta, J. (2001). A prospective comparison of developmental outcome of children with in utero cocaine exposure and controls using the Battelle Developmental Inventory. *Journal of Developmental & Behavioral Pediatrics, 22*(1), 27–34.

Husak, D. N. (2004). The moral relevance of addiction. *Substance Use & Misuse, 39*(3), 399–436. doi:10.1081/JA-120029984

Hussong, A. M., Wong, M. M., Fitzgerald, H. E., Puttler, L. I. & Zucker, R. A. (2005). Social competence in children of alcoholic parents over time. *Developmental Psychology, 41*(5), 747–759. doi:10.1037/0012-1649.41.5.747

Hyshka, E. (2009). The saga continues: Canadian legislative attempts to reform cannabis law in the twenty-first century. *Canadian Journal of Criminology and Criminal Justice, 51*(1), 73–91. doi:10.1353/ccj.0.0043

Hyshka, E. M. A., Butler-McPhee, J. M., Elliott, R. L. L. M., Wood, E. P. & Kerr, T. P. (2012). Canada moving backwards on illegal Drugs. *Canadian Journal of Public Health, 103*(2), 125–127. doi:http://dx.doi.org/10.17269/cjph.103.2926

International Narcotics Control Board. (2014). *2013 Annual Report.* New York, NY: United Nations.

Iparraguirre, J. (2015, 9 October). Socioeconomic determinants of risk of harmful alcohol drinking among people aged 50 or over in England. *BMJ Open, 5*(7). doi:10.1136/bmjopen-2015-007684

Iran Human Rights. (2015). Deadly injustice: Visualizing executions in Iran 2011–2015. *Small Media.* Retrieved from https://iranhr.net/media/files/DeadlyInjustice.pdf

Ireland, C., Berg, B. L. & Mutchnick, R. J. (2010). *Research methods for criminal justice and the social sciences: Practice and applications.* Upper Saddle River, NJ: Pearson Education Inc.

Irniger, M. M., Mutisya, S. & Harrison, T. (2009). Club drugs. In G. L. Fisher & N. A. Roget (Eds.), *Encyclopedia of substance abuse prevention, treatment, & recovery* (pp. 191–194). Thousand Oaks, CA: Sage Publications.

Jeeves, M. & Brown, W. (2009). Neuroscience, psychology and religion: Illusions, delusions and realities about human nature. West Conshohocken, PA: Templeton Foundation Press.

Jensen, E. L. & Gerber, J. (1993). State efforts to construct a social problem: The 1986 war on drugs in Canada. *Canadian Journal of Sociology, 18*(4), 453–462. doi:10.2307/3340900

Jensen, G. F. & Brownfield, D. (1986). Gender, lifestyles, and victimization: Beyond routine activity. *Violence and victims, 1*(2), 85–99.

Jessor, R. & Jessor, S. L. (1977). *Problem behavior and psychosocial development: A longitudinal study of youth.* New York, NY: Academic Press.

Jha, P. & Peto, R. (2014). Global health: Global effects of smoking, of quitting, and of taxing tobacco. *New England Journal of Medicine, 370*(1), 60–68. doi:10.1056/NEJMra1308383

Johnson, M. W. (2011). Cocaine. *Encyclopedia of drug dolicy.* Retrieved from doi:10.4135/9781412976961

Johnston, L. D., O'Malley, P. M., Bachman, J. G. & Schulenberg, J. E. (2006). *Monitoring the future: National results on adolescent drug use: Overview of Key Findings 2005.* NIH Publication No. 06-5882. Rockville, MD: National Institute on Drug Abuse.

Jones, C. (2010). Good politics, bad policy: Drug prohibition ignores science, compassion, experience and logic. *Inroads: A Journal of Opinion, 26*, 85–97.

Jones, J. D., Ehrlich, K. B., Lejuez, C. W. & Cassidy, J. (2015). Parental knowledge of adolescent activities: Links with parental attachment style and adolescent substance use. *Journal of Family Psychology, 29*(2), 191–200. doi:10.1037/fam0000070

Jones, J. M. (2015, 27 July). Drinking highest among educated, upper-income Americans. *Gallup News.* Retrieved from http://www.gallup.com/poll/184358/drinking-highest-among-educated-upper-income-americans.aspx

Kallant, H. (2009). What neurobiology cannot tell us about addiction. *Addiction, 105*(5), 780-789. doi:10.1111/j.1360-0443.2009.02739.x

Kamoouh, C. (1996). Is the problem drug addiction or society? Amoral reflections on the postmodern. *Telos, 1996*(108), 105–116.

Kandel, D. B., Rosenbaum, E. & Chen, K. (1994). Impact of maternal drug use and life experiences on pre-adolescent children born to teenage mothers. *Journal of Marriage and the Family, 56*(2), 325–340.

Kaplan, H. B. (1975). Sequelae of self-derogation: Predicting from a general theory of deviant behavior. *Youth and Society, 7*(2), 171–197.

Kaplan, H. B., Martin, S. S. & Robbins, C. (1984). Pathways to adolescent drug use: Self-derogation, peer influence, weakening of social controls, and early substance use. *Journal of Health and Social Behavior, 25*(3), 270–289.

Karazsia, B. T., Crowther, J. H. & Galioto, R. (2013). Undergraduate men's use of performance-and appearance-enhancing substances: An examination of the gateway hypothesis. *Psychology of Men & Masculinity, 14*(2), 129–137.

Kassam, A. (2005). *Benzodiazepine and similar sedative-hypnotic use in Canada.* Dissertation, ProQuest, UMI Dissertations Publishing.

Kellen, A., Powers, L. & Birnbaum, R. (2017). Drug use, addiction and the criminal justice system. In R. Csiernik & W. S. Rowe (Eds.) *Responding to the oppression of addiction: Canadian social work perspectives* (3rd ed., pp. 250–280). Toronto, ON: Canadian Scholars.

Kenny, C. & P. C. Nolin (2002). *Cannabis: Our position for a Canadian public policy: Report of the Senate Special Committee on Illegal Drugs.* Retrieved from https://sencanada.ca/Content/SEN/Committee/371/ille/rep/summary-e.pdf

Kerrigan, S. & Lindsey, T. (2005). Fatal caffeine overdose: Two case reports. *Forensic Science International, 153*(1), 67–69. doi:10.1016/j.forsciint.2005.04.016

Khanna, J. M. (2009). Barbiturates: Complications. In P. Korsmeyer & H. R. Kranzler (Eds.), *Encyclopedia of drugs, alcohol & addictive behavior* (3rd ed., Vol. 1, pp. 207–208). Detroit, MI: Macmillan Reference USA.

Khanna, N. (2012). Multiracial Americans: Racial identity choices and implications for the collection of race data. *Sociology Compass, 6*(4), 361–331. doi:10.1111/j.1751-9020.2011.00454.x

Khantzian, E. J. (1985). The self-medication hypothesis of addictive disorders: Focus on heroin and cocaine dependence. *American Journal of Psychiatry, 142*, 1259–1264.

Khantzian, E. J. (1997). The self-medication hypothesis of substance use disorders: A reconsideration and recent applications. *Harvard Review of Psychiatry, 4*, 231–244. doi:10.3109/10673229709030550

Khenti, A. (2014). The Canadian war on drugs: Structural violence and unequal treatment of Black Canadians. *International Journal of Drug Policy, 25*(2), 190–195. doi:10.1016/j.drugpo.2013.12.001

Kim, H. K., Kim H. K., Tiberio, S. S., Pears, K. C. & Capaldi, D. M. (2013). Growth of men's alcohol use in early adulthood: Intimate partners' influence. *Psychology of Addictive Behaviors, 27*(4), 1167–1174. doi:10.1037/a0033502

Kim, Y.-M. (2004). *A structural equation modeling analysis of the direct and indirect effects of parental influence upon adolescent alcohol use.* Dissertation, ProQuest, UMI Dissertations Publishing.

Kimberley, D. & Osmond, L. (2017). Concurrent disorders and social work interventions. In R. Csiernik and W. S. Rowe. *Responding to the oppression of addiction: Canadian social work perspectives* (3rd ed., pp. 363–394). Toronto, ON: Canadian Scholars.

Kiuru, N., Burk, W. J., Laursen, B., Salmela-Aro, K. & Nurmi, J.-E. (2010). Pressure to drink but not to smoke: Disentangling selection and socialization in adolescent peer networks and peer groups. *Journal of Adolescence, 33*(6), 801–812. doi:10.1016/j.adolescence.2010.07.006

Kleiman, M. A. R., Caulkins, J. P. & Hawken, A. (2011). *Drugs and drug policy: What everyone needs to know.* New York, NY: Oxford University Press.

Knop, J., Goodwin, D. W., Jensen, P. & Penick, E. (1993). A 30-year follow-up study of the sons of alcoholic men. *Acta Psychiatrica Scandinavica, 87*, 48–53.

Kobayashi, M. (2014). Marked asymmetry of white matter lesions caused by chronic toluene exposure. *Neurological Sciences, 35*(3), 495–497.

Koposov, R. A., Ruchkin, V. V., Eisemann, M. & Sidorov, P. I. (2002). Alcohol use in adolescents from northern Russia: The role of the social context. *Alcohol and Alcoholism, 37*(3), 297–303. doi:10.1093/alcalc/37.3.297

Kornhauser, R. R. (1978). *Social sources of delinquency: An appraisal of analytic models.* Chicago, IL: University of Chicago Press.

Korotkikh, M. (2008). Risk factors for marijuana use among Russian and Canadian adolescents: A comparative analysis. *Masters Abstracts International, 46*(04), 1917. Proquest, UMI Dissertations Publishing.

Koski, A., Sirén, R., Vuori, E. & Poikolainen, K. (2007). Alcohol tax cuts and increase in alcohol positive sudden deaths—a time series intervention analysis. *Addiction, 102*(3), 362–368. doi:10.1111/j.1360-0443.2006.01715.x

Kosten, T., Rounsaville, B. & Kleber, H. (1985). Parental alcoholism in opioid addicts. *Journal of Nervous & Mental Disease, 173*(8), 461–469.

Kothari, B. H., Sorenson, P., Bank, L. & Snyder, J. (2014). Alcohol and substance use in adolescence and young adulthood: The role of siblings. *Journal of Family Social Work, 17*(4), 324–343. doi:10.1080/10522158.2014.924457

Kramer, J. M. (2011). Drug abuse in Russia. *Problems of Post-Communism, 58*(1), 31–43. doi:10.2753/PPC1075-8216580103

Kreager, D. A., Haynie, D. L. & Hopfer, S. (2012). Dating and substance use in adolescent peer networks: A replication and extension. *Addiction, 108*(3), 638–647. doi:10.1111/j.1360-0443.2012.04095.x

Kroll, B. (2004). Living with an elephant: Growing up with parental substance misuse. *Child & Family Social Work, 9*(2), 129–140. doi:10.1111/j.1365-2206.2004.00325.x

Kulbok, P., Thatcher, E., Park, E. & Meszaros, P. (2012). Evolving public health nursing roles: Focus on community participatory health promotion and prevention. *The Online Journal of Issues in Nursing, 17*(2), 1.

Kunic, D. (2006). The Computerized Assessment of Substance Abuse (CASA). *Forum on Corrections Research, 18*(1), 19–23.

Kyrrestad Strøm, H., Adolfsen, F., Fossum, S., Kaiser, S. & Martinussen, M. (2014). Effectiveness of school-based preventive interventions on adolescent alcohol use: A meta-analysis of randomized controlled trials. *Substance Abuse Treatment, Prevention, and Policy, 9*(48), 1–11. doi:10.1186/1747-597X-9-48

Lalone, L. V. (2000). *The personality of alcoholism: Merging the five-factor model of personality with a typologic model of alcohol dependence.* Dissertation, ProQuest, UMI Dissertations Publishing.

Lancet. (2011). Russia's punitive drug laws. *The Lancet, 377*(9783), 2056–2056.

Lane, C. P., Graham, N. A. & Ovson, E. A. (2006). Nicotine. *Journal of Addictive Diseases, 25*, 17–31.

Lankenau, S. E. (2009). OxyContin. In P. Korsmeyer & H. R. Kranzler (Eds.), *Encyclopedia of drugs, alcohol & addictive behavior* (3rd ed., Vol. 3, p. 193). Detroit, MI: Macmillan Reference USA.

Laqueur, H. (2015). Uses and abuses of drug decriminalization in Portugal. *Law & Social Inquiry, 40*(3), 746–781. doi:10.1111/lsi.12104

Larsen, H., Engels, R. C. M. E., Souren, P. M., Granic, I. & Overbeek, G. (2010). Peer influence in a micro-perspective: Imitation of alcoholic and non-alcoholic beverages. *Addictive Behaviors, 35*(1), 49–52. doi:10.1016/j.addbeh.2009.08.002

Larsen, H., Overbeek, G., Granic, I. & Engels, R. C. M. E. (2012). The strong effect of other people's drinking: Two experimental observational studies in a real bar. *The American Journal on Addictions, 21*(2), 168–175. doi:10.1111/j.1521-0391.2011.00200.x

LaRusso, M. D., Romer, D. & Selman, R. L. (2008). Teachers as builders of respectful school climates: Implications for adolescent drug use norms and depressive symptoms in high school. *Journal of Youth and Adolescence, 37*(4), 386–398. doi:10.1007/s10964-007-9212-4

Laslett, A., Mugavin, J., Jiang, H., Manton, E., Callinan, S., MacLean, S. & Room, R. (2015). *The hidden harm: Alcohol's impact on children and families.* Canberra, Australia: Foundation for Alcohol Research and Education.

Lasnier, B., Brochu, S., Boyd, N. & Fischer, B. (2010). A heroin prescription trial: Case studies from Montreal and Vancouver on crime and disorder in the surrounding neighbourhoods. *International Journal of Drug Policy, 21*(1), 28–35.

Lawrence, R. E., Rasinski, K. A., Yoon, J. D. & Curlin, F. A. (2013). Physicians' beliefs about the nature of addiction: A survey of primary care physicians and psychiatrists. *American Journal on Addictions, 22*(3), 255–260. doi:10.1111/j.1521-0391.2012.00332.x

Le Dain Commission. (1970). *Interim report.* Ottawa, ON: Information Canada.

Le Dain Commission. (1973). *Final report: Commission of Inquiry into the non-medical use of drugs.* Ottawa, ON: Information Canada.

Leblanc, D. (2016, 7 February). Liberals' vow to legalize pot creating chaos, police say. *Globe and Mail.* Retrieved from http://www.theglobeandmail.com/news/politics/liberals-vow-to-legalize-pot-creating-chaos-police-say/article28641321

Ledermann, S. (1956). *Alcohol, alcoholisme, alcoolisation* (Vol. 1). Paris, France: Presses Universitaires de France.

Lee, M. A. & Shlain, B. (1992). *Acid dreams: The complete social history of LSD: The CIA, the sixties, and beyond.* New York, NY: Grove Press.

Leon, D. A., Saburova, L., Tomkins, S., Andreev, E., Kiryanov, N., McKee, M. & Shkolnikov, V. M. (2007). Hazardous alcohol drinking and premature mortality in Russia: A population based case-control study. *The Lancet, 369*(9578), 2001–2009. doi:10.1016/S0140-6736(07)60941-6

Leshner, A. I. (1997). Addiction is a brain disease, and it matters. *Science, 278*(5335), 45–47. doi:10.1126/science.278.5335.45

Leukefeld, C. G. & Stoops, W. W. (2009). OxyContin. In G. L. Fisher & N. A. Roget (Eds.), *Encyclopedia of substance abuse prevention, treatment, & recovery* (pp. 675–678). Thousand Oaks, CA: Sage Publications.

Levine, H. G. (1978). The discovery of addiction: Changing conceptions of habitual drunkenness in America. *Journal of Studies on Alcohol, 39*(1): 143–174. doi:10.15288/jsa.1978.39.143

Levinthal, C. (2014). *Drugs, behavior, and modern society* (8th ed.). Upper Saddle River, NJ: Pearson Education.

Levy, N. (2013). Addiction is not a brain disease (and it matters). *Frontiers in psychiatry, 4*, 24. doi:10.3389/fpsyt.2013.00024

Liberal Party of Canada (2016). Marijuana. Retrieved from https://www.liberal.ca/realchange/marijuana/

Liebregts, N., van der Pol, P., van Lar, M., de Graaf, R., van den Brink, W. & Korf, D. J. (2013). The role of parents, peers and partners in cannabis use and dependence trajectories among young adult frequent users. *Contemporary Drug Problems, 40*(4), 531–568. doi:10.1177/009145091304000405

Link, T. & Smith, K. (2014). Age and drug use. In C. Forsyth & H. Copes (Eds.), *Encyclopedia of social deviance* (pp. 11–13). Thousand Oaks, CA: Sage Publications.

Lloyd, C., Joyce, R., Hurry, J. & Ashton, M. (2000). The effectiveness of primary school drug education. *Drugs: Education, Prevention & Policy, 7*(2), 109–126. doi:10.1080/dep.7.2.109.126

Loke, A. Y. & Mak, Y.-W. (2013). Family process and peer influences on substance use by adolescents. *International Journal of Environmental Research and Public Health, 10*, 3868–3885. doi:10.3390/ijerph10093868

Lu, H. & Miethe, T. D. & Liang, B. (2009). *China's drug practices and policies*: Surrey, UK: Ashgate.

Lucas, P. (2009). Moral regulation and the presumption of guilt in Health Canada's medical cannabis policy and practice. *International Journal of Drug Policy, 20*(4), 296–303. doi:10.1016/j.drugpo.2008.09.007

MacCoun, R. & Reuter, P. (2002). Preface: The varieties of drug control at the dawn of the twenty-first century. *The Annals of the American Academy of Political and Social Science, 582*, 7–19.

MacCoun, R. J. & Reuter, P. (2011). Assessing drug prohibition and its alternatives: A guide for agnostics. *Annual Review of Law and Social Science, 7*, 61–78. doi:10.1146/annurev-lawsocsci-102510-105442

Mackie, C. J., Conrod, P. & Brady, K. (2012). Depression and substance use. In J. C. Verster, K. Brady, M. Galanter & P. Conrod (Eds.), *Drug abuse and addiction in medical illness* (pp. 275–284). New York, NY: Springer.

MacQueen, K. (2013, 10 June). Why it's time to legalize marijuana. *Macleans*. Retrieved from http://www.macleans.ca/news/canada/why-its-time-to-legalize-marijuana

MADD Canada. (2015). *Mothers against drunk driving (MADD Canada)*. Retrieved from http://madd.ca/pages

Malleck, D. J. (1999). *Refining poison, defining power: Medical authority and the creation of Canadian drug prohibition laws, 1800–1908*. Dissertation, ProQuest, UMI Dissertations Publishing

Malleck, D. J. (2003). Federal prohibition (Canada). In J. S. Blocker, I. R. Tyrrell & D. M. Fahey (Eds.), *Alcohol and temperance in modern history: A global encyclopedia*. Santa Barbara, CA: ABC-CLIO.

Månsson, J. & Ekendahl, M. (2015). Protecting prohibition. *Contemporary Drug Problems, 42*(3), 209–225. doi:10.1177/0091450915599348

Marcos, A. C., Bahr, S. J. & Johnson, R. E. (1986). Test of a bonding/association theory of adolescent drug use. *Social Forces, 65*(1), 135–161. doi:10.1093/sf/65.1.135

Marlatt, G. A., Larimer, M. E. & Witkiewitz, K. (2012). *Harm reduction: Pragmatic strategies for managing high-risk behaviors* (2nd ed.). New York, NY: Guilford Press.

Marshall, S. G. (2015). Canadian drug policy and the reproduction of indigenous inequities. *International Indigenous Policy Journal, 6*(1), article 7. doi:10.18584/iipj.2015.6.1.7

Martin, J. & Govender, K. (2011). "Making muscle junkies": Investigating traditional masculine ideology, body image discrepancy, and the pursuit of muscularity in adolescent males. *International Journal of Men's Health, 10*(3), 220–239.

Martino, S. C., Collins, R. L., Ellickson, P. L., Schell, T. L. & McCaffrey, D. (2006). Socio-environmental influences on adolescents' alcohol outcome expectancies: a prospective analysis. *Addiction, 101*(7), 971–983. doi:10.1111/j.1360-0443.2006.01445.x

Marulanda, N. & Colegial, C. (2005). Neurotoxicity of solvents in brain of glue abusers. *Environmental Toxicology and Pharmacology, 19*(3), 671–675.

Mason, M. J., Mennis, J., Linker, J., Bares, C. & Zaharakis, N. (2014). Peer attitudes effects on adolescent substance use: The moderating role of race and gender. *Prevention Science, 15*, 56–64. doi:10.1007/s11121-012-0353-7

Mason, M., Mennis, J., Way, T., Light, J., Rusby, J., Westling, E., Crewe, S., Flay, B., Campbell, L., Zaharakis, N. & McHenry, C. (2015). Young adolescents' perceived activity space risk, peer networks, and substance use. *Health & Place, 34*, 143–149. doi:10.1016/j.healthplace.2015.04.005

Massey, J. L. & Krohn, M. D. (1986). A longitudinal examination of an integrated social process model of deviant behavior. *Social Forces, 65*(1), 106–134.

Matuszak, J. & Rajendren, M. (2011). Amphetamines. In M. A. Kleiman. & J. E. Hawdon (Eds.), *Encyclopedia of drug policy* (pp. 22–26). Thousand Oak, CA: Sage Publications.

Matza, D. (1964). *Delinquency and drift*. New York, NY: John Wiley & Sons.

McCabe, S. E., Teter, C. J. & Boyd, C. J. (2006). Medical use, illicit use and diversion of prescription stimulant medication. *Journal of Psychoactive Drugs, 38*(1), 43–56. doi:10.1080/02791072.2006.10399827

McCaffrey, H. (2010). A bitter pill to swallow: Portugal's lessons for drug law reform in New Zealand. *Law Review, 40*(4), 771–830.

McClure, E. A., Lydiard, J. B., Goddard, S. D. & Gray, K. M. (2015). Objective and subjective memory ratings in cannabis-dependent adolescents. *The American Journal on Addictions, 24*(1), 47–52.

McCrae, R. R. & John, O. P. (1992). An introduction to the five-factor model and its applications. *Journal of Personality, 60*(2), 175–215. doi:10.1111/j.1467-6494.1992.tb00970.x

McKenna, D. & Riba, J. (2015). New world tryptamine hallucinogens and the neuroscience of ayahuasca. *Current Topics in Behavioral Neurosciences, 29*, 1–27.

McNeil, R., Kerr, T., Lampkin, H. & Small, W. (2015). "We need somewhere to smoke crack": An ethnographic study of an unsanctioned safer smoking room in Vancouver, Canada. *The International Journal on Drug Policy, 26*(7), 645–652. doi:10.1016/j.drugpo.2015.01.015

Mehler Papherny, A. (2009, 8 December). Painkiller deaths double in Ontario. *Globe and Mail*. Retrieved from http://www.theglobeandmail.com/life/painkiller-deaths-double-in-ontario/article1205696

Merton, R. K. (1938). Social structure and anomie. *American Sociological Review, 3*(5), 672–682.

Midford, R. (2000). Does drug education work? *Drug & Alcohol Review, 19*(4), 441–446. doi:10.1080/09595230020004939

Miller, B. A., Downs, W. R., Gondoli, D. M. & Keil, A. (1987). The role of childhood sexual abuse in the development of alcoholism in women. *Violence and Victims, 2*(3), 157–172.

Miller, D. C. & Salkind, N. J. (2002). *Handbook of research design and social measurement* (6th ed.). Thousand Oaks, CA: Sage Publications.

Mithoefer, M. C., Grob, C. S. & Brewerton, T. D. (2016). Novel psychopharmacological therapies for psychiatric disorders: psilocybin and MDMA. *The Lancet Psychiatry, 3*(5), 481–488.

Moreno, M. A. & Whitehill, J. M. (2014). Influence of social media on alcohol use in adolescents and young adults. *Alcohol Research, 36*(1), 91–100.

Morrell, A. (2015, 1 July). The OxyContin clan: The $14 billion newcomer to Forbes 2015 list of richest U.S. families. *Forbes*. Retrieved from http://www.forbes.com/sites/alexmorrell/2015/07/01/the-oxycontin-clan-the-14-billion-newcomer-to-forbes-2015-list-of-richest-u-s-families/#4695d3afc0e2

Moser, R. P. & Jacob, T. (1997). Parent-child interactions and child outcomes as related to gender of alcoholic parent. *Journal of Substance Abuse, 9*, 189–208. doi:10.1016/S0899-3289(97)90016-X

Mosher, C. (1999). *Imperialism, irrationality, and illegality: The first 90 years of Canadian drug policy, 1908–1998*. Seattle, WA: Canadian Studies Center, University of Washington.

Mosher, C. (2001). Predicting Drug Arrest Rates: Conflict and social disorganization perspectives. *Crime & Delinquency, 47*(1), 84–104.

Mosher, C. (2011). Convergence or divergence? Recent developments in drug policies in Canada and the United States. *American Review of Canadian Studies, 41*(4), 370–386. doi:10.1080/02722011.2011.623409

Mosher, C. J. & Akins, S. M. (2014). *Drugs and drug policy: The control of consciousness alteration* (2nd ed.). Thousand Oaks, CA: Sage Publications.

Mulder, R. T. (2002). Alcoholism and personality. *Australasian Psychiatry, 36*(1), 46–51. doi:10.1046/j.1440-1614.2002.00958.x

Mullally, U. (2014, 14 June). Warning about PMA/PMMA drug after six deaths in Ireland. *The Irish Times*. Retrieved from http://www.irishtimes.com/news/health/warning-about-pma-pmma-drug-after-six-deaths-in-ireland-1.1832118

Murphy, C. M. & Ting, L. (2010). The effects of treatment for substance use problems on intimate partner violence: A review of empirical data. *Aggression and Violent Behavior, 15*(5), 325–333. doi:10.1016/j.avb.2010.01.006

Murphy, E. (1922). *The black candle*. Toronto, ON: Thomas Allen.

Murray, G. F. (1987). Cocaine use in the era of social reform: The natural history of a social problem in Canada, 1880–1911. *Canadian Journal of Law and Society, 2*, 29–43. doi:10.1017/S0829320100001149

Mylant, M., Ide, B., Cuevas, E. & Meehan, M. (2002). Adolescent children of alcoholics: Vulnerable or resilient? *Journal of the American Psychiatric Nurses Association, 8*(2), 57–64. doi:10.1067/mpn.2002.125037

Nadelmann, E. A. (1988). The case for legalization. *The Public Interest, 92*, 3–31.

Nadelmann, E. A. (1989). Drug prohibition in the United States: Costs, consequences, and alternatives. *Science, 245*(4921), 939–947. doi:10.2307/1704189

National Centre on Addiction and Substance Abuse. (2009). *The importance of family dinners V.* New York, NY: Columbia University.

National Centre on Addiction and Substance Abuse. (2012). *The importance of family dinners VIII.* New York, NY: Columbia University.

National Crime Prevention Centre. (2009). *School-based drug abuse prevention: Promising and successful programs.* Ottawa, ON: Public Safety Canada.

Newport, D. J., Carpenter, L. L., McDonald, W. M., Potash, J. B., Tohen, M. & Nemeroff, C. B. (2015). Ketamine and other NMDA antagonists: Early clinical trials and possible mechanisms in depression. *American Journal of Psychiatry, 172*(10), 950–966.

Nissaramanesh, B., Trace, M. & Roberts, M. (2005). *The rise of harm reduction in the Islamic Republic of Iran.* Briefing Paper Eight. Oxford, UK: Beckley Foundation Drug Policy Programme.

Nosyk, B., Geller, J., Guh, D., Oviedo-Joekes, E., Briquette, S., March, D., Schechter, M. T., Anis, A. (2010). The effect of motivational status on treatment outcome in the North American Opiate Medication Initiative (NAOMI) study. *Drug and Alcohol Dependence, 111*(1–2), 161–165. doi:10.1016/j.drugalcdep.2010.03.019

Nosyk, B., Guh, D., Bansback, N., Oviedo-Joekes, E., Brissette, S., Marsh, D. C., Meikleham, E., Schechter, M. & Anis, A. (2012). Cost-effectiveness of diacetylmorphine versus methadone for chronic opioid dependence refractory to treatment. *Canadian Medical Association Journal, 184*(6), E317–E328.

Nye, F. I. (1958). *Family relationships and delinquent behavior.* Westport, CT: Greenwood Press.

O'Brien, C. (2010). Addiction and dependence in DSM-V. *Addiction, 106*(5), 866–867. doi:10.1111/j.1360-0443.2010.03144.x

Ogborne, A. (2000). Use of cannabis in self-treatment. *Journal of Psychoactive Drugs, 32*(4), 435–443.

Oksanen, A. (2013). Deleuze and the theory of addiction. *Journal of Psychoactive Drugs, 45*(1), 57–67.

Olsen, A. & Mooney-Somers, J. (2014). Is there a problem with the status quo? Debating the need for standalone ethical guidelines for research with people who use alcohol and other drugs. *Drug and Alcohol Review, 33*(6), 637–642.

Osgood, D. W. & Anderson, A. L. (2004). Unstructured socializing and rates of delinquency. *Criminology, 42*(3), 519–549. doi:10.1111/j.1745-9125.2004.tb00528.x

Osgood, D. W., Wilson, J. K., O'Malley, P. M., Bachman, J. G. & Johnston, L. D. (1996). Routine activities and individual deviant behavior. *American Sociological Review, 61*(4), 635–655. doi:10.2307/2096397

Oviedo-Joekes, E., Brissette, S., Marsh, D., Lauzon, P., Guh, D., Anis, A. & Schechter, M. (2009). Diacetylmorphine versus methadone for the treatment of opioid addiction. *The New England Journal of Medicine, 361*(8), 777–786.

Oviedo-Joekes, E., Marchand, K., Lock, K., Chettiar, J., Marsh, D. C., Brissette, S., Anis, A. & Schechter, M. T. (2014). A chance to stop and breathe: participants' experiences in the North American Opiate Medication Initiative clinical trial. *Addiction Science & Clinical Practice, 9*(21), 21. doi:10.1186/1940-0640-9-21

Oviedo-Joekes, E., Nosyk, B., Brissette, S., Chettiar, J., Schneeberger, P., Marsh, D. C., Krausz, M., Anis, A. & Schechter, M. T. (2008). The North American opiate medication initiative (NAOMI): Profile of participants in North America's first trial of heroin-assisted treatment. *Journal of Urban Health: Bulletin of the New York Academy of Medicine, 85*(6), 812–825. doi:10.1007/s11524-008-9312-9

Pacula, R. L., MacCoun, R., Reuter, P., Chriqui, J., Kilmer, B., Harris, K., Paoli, L. & Schäfer, C. (2005). What does it mean to decriminalize marijuana? A cross-national empirical examination. *Advances in Health Economics and Health Services Research, 16*, 347–369.

Paoli, L. (2002). The price of freedom: Illegal drug markets and policies in post-Soviet Russia. *Annals of the American Academy of Political and Social Science, 582*, 167–180.

Parker, H., Aldridge, P. & Measham, F. (1998). *Illegal leisure: The normalization of adolescent recreational drug use*. New York, NY: Routledge.

Parsai, M., Marsiglia, F. F. & Kulis, S. (2010). Parental monitoring, religious involvement and drug use among Latino and non-Latino youth in the Southwestern United States. *British Journal of Social Work, 40*(1), 100–114. doi:10.1093/bjsw/bcn100

Pasternak, G. W. (2009a). Codeine. In P. Korsmeyer & H. R. Kranzler (Eds.), *Encyclopedia of drugs, alcohol & addictive behaviour* (3rd ed., Vol. 1, pp. 331). Detroit, MI: Macmillan Reference USA.

Pasternak, G. W. (2009b). Morphine. In P. Korsmeyer & H. R. Kranzler (Eds.), *Encyclopedia of drugs, alcohol & addictive behavior* (3rd ed., Vol. 3, pp. 79–81). Detroit, MI: Macmillan Reference USA.

Peele, S. (1985a). *The meaning of addiction: An unconventional view*. San Francisco, CA: Jossey-Bass.

Peele, S. (1985b). *The meaning of addiction: Compulsive experience and its interpretation*. Lexington, MA: Lexington Books.

Perez, V. W. (2007). *The social production of risk: Perceived risk and disapproval as mechanisms of social control in a social influence model of youth marijuana use*. Dissertation, ProQuest, UMI Dissertations Publishing.

Pergolizzi, J., Böger, R. H., Budd, K., Dahan, A., Erdine, S., Hans, G., Kress, H. G., Langford, R., Likar, R., Raffa, R. B. & Sacerdote, P. (2008). Opioids and the management of chronic severe pain in the elderly: Consensus statement of an international expert panel with focus on the six clinically most often used World Health Organization Step III opioids (buprenorphine, fentanyl, hydromorphone, methadone, morphine, oxycodone). *Pain Practice, 8*(4), 287–313.

Petrosino, A., Turpin-Petrosino, C. & Buehler, J. (2013). "Scared straight" and other juvenile awareness programs for preventing juvenile delinquency. *Cochrane Database of Systematic Reviews, 4*, 1–44. doi: 10.1002/14651858.CD002796.pub2

Plourde, C., Gendron, A. & Brunelle, N. (2012). Profile of substance use and perspectives on substance use pathways among incarcerated aboriginal women. *Journal of Aboriginal and Indigenous Community Health, 10*(1), 83–95.

Pope, M., Chaiton, M. & Schwartz, R. (2015). Raising the minimum age for access to tobacco to 21. Toronto, ON: Ontario Tobacco Research Unit. Retrieved from http://otru.org/wp-content/uploads/2015/08/update_august2015.pdf

Préville, M., Vasiliadis, H.-M., Bossé, C., Dionne, P.-A., Voyer, P. & Brassard, J. (2011). Pattern of psychotropic drug use among older adults having a depression or an anxiety disorder: Results from the longitudinal ESA study. *Canadian Journal of Psychiatry, 56*(6), 348–357.

Prochaska, J., Norcross, J. & DiClimente, C. (1994). *Changing for good.* New York, NY: William Morrow.

Public Health Agency of Canada. (2007). *Canadian street youth and substance use: Findings from enhanced surveillance of Canadian street youth, 1999–2003.* No. HP5-23/2007. Ottawa, ON: Minister of Health. Retrieved from http://www.phac-aspc.gc.ca/std-mts/reports_06/pdf/street_youth_e.pdf

Quinney, R. (1977). *Class, state and crime.* New York, NY: David McKay.

Raj, H., Kumar, K., Sinha, V. K. & Dogra, R. (2012). A comparative study on behavioural problems in children of alcohol dependent parents. *Dysphrenia, 3*(2), 137–143.

RCMP. (2012). *Racing against drugs.* Retrieved from http://www.rcmp-grc.gc.ca/on/prog-serv/rad-ccld-eng.htm

Reckless, W. C. (1967). *The crime problem* (4th ed.). New York, NY: Appleton-Century-Crofts.

Rehm, J., Ballunas, D., Brochu, S., Fischer, B., Gnam, W., Patra, J., Popova, S., Sarnocinska-Hart, A. & Taylor, B. (2006). *The costs of substance abuse in Canada 2002: Highlights.* Ottawa, ON: Canadian Centre on Substance Abuse.

Rehm, J., Mathers, C., Popova, S., Thavorncharoensap, M., Teerawattananon, Y. & Patra, J. (2009). Alcohol and global health 1: Global burden of disease and injury and economic cost attributable to alcohol use and alcohol-use disorders. *The Lancet, 373*(9682), 2223–2233.

Reinarman, C. (1988). The social construction of an alcohol problem. *Theory and Society, 17*(1), 91–120.

Reinarman, C. (2004). Public health and human rights: The virtues of ambiguity. *International Journal of Drug Policy, 15*(4), 239–241. doi:10.1016/j.drugpo.2004.06.004

Reinarman, C. (2005). Addiction as accomplishment: The discursive construction of disease. *Addiction Research & Theory, 13*(4), 307–320. doi:10.1080/16066350500077728

Reinarman, C. & Levine, H. G. (1997). *Crack in America: Demon drugs and social justice.* Berkeley, CA: University of California Press.

Reiss, A. J., Jr. (1951). Delinquency as the failure of personal and social controls. *American Sociological Review, 16*(2), 196–207. doi:10.2307/2087693

Reith, G. (2004). Consumption and its discontents: Addiction, identity and the problems of freedom. *The British journal of sociology, 55*(2), 283–300.

Renard, J., Loureiro, M., Rosen, L. G., Zunder, J., de Oliveira, C., Schmid, S., Rushlow, W. J. & Laviolette, S. R. (2016). Cannabidiol counteracts amphetamine-induced neuronal and behavioral sensitization of the mesolimbic dopamine pathway through a novel mTOR/p70S6 kinase signaling pathway. *The Journal of Neuroscience, 36*(18), 5160–5169.

Renard, J., Rosen, L. G., Loureiro, M., De Oliveira, C., Schmid, S., Rushlow, W. J. & Laviolette, S. R. (2017). Adolescent cannabinoid exposure induces a persistent sub-cortical hyper-dopaminergic state and associated molecular adaptations in the prefrontal cortex. *Cerebral Cortex, 27*(2), 1297–1310. doi:10.1093/cercor/bhv335

Rigter, H. (2006). What drug policies cost: Drug policy spending in the Netherlands in 2003. *Addiction,* *101*(3), 323–329.

Ringwalt, C., Ennett, S. T. & Holt, K. D. (1991). An outcome evaluation of Project DARE (Drug Abuse Resistance Education). *Health Education Research, 6*(3), 327–337. doi:10.1093/her/6.3.327

Ritter, A. (2011). Methadone. In M. A. Kleiman. & J. E. Hawdon (Eds.), *Encyclopedia of drug policy* (pp. 507–509). Thousand Oak, CA: Sage Publications.

Roberts, G., McCall, D., Stevens-Lavigne, A., Anderson, J., Paglia, A., Bollenbach, S., Wiehe, J. & Gilksman, L. (2009). Preventing substance use problems among young people: A compendium of best practices. Ottawa, ON: Health Canada. Retrieved from http://www.hc-sc.gc.ca/hc-ps/alt_formats/hecs-sesc/pdf/pubs/adp-apd/prevent/young-jeune-eng.pdf

Room, R. (1997). Alcohol, the individual and society: What history teaches us. *Addiction* 92(1): 7–11. doi:10.1046/j.1360-0443.92.3s1.15.x

Room, R. (2003). Preventing alcohol problems: Popular approaches are ineffective, effective approaches are politically impossible. Paper presented at the 13th Alcohol Policy Conference, Boston, MA.

Room, R. (2012). Reform by subtraction: The path of denunciation of international drug treaties and re-accession with reservations. *International Journal of Drug Policy, 23*(2012), 401–406. doi:10.1016/j.drugpo.2012.04.001

Room, R. (2014). Legalizing a market for cannabis for pleasure: Colorado, Washington, Uruguay and beyond. *Addiction, 109*(3), 345–351. doi:10.1111/add.12355

Room, R. & Reuter, P. (2012). How well do international drug conventions protect public health? *The Lancet, 379*(9810), 84–91. doi:10.1016/S0140-6736(11)61423-2

Rose, N., O'Malley, P. & Valverde, M. (2006). Governmentality. *Annual Review of Law and Social Science, 2*(1), 83–104. doi:10.1146/annurev.lawsocsci.2.081805.105900

Rossow, I. & Norström, T. (2012). The impact of small changes in bar closing hours on violence: The Norwegian experience from 18 cities. *Addictions, 107*(3), 530–537. doi:10.1111/j.1360-0443.2011.03643.x

Rothwell, V. L. (2011). Heroin. In M. A. Kleiman. & J. E. Hawdon (Eds.), *Encyclopedia of drug policy* (pp. 357–361). Thousand Oak, CA: Sage Publications.

Rowan, M., Poole, N., Shea, B., Gone, J. P., Mykota, D., Farag, M., Hopkins, C., Hall, L., Mushquash, C. & Dell, C. (2014). Cultural interventions to treat addictions in Indigenous populations: Findings from a scoping study. *Substance Abuse Treatment, Prevention, and Policy, 9*, 34. doi:10.1186/1747-597X-9-34

Rubino, T. & Parolaro, D. (2008). Long lasting consequences of cannabis exposure in adolescence. *Molecular and cellular endocrinology, 286*(1), S108–S113.

Russoniello, K. (2012). The devil (and drugs) in the details: Portugal's focus on public health as a model for decriminalization of drugs in Mexico. *Yale Journal of Health Policy, Law, and Ethics, 12*(2), 371–431.

Ryan, D. (2014, 30 May). Heroin addiction on the rise among young drug users. *Vancouver Sun.* Retrieved from http://www.vancouversun.com/health/Part+Heroin+addiction+rise+among+young+drug+users+with+video/9894355/story.html

Samek, D. R. & Rueter, M. A. (2011). Considerations of elder sibling closeness in predicting younger sibling substance use: Social learning versus social bonding explanations. *Journal of Family Psychology, 25*(6), 931–941.

Sandberg, S. (2011). Is cannabis use normalized, celebrated or neutralized? Analysing talk as action. *Addiction Research and Theory, 20*(5), 372–381.

Sarang, A., Rhodes, T., Sheon, N. & Page, K. (2010). Policing drug users in Russia: Risk, fear, and structural violence. *Substance Use & Misuse, 45*(6), 813–864. doi:10.3109/10826081003590938

Schechter, M. & Kendall, P. (2011). Is there a need for heroin substitution treatment in Vancouver's Downtown Eastside? Yes there is, and in many other places too. *Canadian Journal of Public Health, 102*(2), 87–89.

Schneider, S. (2009). *Iced: The story of organized crime in Canada.* Mississauga, ON: John Wiley & Sons Canada.

Scott, D. M. & Taylor, R. E. (2007). Health-related effects of genetic variations of alcohol-metabolizing enzymes in African Americans. *Alcohol Research & Health, 30*(1), 18–21.

Sen, B. (2010). The relationship between frequency of family dinner and adolescent problem behaviors after adjusting for other family characteristics. *Journal of Adolescence, 33*(1), 187–196. doi:10.1016/j.adolescence.2009.03.011

Sigler, R. T. & Talley, G. B. (1995). Drug abuse resistance education program effectiveness. *American Journal of Police, 14*(3/4), 111–121.

Singh, R. D., Jimerson, S. R., Renshaw, T., Saeki, E., Hart, S. R., Earhart, J. & Stewart, K. (2011). A summary and synthesis of contemporary empirical evidence regarding the effects of the drug abuse resistance education program (D.A.R.E.). *Contemporary School Psychology: Formerly "The California School Psychologist," 15*(1), 93–102.

Single, E. (1995). Defining harm reduction. *Drug and Alcohol Review, 14*(3), 287–290. doi:10.1080/09595239500185371

Single, E., Brewster, J., MacNeil, P., Hatcher, J. & Trainor, C. (1995). *Alcohol and drug use: Results from the 1993 general social survey.* Ottawa, ON: Canadian Centre on Substance Abuse.

Skinner, B. F. (1953). *Science and human behavior.* New York, NY: MacMillan.

Small, W., Shoveller, J., Moore, D., Tyndall, M., Wood, E. & Kerr, T. (2011). Injection drug users' access to a supervised injection facility in Vancouver, Canada: The influence of operating policies and local drug culture. *Qualitative Health Research, 21*(6), 743–756. doi:10.1177/1049732311400919

Smart, R. G. & Storm, T. (1964). The efficacy of LSD in the treatment of Alcoholism. *Quarterly Journal of Studies on Alcohol, 25*, 333–338.

Smith, H. S. (1996). *Opioid therapy in the 21st century.* New York, NY: Oxford University Press.

Solomon, R. & Green, M. (1982). The first century: The history of non-medical opiate use and control policies in Canada. *The University of Western Ontario Law Review, 20*(2), 307–336.

Solowij, N. & Battisti, R. (2008). The chronic effects of cannabis on memory in humans: A review. *Current Drug Abuse Reviews, 1*(1), 81–98.

Sonne, S. (2009). Fentanyl. In G. L. Fisher & N. A. Roget (Eds.), *Encyclopedia of substance abuse prevention, treatment, & recovery* (pp. 401–403). Thousand Oaks, CA: Sage Publications.

Spapens, T., Müller, T. & van de Bunt, H. (2015). The Dutch drug policy from a regulatory perspective. *European Journal on Criminal Policy and Research, 21*(1), 191–205. doi:10.1007/s10610-014-9249-3

Spencer, N. (2007, 19 May). OxyContin manufacturer reaches $600 million plea deal over false marketing practices. *World Socialist Web Site.* Retrieved from http://www.wsws.org/en/articles/2007/05/oxy-m19.html

Spithoff, S., Emerson, B. & Spithoff, A. (2015). Cannabis legalization: Adhering to public health best practice. *Canadian Medical Association Journal, 187*(16), 1211–1216.

Spivak, A. L. & Monnat, S. M. (2015). Prohibiting juvenile access to tobacco: Violation rates, cigarette sales, and youth smoking. *International Journal of Drug Policy, 26*(9), 851–859. doi:10.1016/j.drugpo.2015.03.006

Stack, S. J. (2016). Confronting a crisis: An open letter to America's physicians on the opioid epidemic. *West Virginia Medical Journal, 112*(4), 9–10.

Stanhope, M. & Lancaster, J. (2013). *Population centred health care in the community* (8 ed.). Maryland Heights, MO: Elsevier Health Sciences.

Statistics Canada. (2010). *National longitudinal survey of children and youth.* Retrieved from http://www23.statcan.gc.ca/imdb/p2SV.pl?Function=getSurvey&SDDS=4450

Statistics Canada (2014). *Canadian community health survey.* Retrieved from http://www.statcan.gc.ca/eng/survey/household/3226

Statistics Canada. (2015a). *Heavy drinking, by sex, provinces and territories* Retrieved from http://www.statcan.gc.ca/tables-tableaux/sum-som/l01/cst01/health80a-eng.htm

Statistics Canada. (2015b). *Smokers, by sex, provinces and territories.* Retrieved from http://www.statcan.gc.ca/tables-tableaux/sum-som/l01/cst01/health74b-eng.htm

Statistics Canada. (2015c). *Estimates of population, by age group and sex for July 1, Canada, provinces and territories, annual.* CANSIM database. Retrieved from http://www5.statcan.gc.ca/cansim/a26

Stewart, S. H. & Conrod, P. J. (2008). *Anxiety and substance use disorders: The vicious cycle of comorbidity.* New York, NY: Springer.

Stockwell, T., Zhao, J., MacDonald, S., Vallance, K., Gruenwald, P., Ponicki, W., Holder, H., Treno, A. (2011). Impact on alcohol-related mortality of a rapid rise in the density of private liquor outlets in British Columbia: A local area multi-level analysis. *Addictions, 106*(4), 768–776. doi:10.1111/j.1360-0443.2010.03331.x

Stolberg, V. B. (2009). Morphine. In G. L. Fisher & N. A. Roget (Eds.), *Encyclopedia of substance abuse prevention, treatment, & recovery* (pp. 564–566). Thousand Oaks, CA: Sage Publications.

Stolberg, V. B. (2011). Synthetic Narcotics. In M. A. Kleiman. & J. E. Hawdon (Eds.), *Encyclopedia of drug policy* (pp. 756–761). Thousand Oak, CA: Sage Publications.

Strassels, S. A., McNicol, E. & Suleman, R. (2008). Pharmacotherapy of pain in older adults. *Clinics in Geriatric Medicine, 24*(2), 275–298.

Studlar, D. T. (2002). *Tobacco control: Comparative politics in the United States and Canada.* Peterborough, ON: Broadview Press.

Sutherland, E. (1947). *Principles of criminology* (Vol. 4). Philadelphia, PA: J. B. Lippincott.

Svensson, R. (2003). Gender differences in adolescent drug use. *Youth & Society, 34*(3), 300–329. doi:10.1177/0044118X02250095

Sykes, G. M. & Matza, D. (1957). Techniques of neutralization: A theory of delinquency. *American Sociological Review, 22*(6), 664–670.

Szasz, T. (1992). *Our right to drugs: The case for a free market.* Westport, CN: Praeger.

Tang, J. & Dani, J. (2009). Dopamine enables in vivo synaptic plasticity associated with the addictive drug nicotine. *Neuron, 63*(5), 673–682. doi:10.1016/j.neuron.2009.07.025

Tang, Z. & Orwin, R. G. (2009). Marijuana initiation among American youth and its risks as dynamic processes: Prospective findings from a national longitudinal study. *Substance Use & Misuse, 44*(2), 195–211. doi:10.1080/10826080802347636

Tanner, L. (2009, 27 April). ADHD medication study shows academic benefits. *Tulsa World.*

Taplin, C., Saddichha, S., Li, K. & Krausz, M. R. (2014). Family history of alcohol and drug abuse, childhood trauma, and age of first drug injection. *Substance Use & Misuse, 49*(10), 1311–1316. doi:10.3109/10826084.2014.90138

Taylor, S., Buchanan, J. & Ayres, T. (2016). Prohibition, privilege and the drug apartheid: The failure of drug policy reform to address the underlying fallacies of drug prohibition. *Criminology & Criminal Justice, 16*(4), 452–469. doi:10.1177/1748895816633274

Thapar, A., Fowler, T., Rice, F., Scourfield, J., van den Bree, M., Thomas, H., Harold, G. & Hay, D. (2003). Maternal smoking during pregnancy and attention deficit hyperactivity disorder symptoms in offspring. *The American Journal of Psychiatry, 160*(11), 1985–1989.

Thavorncharoensap, M., Teerawattananon, Y., Yothasamut, J. Lertpitakpong, C. & Chaikledkaew, U. (2009). The economic impact of alcohol consumption: A systematic review. *Substance Abuse Treatment, Prevention, and Policy, 4*(20). doi:10.1186/1747-597X-4-20

Thomas, G. (2012). *Analysis of beverage alcohol sales in Canada.* Ottawa, ON: Canadian Centre on Substance Abuse. Retrieved from http://www.ccsa.ca/Resource%20Library/CCSA-Analysis-Alcohol-Sales-Policies-Canada-2012-en.pdf

Thorlindsson, T. & Bernburg, J. G. (2006). Peer groups and substance use: Examining the direct and interactive effect of leisure activity. *Adolescence, 41*(162), 321–339.

Thornton, M. (2007). Prohibition versus legalization: Do economists reach a conclusion on drug policy? *Independent Review, 11*(3), 417–433.

Tobler, N. S. & Stratton, H. H. (1997). Effectiveness of school-based drug prevention programs: A meta-analysis of the research. *The Journal of Primary Prevention, 18*(1), 71–128. doi:10.1023/A:1024630205999

Tri-Council Policy Statement: Ethical Conduct for Research Involving Humans, (December 2014).

Tupper, K. W. (2008a). Drugs, discourses and education: A critical discourse analysis of a high school drug education text. *Discourse: Studies in the Cultural Politics of Education, 29*(2), 223–238. doi:10.1080/01596300801966864

Tupper, K. W. (2008b). Teaching teachers to just say "know": Reflections on drug education. *Teaching and Teacher Education, 24*(2), 356–367. doi:10.1016/j.tate.2007.08.007

Tupper, K. W. (2008c). The globalization of ayahuasca: Harm reduction or benefit maximization?. *International Journal of Drug Policy, 19*(4), 297–303.

Tupper, K. (2009). Ayahuasca healing beyond the Amazon: The globalization of a traditional indigenous entheogenic practice. *Global Networks, 9*(1), 117–136.

Tupper, K. (2011). Ayahuasca in Canada: Cultural phenomenon and policy issue. In B. C. Labate and H. Jungaberle (Eds.), *The internationalization of ayahuasca* (pp. 319–325). Zurich, Switzerland: Lit Verlag.

Turiano, N. A., Whiteman, S. D., Hampson, S. E., Roberts, B. W. & Mroczek, D. K. (2012). Personality and substance use in midlife: Conscientiousness as a moderator and the effects of trait change. *Journal of Research in Personality, 46*(3), 295–305. doi:10.1016/j.jrp.2012.02.009

Turner, C. (2013). *War on science: Muzzled scientists and willful blindness in Stephen Harper's Canada.* Vancouver, BC: Greystone Books.

Tweed, S. H. & Ryff, C. D. (1991). Adult children of alcoholics: Profiles of wellness amidst distress. *Journal of Studies on Alcohol, 52*(2), 133–141.

Twombly, E. C., Holtz, K. D. & Tessman, G. K. (2008). Multimedia science education on drugs of abuse: A preliminary evaluation of effectiveness for adolescents. *Journal of Alcohol and Drug Education, 52*(1), 8–18.

United Nations (1988). *United Nations convention against illicit traffic in narcotic drugs and psychotropic substances.* Vienna, Austria: United Nations.

United Nations Office on Drugs and Crimes. (2009). *Guide to implementing family skills training programmes for drug abuse prevention.* Vienna, Austria: United Nations.

United Nations. (1971). *Convention on psychotropic substances.* Vienna, Austria: United Nations.

United Nations. (1972). *The single convention on narcotic drugs, 1961, as amended by the 1972 protocol amending the single convention on narcotic drugs, 1961.* Retrieved from http://www.unodc.org/pdf/convention_1961_en.pdf

United Nations. (2009). *This day in history: The Shanghai opium commission, 1909.* Retrieved from http://www.unodc.org/unodc/en/frontpage/this-day-in-history-the-shanghai-opium-commission-1909.html

UNODC. (2012). *World Drug Report 2012.* No. E.12.XI.1. New York, NY: United Nations Office on Drugs and Crime. Retrieved from http://www.unodc.org/unodc/data-and-analysis/WDR-2012.html

UNODC. (2013). *World Drug Report 2013.* New York, NY: United Nations Office on Drugs and Crime. Retrieved from www.unodc.org/wdr2013

UNODC. (2014). *World Drug Report 2014.* No. E.14.XI.7. New York, NY: United Nations Office on Drugs and Crime. Retrieved from www.unodc.org/wdr2014

Urberg, K. A., Luo, Q., Pilgrim, C. & Degirmencioglu, S. M. (2003). A two-stage model of peer influence in adolescent substance use: Individual and relationship-specific differences in susceptibility to influence. *Addictive Behaviors, 28*(7), 1243–1256.

Valleriani, J. & MacPherson, D. (2015, 27 February). Why Canada is no longer a leader in global drug policy. *Globe and Mail.* Toronto, ON: Phillip Crawley.

van Beusekom, I., van het Loo, M. & Kahan, J. P. (2002). *Guidelines for implementing and evaluating the Portuguese drug strategy.* Santa Monica, CA: Rand Europe.

van het Loo, M., van Beusekom, I. & Kahan, J. (2002). Decriminalization of drug use in Portugal: The development of a policy. *The Annals of the American Academy of Political and Social Science, 582*(1), 49–63.

van Ooyen-Houben, M. & Kleemans, E. (2015). Drug policy: The 'Dutch model.' *Crime & Justice, 44*(1), 165–226.

Van Ryzin, M. J., Fosco, G. M. & Dishion, T. J. (2012). Family and peer predictors of substance use from early adolescence to early adulthood: An 11-year prospective analysis. *Addictive Behaviors, 37*, 1314–1324. doi:10.1016/j.addbeh.2012.06.020

Virani, A., Bezchlibnyk-Butler, K. Z. & Jeffies, J. (2009). *Clinical handbook of psychotropic drugs* (18th ed.). Toronto, ON: Hogrefe & Huber Publishers.

Visser, J. (2012, 26 June). Bath salts drug believed to be behind violent assault on Toronto cops, arrests in Calgary. *National Post.* Retrieved from http://news.nationalpost.com/2012/06/26/bath-salts-drug-believed-to-be-behind-violent-assault-on-toronto-cops-arrests-in-calgary

Volkow, N. D., Swanson, J. M., Evins, A. E., DeLisi, L. E., Meier, M. H., Gonzalez, R., Bloomfield, M., Curran, V. & Baler, R. (2016). Effects of cannabis use on human behavior, including cognition, motivation, and psychosis: A review. *JAMA psychiatry, 73*(3), 292–297.

Walls, M., Sittner Hartshorn, K. J. & Whitbeck, L. B. (2013). North American Indigenous adolescent substance use. *Addictive Behaviors, 38*(5), 2103–2109. doi:10.1016/j.addbeh.2013.01.004

Walsh, A., Callaway, R., Belle-Isle, L., Capier, R., Kay, R., Lucas, P. & Holtzman S. (2013). Cannabis for therapeutic purposes: Patient characteristics, access, and reasons for use. *International Journal of Drug Policy,* 24(6), 511–516. doi:10.1016/j.drugpo.2013.08.010

Walters, G. D. (2002). Lessons learned from project MATCH. *Addictive Disorders & Their Treatment, 1*(4), 135–139. doi:10.1097/00132576-200211000-00004

Walton, D. (2001, 7, April). Children trafficking in Ritalin, Dexedrine. *Globe and Mail.*

Watkin, J., Rowe, W. S. & Csiernik, R. (2010). Prevention as controversy: Harm reduction. In R. Csiernik & W. S. Rowe (Eds.), *Responding to the oppression of addiction: Canadian social work perspectives,* (2nd ed., pp. 19–36). Toronto, ON: Canadian Scholars' Press.

Waxman, M. & Csiernik R. (2010). Culture as prevention: A case study of urban Canadian Jewish male students. In R. Csiernik & W. S. Rowe (Eds.) *Responding to the oppression of addiction: Canadian social work perspectives* (2nd ed., pp 47–62). Toronto, ON: Canadian Scholars' Press.

Weatherburn, D. (2014). The pros and cons of prohibiting drugs. *Australian & New Zealand Journal of Criminology, 47*(2), 176–189. doi:10.1177/0004865814524423

Webster, P. C. (2014). Canada opposes harm reduction policies for drug users. *Canadian Medical Association Journal, 186*(4), 256–256. doi:10.1503/cmaj.109-4714

Weekes, J., Thomas, G. & Graves, G. (2004). *Substance abuse in corrections: FAQs.* Ottawa, ON: Canadian Centre on Substance Abuse.

Weil, A. & Rosen, W. (2004). *From chocolate to morphine: Everything you need to know about mind-altering drugs.* New York, NY: Houghton Mifflin Company.

Wen, H. (2014). Ethical challenges to punitive law on drug users in China. *Asian Bioethics Review, 6*(2), 158–173.

Werb, D., Rowell, G., Guyatt, G., Kerr, T., Montaner, J. & Wood, E. (2011). Effect of drug law enforcement on drug market violence: A systematic review. *International Journal of Drug Policy, 22*(2), 87–94. doi:10.1016/j.drugpo.2011.02.002

West, S. L. & O'Neal, K. K. (2004). Project D.A.R.E. Outcome effectiveness revisited. *American Journal of Public Health, 94*(6), 1027–1029. doi:10.2105/AJPH.94.6.1027

White, J. (2007). Missouri legislator wants to ban baking soda. *The High Road.* Retrieved from http://www.thehighroad.org/archive/index.php/t-267588.html

Whitehead, C., Shaw, R. & Giles, D. (2010). 'Crack down on the celebrity junkies': Does media coverage of celebrity drug use pose a risk to young people? *Health, Risk & Society, 12*(6), 575–589. doi:10.1080/13 698575.2010.515736

Whiteman, S. D., Jensen, A. C. & Maggs, J. L. (2013). Similarities in adolescent siblings' substance use: Testing competing pathways of influence. *Journal of Studies on Alcohol and Drugs, 74*(1), 104–113. doi:http://dx.doi.org/10.15288/jsad.2013.74.104

Wiens, T. K. & Walker, L. J. (2015). The chronic disease concept of addiction: Helpful or harmful? *Addiction Research & Theory, 23*(4), 309–321. doi:10.3109/16066359.2014.987760

Wigmore, T. & Farquhar-Smith, P. (2016). Opioids and cancer: Friend or foe? *Current Opinion in Supportive and Palliative Care, 10*(2), 109–118.

Williams, G. (2010). *The criminalization of recreational marijuana use in Canada: A scientific, social, legal and philosophical analysis based on the work of Douglas Husak.* Dissertation, ProQuest UMI Dissertations Publishing.

Winkelman, M. (2014). Psychedelics as medicines for substance abuse rehabilitation: Evaluating treatments with LSD, peyote, ibogaine and ayahuasca. *Current Drug Abuse Reviews, 7*(2), 101–116.

Wong, S. K. (2005). The effects of adolescent activities on delinquency: A differential involvement approach. *Journal of Youth and Adolescence, 34*(4), 321–333. doi:10.1007/s10964-005-5755-4

Woo, A. (2014, 22 November). Vancouver addicts soon to receive prescription heroin. *Globe and Mail.* Retrieved from http://www.theglobeandmail.com/news/british-columbia/vancouver-heroin-addicts-authorized-to-get-drug/article21717642

World Health Organization. (2014). *Health behaviour in school-aged children.* Retrieved from http://www.hbsc.org/membership/countries/canada.html

Wray, R., Hyman, I., Agic, B., Bennett-Abu-Ayyash, C., Kanee, M., Lam, R., Mohamed, A. & Tuck, A. (2013). We ask because we care: The Tri-Hospital and TPH health equity data collection research project report. Toronto, ON: Centre for Addiction and Mental Health.

Xiao, S., Yang, M., Zhou, L. & Hao, W. (2015). Transition of China's drug policy: Problems in practice. *Addiction, 110*(2), 193–194.

Yang, M., Zhou, L., Hao, W. & Xiao, S.-Y. (2014). Drug policy in China: Progress and challenges. *The Lancet, 383*(9916), 509–509.

Young, M. M., Saewyc, E., Boak, A., Jahrig, J., Anderson, B., Doiron, Y.,Taylor, S., Pica, L., Laprise, P. & Clark, H. (2011). *Cross-Canada report on student alcohol and drug use: Technical report.* Ottawa, ON: Canadian Centre on Substance Abuse. Retrieved from http://www.ccsa.ca/Resource%20 Library/2011_CCSA_Student_Alcohol_and_Drug_Use_en.pdf

Zagaria, M. A. E. (2008). Antipsychotics in seniors: Warnings to prevent misuse. *U.S. Pharmacist*, 33(11), 20–22.

Zaric, G., Brennan, A., Varenbut, M. & Daiter, J. (2012). The cost of providing methadone maintenance treatment in Ontario, Canada. *The American Journal of Drug and Alcohol Abuse,* 38(6), 559–566.

Zucker, J. P. & Piasecki, M. (2009). Tobacco. In G. L. Fisher & N. A. Roget (Eds.), *Encyclopedia of substance abuse prevention, treatment, & recovery* (pp. 905–909). Thousand Oaks, CA: Sage Publications.

INDEX